How does a large population of neurons in the brain work? How can synchronized firing be achieved? What factors regulate how many and which neurons will fire under different conditions? These questions form the central theme of this book. Using a combined experimental-theoretical approach that is new to neuroscience, the authors present important new techniques for the physiological reconstruction of a large biological neuronal network. They begin by discussing experimental studies of the CA3 hippocampal region in vitro, focusing on single-cell and synaptic electrophysiology, particularly the effects one single neuron is able to exert on its connected followers. This is followed by a description of a computer model of the system, first for individual cells, and then for the entire detailed network. The model behavior is compared with experiments under a variety of conditions. The results shed significant light on the mechanisms of epilepsy, EEG, and biological oscillations and provide an excellent "test case" for theories of neural networks.

Researchers in neurophysiology and physiological psychology, physicians concerned with epilepsy and related disorders, and students and researchers in computational neuroscience will find this book an invaluable resource.

T0275776

Neuronal networks of the hippocampus

Neuronal networks
of the hippocampus

ROGER D. TRAUB
Thomas J. Watson Research Center, I.B.M.
Department of Neurology, Columbia University

RICHARD MILES
Department of Neurology, Columbia University
Pasteur Institute, Paris

appendix by
Lawrence S. Schulman
Department of Physics
Clarkson University

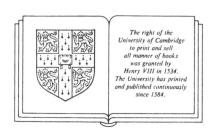

The right of the
University of Cambridge
to print and sell
all manner of books
was granted by
Henry VIII in 1534.
The University has printed
and published continuously
since 1584.

CAMBRIDGE UNIVERSITY PRESS

Cambridge
New York   Port Chester
Melbourne   Sydney

CAMBRIDGE UNIVERSITY PRESS
Cambridge, New York, Melbourne, Madrid, Cape Town, Singapore, São Paulo

Cambridge University Press
The Edinburgh Building, Cambridge CB2 8RU, UK

Published in the United States of America by Cambridge University Press, New York

www.cambridge.org
Information on this title: www.cambridge.org/9780521364812

First published 1991
This digitally printed version 2008

A catalogue record for this publication is available from the British Library

Library of Congress Cataloguing in Publication data
Traub, Roger D.
Neuronal networks of the hippocampus / Roger D. Traub, Richard
Miles : appendix by Lawrence S. Schulman.
p. cm.
Includes bibliographical references.
ISBN 0-521-36481-7
1. Hippocampus – Computer simulation. 2. Neural networks.
I. Miles, Richard, 1951– . II. Title.
[DNLM: 1. Computer Simulation. 2. Hippocampus – physiology.
3. Models, Neurological. 4. Neurons – physiology. WL 314 T777n]
QP383.25.T73 1991
599'.0188 – dc20
DNLM/DLC
for Library of Congress   90-2675

ISBN 978-0-521-36481-2 hardback
ISBN 978-0-521-06331-9 paperback

Du siehst, mein Sohn, zum Raum wird hier die Zeit.

– Richard Wagner, *Parsifal*

Contents

Acknowledgments

We would like to thank our many colleagues, most especially Robert K. S. Wong, without whom neither of the authors would ever have worked on the hippocampus. Bob Wong posed many of the questions addressed here, often guessed the answers, and was deeply involved in much of the actual research, as a quick perusal of the references will readily show. György Buzsáki, Lawrence Schulman, Geoffrey Grinstein, F. Edward Dudek, and John G. R. Jefferys have provided important criticisms of portions of the manuscript, and Dr. Schulman contributed the appendix to Chapter 9 on percolation theory. Lawrence Schulman and Ralph Siegel provided numerous helpful suggestions for the section on chaos in Chapter 7. Our collaborators have also included W. D. Knowles, C. P. Taylor, R. Snow, R. Llinás, J. H. Schneiderman, B. Strowbridge, T. A. Pedley, A. R. Kay, R. Numann, A. Stelzer, N. Chamberlin, and R. Dingledine. RDT received invaluable assistance from the Computing Systems Department of the IBM T. J. Watson Research Center and wishes to express special thanks to Angelo Rossi and W. G. Pope. RDT wishes to thank Benoit Mandelbrot for recruiting him on behalf of IBM. The original work described here was supported in part by IBM, the Esther A. and Joseph Klingenstein Fund, the National Institutes of Health, and the Epilepsy Society.

We also wish to remember the earlier inspiration provided by the late Leon G. Barnhart, Joseph H. Wegstein, and Jeannette R. Decker.

Prologue

Our approach to modeling the brain

What makes the brain so difficult to understand? This question has no simple answer. Many aspects of brain structure obviously contribute to its complexity. There are the large numbers of cells that have different shapes and electrical properties. There are the bewildering connection patterns within and between hundreds of nuclear regions. Dozens of neurotransmitters and modulators exist, each with its own repertoire of receptors and synaptic actions. Data on all of these issues are being and will continue to be pursued with tenacity and persistence, yet, in our opinion, there persists a nagging uncertainty as to what underlying principles, if any, are at work in the brain.

Our doubt exists because the function and behavior of the brain are clearly dependent on the simultaneous activities of many, perhaps all, of its elements. How can activity in so many cells be measured and understood when most experimental techniques allow access to only a few? Just as compelling, what conceptual framework is appropriate for thinking about the simultaneous, coupled activities of large populations of neurons?

In this monograph we shall describe our own approach to a small part of this imposing problem. No single aspect of our approach is mysterious or unique, yet the different aspects may provide new insight into the functioning of the mammalian cortex. We are interested in neuronal population activities generated within small networks of cortical neurons. We shall show how recurrent excitatory and inhibitory connections between cells in a single region are crucial in shaping spontaneous population activities. In our view, these intrinsically generated collective activities of the cortex are relevant to its function. This differs from the view that the cortex is a computational machine whose only function is to transform afferent information into neuronal output or into perception; such a view usually assumes the unstimulated cortex to be at rest. It is clear, however, that activity evoked by afferent stimuli must always be superimposed on autonomous, spontaneous brain activity.

We attempt to synthesize neuronal population activities from our best estimates of cellular currents, unitary synaptic properties, and anatomical connectivities. We suspect that this approach will be more relevant than reductionist attempts to explain complex attributes of the brain, such as memory, strictly in terms of the properties of single membrane proteins or synaptic elements.

Our general method utilizes these ideas: First, we study a small region of brain that generates interesting collective behaviors. We study the in vitro hippocampal CA3 region, a preparation that may contain 1,000 to 20,000 neurons (depending on how the tissue is prepared). Our preparation is small compared with an entire hippocampus (of order 1 million neurons, see Table 1.1) and minuscule compared with an entire human brain (estimates of 10^{11} neurons are in vogue). Nevertheless, we shall show that the in vitro CA3 region contains enough synaptic circuitry to produce a challenging variety of population activities. Second, we try to study the system at multiple levels of organization. That is, we and our colleagues perform experiments to characterize single membrane currents in isolated neurons, the firing properties of individual neurons within brain slices, the synaptic interactions between neurons within a slice, and finally the responses of populations of neurons either spontaneously active or subjected to localized stimulation. Our ideas must span our own data, together with those of numerous other investigators. Third, we construct computer models using these data. Each model is an embodiment of a set of ideas about how the CA3 region is put together. To an extent limited by our confidence in these ideas and our technical ability in simulation, we can perform experiments on the models. These computational experiments test the ideas embodied into the model for internal consistency and for another kind of consistency: The model is defined only by what we know of hippocampal *structure,* including unitary synaptic interactions, network topology, and single-cell physiology, but the model's actual behavior is not built in, nor can it often be guessed until a simulation is indeed run on the computer. The behavior each model generates should agree with the behavior of the real biological system. Because a computer model allows us, in principle, to observe the behavior of all of the thousands of cells in the model, and because we know the model's exact structure (e.g., precisely which cells are connected), we hope that it will lead us to a better framework for thinking about how populations of real neurons work. We hope also that simulations will generate interesting testable predictions. For those accustomed to thinking about idealized, abstract neural networks, several surprises are in store.

Why the hippocampus? We have studied the hippocampal slice because of the anatomical simplicity and technical advantages of this system.[1]

There are two criteria to use in selecting a portion of the brain for modeling. One criterion is that a so-called computational model can be established. The behavior of the model should illuminate a transformation carried out between one set of neurons that encodes a characterizable "input" and another set (or perhaps the same set) that encodes an output. Such models have been proposed for aspects of visual function (Zipser and Andersen, 1988), for more general memorylike properties of networks of neuronlike elements (Carpenter and Grossberg, 1987; Hopfield and Tank, 1986), and for schemes of development or plasticity in networks that learn to discriminate form (Lehky and Sejnowski, 1988; Linsker, 1988). Although the physical/computational features of such models may be analyzable, and may perhaps have practical engineering applications, they are not intended to represent in detail actual networks of neurons within the brain, but rather to shed light on general principles.

A second criterion one might use in selecting a brain portion is that experiments be feasible. Can data be obtained for single-cell properties, characteristics of single synapses and network connectivity, that are critical for building a detailed model of the system? Such experimental data are readily obtained from the hippocampal slice and more recently are being obtained from neocortical slices as well (Mason et al., 1989).

Only for invertebrate networks (Getting and Dekin, 1985a,b; Heinzel, 1988a,b; Heinzel and Selverston, 1988) has it proved possible to reconstruct from first principles a neuronal network of known function. For the mammalian brain, it is not easy to find a region that can be studied both as a network and as a computational system. That is, it is difficult to find a brain region of known and relatively straightforward function where one can also determine the cellular properties and unitary synaptic interactions.[2] In this book we shall emphasize network aspects of the hippocampus and present a model of a hippocampal subregion that is based on first principles and that reproduces numerous observable experimental phenomena. This still does not tell us what "computation" the hippocampus performs. It will not tell us why the hippocampus is important for the formation of long-term memories, why there are place-responsive cells in it, or what biological role theta rhythm (rhythmic slow activity) plays or why sniffing in rats is phase-locked to theta (Komisaruk, 1970). Nevertheless, our model may be useful for those interested in larger questions of nervous system function, but who are not necessarily interested in the structural details of the hippocampus, in providing a set of constraints on any "computational theory" for the hippocampus. We know, with reasonable accuracy, the pattern of the synaptic connections and many of the synaptic actions in the hippocampus. We know the types of collective behaviors this system can generate, and we can predict how these behaviors will change after the synapses have been modified in specified ways. This model could thus serve as a basis for more theoretical and abstract models of the hippocampus (and perhaps of cortex in general) and could help to generate a set of rules to limit how such abstract models can be constructed.

How a model of cortex differs from models of invertebrate systems. There are crucial differences between the hippocampus and invertebrate pattern-generating neural systems. It is well to address these differences at the outset. Many of the neurons in invertebrates possess individual identities and distinctive physiological properties. The neurons can be studied in relative isolation from each other, and *all* pairwise interactions can, in principle, be described. In a model of the invertebrate network, each neuron in the network can correspond to a particular neuron in the animal, and each synapse in the model to a particular synapse in the animal.[3] Such a model has a satisfying, tangible quality to it, even if the behaviors generated by the model are exceedingly complicated.

In cortex, such an approach must be modified. There are far too many neurons to study each one as an individual. It does not appear likely that individual neurons have an identity across different members of the species in a manner analogous, say, to cell R2 of *Aplysia*. Nor is it likely that the precise details of connections between cells are the same across different members of the species. Thus, the properties of hippocampal pyramidal cells are properties of a "generic" pyramidal cell. The brain seems to consist of a number of distinct neuronal classes. Until we know better, it is possible to assume that two neurons from the same class have similar physiological properties. Similarly, we cannot expect to reconstruct a complete "wiring diagram" of all the connections in a given slice. Rather, from many experiments we hope to arrive at a statistical description of the connectivity patterns and the synaptic actions. Although our model of a hippocampal network has as many cells in it (to within an order of magnitude) as the actual experimental system, there is no well-defined isomorphism between the cells and synapses in the model and the cells and synapses in a particular slice. We are thus looking at "average" properties of the network, even though we do not model populations of cells by lumping the cells together, as discussed later. Here, "average" should be taken to mean "typical" or "generic," rather than "arithmetical average."

It follows that the network properties that we can legitimately analyze are only those properties that do not depend on a precise network connectivity. This is true even if, in a particular computer simulation, the details of the simulation depend on the connectivity pattern of the model network as it exists in the computer! Thus, we can analyze, for example, the number of cells firing bursts after one cell is stimulated and how this number is influenced by the efficacy of the inhibitory synapses.

As one example of the relation between network structure and its behavior, we can show how the propagation of activity along excitatory chains is influenced by the timing and strength of inhibitory inputs to cells along the chain. But we cannot predict that a particular group of 12 cells in a slice will fire at a given time. Indeed, to run a simulation at all requires construction of a specific network, but the information is not available to make sure that the sample network matches any sample slice in all its details. On the other hand, experimentally demonstrating that a particular set of 12 cells (arbitrarily chosen) will fire at some time is impossible anyway, with our current apparatus, just as impossible as it is to reconstruct the precise wiring pattern of the slice. Thus, the statistical character of our modeling approach does not yet have observable consequences. By allowing simultaneous functional recordings from large numbers of neurons, advances in optical recording methodology may change this (Grinvald, 1985).

On the notion of scaling to infinite size: a further distinction between finite pattern generators and large networks with statistical descriptions. Invertebrate central pattern-generating networks (CPGs) perform a limited range of reasonably well defined tasks. The complexity of these tasks is limited (e.g., produce particular sets of rhythmic drives to some set of muscles). The task complexity presumably is what determines the number and properties of the neurons and connections required to do the job; there may, in addition, be flexibility in how given neurons contribute to the operation of different interconnected networks (Dickinson and Marder, 1989; Dickinson, Mecsas, and Marder, 1990). Mammalian cortex is more of a "general-purpose machine" – it is not designed merely to proceed through stereotyped motions. The computational problems it faces do not have obvious bounds on their complexity, and these problems are not determined in advance. The anatomical substrates of different parts of the cortex appear similar, whether these parts be devoted to various sensory, motor, or "associational" tasks. We expect, furthermore, that the larger the computational system, the more powerful it is. It is for these reasons that the principles underlying invertebrate CPGs may not generalize to mammalian cortex. An analogy might be to view a CPG as a small, special-purpose machine dedicated to a limited number of completely characterized computations, and to view cortex as a general-purpose supercomputer. It is our hope that hippocampal networks with 10^4 neurons will exhibit principles that will scale upward into networks of arbitrarily large size, just as early digital computers, containing about 10^4 switching devices, were built on principles that still apply to today's machines containing millions of devices. (We do not intend to suggest, however, that the principles at work in the hippocampus have anything to do with digital computers.)

On the difference between distributed-network models and lumped-circuit models. One technical approach to modeling interconnected networks of neurons involves "lumping" together all the neurons of a given type into a single representative neuron. The distributed circuitry is thus compressed into a small network, which, it is hoped, will still capture the essential global behaviors of the system (Freeman, 1979; Leung, 1982). Such an approach offers the advantages of conceptual simplicity and may even allow an analytical characterization of the system, always a desirable feature. Unfortunately, the lumping approach is not applicable to the hippocampal CA3 region, where the interesting behaviors depend on the excitatory interactions between the pyramidal cells. Lumping the pyramidal cells together into a representative pyramidal cell, with an averaged synaptic feedback loop of this element onto itself, would discard the interesting structure and features of the system. A lumped circuit would not allow one to predict that single excitatory synapses would be powerful enough for bursts of action potentials to propagate from one cell to each of its connected followers in the absence of inhibition, nor would it allow an understanding of how inhibition regulates propagation of impulses along excitatory polysynaptic pathways, as discussed later. We have also produced a particular example in which a lumped system equivalent to a given network generates a behavior quite distinct from the network behavior generated when the system parameters are minimally perturbed (see Chapter 7). Thus, the lumping procedure is not a robust approximation of the system for the network phenomena that interest us. We therefore attempt to represent each physical neuron by a model neuron in the computer and to simulate each synaptic connection explicitly. In a way, our computer model is almost as complex as the biological system it is intended to illuminate. What, then, has been gained? There are three rewards. First, one may show that a certain well-defined set of cellular and synaptic properties is necessary and sufficient to account for the experimental observations. Second, numerical experiments, impossible to perform in the biological system, can be explored with the model. For example, we can, in simulations, change the density or spatial distribution of one particular set of synapses. Finally, we hope that the computer model will be part of a series of models of increasing abstraction that, we hope, will illuminate new physical principles while still remaining faithful to the physiology (Pytte, Grinstein, and Traub, in press).

Scope of this work

Physiological studies of slices of the hippocampus in vitro have both motivated and allowed us to construct a distributed cellular model with 9,900 CA3 neurons.[4] Computer simulations can be compared in detail with intracellular recordings from pairs of neurons and with extracellular recordings. We construct a population model from these basic physiological data. This is a prototypical "bottom-up" approach. This model accounts for a variety of collective phenomena whose properties depend on cellular interactions throughout the population. These collective phenomena include synchronized discharges that develop in local regions and then propagate across the tissue, as well as population oscillations in which a population rhythm occurs that is faster than the average period of the irregularly firing individual cells.

In this book, we first present some concepts regarding what the hippocampus does, largely derived from in vivo work. We then review the physiological data from which we have constructed a model of the CA3 region of the hippocampal slice. We next address some general issues involved in modeling individual neurons and present our own particular model of a CA3 pyramidal cell. We consider some of the complex technical problems involved in simulating realistically a network of neurons and describe the detailed structure of our own CA3 population model, emphasizing its basis in experimental data. Finally, we illustrate in detail the interplay between results obtained from simulations and experimental work.

Our interest in the in vitro CA3 region began because this system could mimic a form of epileptic activity called the interictal EEG spike when synaptic inhibition was suppressed. The principles involved in the generation of interictal spikes proved seminal in our understanding of nonepileptic, putatively normal, collective neuronal behavior in this region of the brain. Consistent with this, in vivo recordings suggest the existence of a continuum of population behaviors between the frankly epileptic and the normal (see the section "Synchroniziation and EEG in the Hippocampus" in Chapter 1). Our general paradigm is this: Does our understanding of cellular physiology and synaptic connectivity and circuitry, embodied in a computer model, suffice to account for the behavior of a neuronal population? What predictions can be made and tested? What happens when the model includes not only synaptic interactions between cells but also nonsynaptic interactions, such as electric-field effects?

We have evolved the model by adding cell types, by increasing the number of cells, and by describing (as best we can) the spatial distributions of synaptic connections. As new features are added, we explore the effects of parameter changes, alone and in combination. Parameters of particular importance are the strengths of the synaptic connections and their spatial distributions. Although some parameters can be manipulated experimentally, other factors, such as synaptic connectivity, can be modified more easily in simulations.

We originally studied the CA3 region because it generates in isolation synchronized epileptiform discharges (Schwartzkroin and Prince, 1978;

Wong and Traub, 1983; but see, however, Hablitz, 1984). Under conditions where synchronized events occur in both CA3 and CA1, the CA3 event leads the CA1 event (Traynelis and Dingledine, 1988; Wong and Traub, 1983). Synchronized events in CA1, in vitro, thus appear to be "projected" from CA3 along Schaffer collaterals. It is not clear if dentate granule cells discharge synchronously in the slice, and the hilar/CA4 region has not been studied to the same extent as the other regions (see, however, Ogata and Ueno, 1976). The ability of the CA3 region to generate autonomously synchronized bursts reflects the existence of strong but sparse excitatory connections between pyramidal cells (Ishizuka, Weber, and Amaral, 1990; Lorente de Nó, 1934), as well, perhaps as the particular intrinsic properties of the pyramidal neurons. The problem is to understand more precisely how this is possible. The special synaptic organization of CA3, most dramatically displayed during epileptiform events, also endows the CA3 region with the ability to generate a variety of other nonpathological behaviors in which groups of neurons fire together with greater or lesser degrees of synchrony. The factors that regulate the extent of synchrony and that determine which subgroups of neurons fire together may be of general neurobiological significance.

1   The hippocampus in context

Review of anatomy

In this chapter we shall review some aspects of the anatomy and physiology of the hippocampus, considering the hippocampus as only one component of the whole brain. We shall discuss also some clinical consequences of abnormal hippocampal function (epilepsy, amnestic states).
Our purpose is to provide a biological background for the more detailed
physiological and mathematical material to follow. We wish to define
some of the relevant questions that can be answered in brain slices and
in computer models of brain slices. We shall move freely between observations of the hippocampus from many different species (rodents, nonhu-
man primates, humans, and so on), assuming that the same general
principles apply to all of them.

The hippocampus is a cortical structure that is necessary for the formation of new memories. The detailed mechanisms by which this function
is accomplished are not well understood. The hippocampus in rodents
contains cells that respond to spatial location ("place cells"). It generates characteristic EEG rhythms that depend on the behavioral state of
animal. The hippocampus readily produces seizures in experimental contexts, and epileptic seizures originating in or near the hippocampus pose
an important clinical problem.

The hippocampus forms a rather large part of the rodent brain
(Paxinos and Watson, 1986). There is one hippocampus on each side of
the brain. In humans, there is a hippocampus in each of the two medial
temporal lobes. The hippocampus is anatomically the simplest type of
cortex, with the cell bodies of the principal neurons aligned in a single
layer. This fact is important to its usefulness in physiological experiments.

The "hippocampal formation" consists of the hippocampus proper
together with other nearby structures: the dentate gyrus and the subiculum. The hippocampus proper is sometimes called the cornu Ammonis
("Ammon's horn," abbreviated CA). Lorente de Nó (1934) defined
subdivisions of the CA. The principal subdivisions are denoted CA1,
CA2, and CA3. He used as criteria for his subdivisions the morphology

1

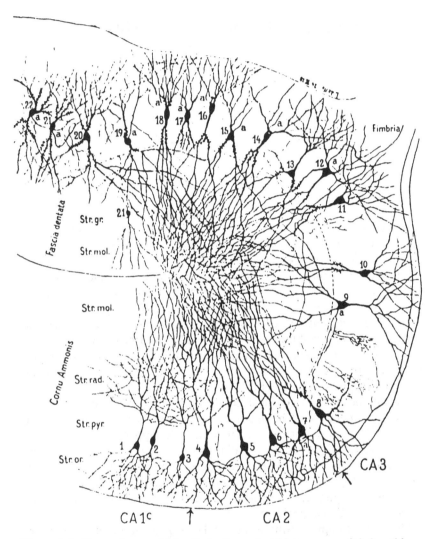

Figure 1.1. Types of pyramidal cells in the rodent hippocampus (12-day-old mouse), stained by the Golgi method; "a" denotes the axon. Cell 12 shows a Schaffer collateral. Cell 7 is a pyramidal cell giving rise to longitudinal associa- tion fibers. Cell 19 is a pyramidal cell without a Schaffer collateral. Cell 9 is a pyramidal basket cell. Cells 21 and 22 are called "modified pyramids" by Lorente de Nó and lie in his region CA4. (From Lorente de Nó, 1934, with permission of the author.)

of the principal cell type (the pyramidal cells), the patterns of termina- tion and distribution of fiber pathways (e.g., the mossy fibers), and the layout of the stratum pyramidale, the layer of cell bodies of the pyrami- dal cells (Figures 1.1 and 1.2). We shall follow the terminology of

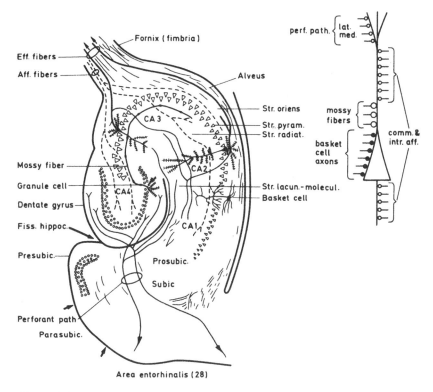

Figure 1.2. Left: Schematic illustration of interconnections within the hippocampus and some afferent and efferent pathways. Right: Schematic illustrating lamination of inputs to a CA3 pyramidal cell. (From Brodal, 1981, with permission.)

Lorente de Nó, with the proviso that the boundaries of CA2 are not always perfectly clear, and noting that CA1 and CA3 are in turn subdivided into subregions. CA1–3 pyramidal cells in the rodent lie in a well-defined visible band; this fact favors anatomical and physiological studies, as does the laminar pattern of the many fiber pathways: the mossy fibers, the Schaffer collaterals to the stratum radiatum of CA1, the commissural inputs to CA1 and CA3, the perforant path to the strata lacunosum and moleculare of CA1 to CA3 and to the denate gyrus, and so on. Some estimates of the numbers of cells in human and rodent hippocampi are listed in Table 1.1.

In comparing the sizes of the human hippocampus and the rodent hippocampus, note that CA1 has increased relatively more than CA2–3. The human stratum pyramidale[1] is relatively thicker, especially in CA1, with the band of cell bodies not as well defined as in rodents (Braak, 1974), and with CA1 somata reaching even to the alevus (Stephan, 1983).

Table 1.1. *Estimates of the numbers of pyramidal or granule cells in various hippocampal regions*

Species	Age	Region	Estimate	Reference
Rat	1 month	CA1	320,000–420,000	Boss et al., 1987
Rat	1 month	CA3	210,000–330,000	Boss et al., 1987
Rat	Adult	CA1–3	260,000	Cassell and Brown, 1977
Human	Adult	CA2–3	2,350,000	Brown and Cassell, 1980
Human	Adult	CA1	4,630,000	Zola-Morgan et al., 1986
Rat	1 month	Dentate	700,000–1,000,000	Boss et al., 1985

In order to put these cell numbers in context for the in vitro studies to be discussed later, we note that the number of cells in the rat CA3 region in vivo is about an order of magnitude larger than the number in the largest in vitro guinea pig preparation that we use. Thus, we estimate that the longitudinal CA3 slice (400 μ thick and 10 mm long) contains about 20,000 pyramidal cells. The CA3 region of a transverse slice may contain 3,000–5,000 cells.

The major cell type in the hippocampus proper is the pyramidal cell (Lorente de Nó, 1934), whereas in the dentate gyrus it is the dentate granule cell. Both of these groups of cells produce excitation in their postsynaptic cells that is fast (milliseconds). Significant minorities of inhibitory cells are recognized by their characteristic locations, morphologies, and axonal distributions; these include basket cells, chandelier cells (Somogyi et al., 1983b), mossy cells (Ribak, Seress, and Amaral, 1985), pyramidal basket cells (Ribak and Seress, 1983), and so on. Inhibitory cells can mediate either fast (lasting milliseconds to tens of milliseconds) or slow (tens to hundreds of milliseconds) types of inhibition. There have been studies that have related the electrical properties of inhibitory cells to their morphological types (Kawaguchi and Hama, 1987, 1988; Lacaille and Schwartzkroin, 1988a,b; Lacaille et al., 1987; Scharfman and Schwartzkroin, 1988b; Schwartzkroin and Kunkel, 1985; Schwartzkroin and Mathers, 1978). Most, but not all, of the nonpyramidal cells are presumed to be inhibitory. This conclusion is based on staining for the inhibitory neurotransmitter γ-aminobutyric acid (GABA) or the GABA-synthesizing enzyme glutamic acid decarboxylase (GAD) (Sloviter and Nilaver, 1987; Somogyi et al., 1983c). In some cases, dual intracellular recording has proved that certain cells are inhibitory (Knowles and Schwartzkroin, 1981a,b; Lacaille and Schwartzkroin, 1988a,b; Lacaille et al., 1987; Miles and Wong, 1984). Most of the long-range intrahippocampal connections, as well as hippocampal inputs and outputs, are excitatory, but there are exceptions. The exceptions include GABA-ergic fibers into the hippocampus that originate in the septum (Freund and Antal, 1988), as well as dentate hilar cells with commissural projections (Ribak et al., 1986).

Some of the major pathways within and involving the hippocampus are these: (i) the *perforant path,* originating in entorhinal cortex (EC); (ii) the *mossy fibers,* suprapyramidal and infrapyramidal, connecting dentate granule cells to CA3 pyramidal cells and hilar neurons (Claiborne, Amaral, and Cowan, 1986; Lorente de Nó, 1934; Yamamoto, 1982); (iii) the *Schaffer collaterals* of CA3 pyramidal axons, making en passant synapses onto CA1 pyramidal cells; (iv) the *commissural connections;* (v) the *recurrent excitatory connections* between CA3 pyramidal cells (MacVicar and Dudek, 1980a; Miles and Wong, 1986) and between CA1 pyramidal cells (Christian and Dudek, 1988b; Dichter, Herman, and Selzer, 1973; Hablitz, 1984); (vi) *inhibitory circuitry,* with inhibitory cells excited either by local pyramidal-cell collaterals or by afferent fibers or both (Alger and Nicoll, 1982a; Anderson, Eccles, and Løyning, 1963; Kehl and McLennan, 1985a,b; Newberry and Nicoll, 1984). The excitatory neurotransmitter used by the perforant-path input to the hippocampus is thought to be glutamate or a related amino acid (White et al., 1977b). The transmitter used by excitatory pathways within the hippocampus is also likely to be an excitatory amino acid (Crunelli, Forda, and Kelly, 1983; Nadler et al., 1976).

The so-called trisynaptic circuit consists of the following excitatory loop: entorhinal cortex to dentate granule cells via the perforant path, granule cells to CA3 pyramidal cells via the mossy fibers, and CA3 pyramidal cells to CA1 pyramidal cells via the Schaffer collaterals. Because CA1 cells project back to the entorhinal cortex via the subiculum, perhaps one should refer to the "tetrasynaptic circuit" or "pentasynaptic circuit." The notion of the trisynaptic circuit is an oversimplification. It omits, for example, collateral connections between CA3 cells, the connections between granule cells that are presumed to be mediated via mossy cells in the hilus, perforant-path synapses onto CA1 and CA3 pyramidal cells, and both feedback and feedforward inhibition.

Some of these hippocampal pathways show clear spatial organization. This is particularly true of the mossy fibers, which tend to stay confined to transverse hippocampal "laminae" (Claiborne et al., 1986). The perforant path is also spatially structured: The lateromedial gradient along layers 2 and 3 of the EC is mapped onto the longitudinal gradient along the hippocampus (Witter and Groenewegen, 1984). In addition, layer 2 of the EC projects to the dentate and CA3, and layer 3 projects to CA1 (Steward and Scoville, 1976). Both CA3 pyramidal and hilar cells contribute to the commissural pathways, but apparently CA1 cells do not (Gottlieb and Cowan, 1973). Schaffer-collateral synapses lie in the stratum radiatum of CA1, and commissural fibers from the contralateral CA3 region synapse in the stratum oriens and stratum radiatum of CA1 (Buzsáki and Eidelberg, 1982; Laurberg, 1979) as well as in CA3. The inputs to the hippocampus can be divided into those from cortical structures (including the opposite hippocampus, the same hippocampus via associational fibers, the dentate gyrus, and the entorhinal cortex) and those from noncortical structures (including the septum/diagonal band, the hypothalamus, the brain-stem raphe nuclei, and the locus ceruleus). The outputs from the hippocampus can also be divided into those proceeding to cortical areas [the hippocampi themselves, the subiculum and entorhinal cortex, the medial frontal cortex, and the cingulate gyrus (Brodal, 1981)] and those proceeding to noncortical areas such as the septum. Most, but not all, of the output is carried via axons of pyramidal cells (Alonso and Köhler, 1982; Chronister and DeFrance, 1979; Finch, Nowlin, and Babb, 1983; Swanson and Cowan, 1977). The projection to the septum originates in both pyramidal and nonpyramidal cells (Alonso and Köhler, 1982). The fimbria/fornix was once considered a major output pathway from the hippocampus to the septum and hypothalamus, but it is now known that most of the fibers in the fimbria/fornix originate from cells in the subiculum rather than the hippocampus proper (Chronister, Sikes, and White, 1976; Meibach and Siegel, 1977a).

It may be possible to make a functional distinction between cortical and subcortical inputs to the hippocampus. The cortical inputs seem likely to carry detailed, time-dependent information driven by external events. In contrast, subcortical inputs serve a modulatory function by permitting or enabling different oscillatory modes of the hippocampal circuitry. This would be analogous to the way that modulators can cause invertebrate central pattern generators to switch between different oscillatory modes (Getting and Dekin, 1985a,b; Heinzel, 1988a,b; Heinzel and Selverston, 1988). This hypothesis regarding the differences between cortical and subcortical inputs is suggested by the differing time courses of the respective neurotransmitters (rapid for cortical inputs, slower for at least some of the subcortical inputs), as well as by the numbers of cells supplying the inputs (large for cortical sources, smaller for subcortical sources, particularly from the locus ceruleus). These distinctions, however, are not absolute, because cortical inputs may co-release peptides along with the usual amino acid transmitter, whereas the subcortical septal inputs include the rapidly acting GABA in addition to the slower-acting acetylcholine.

Let us now consider the nonhippocampal inputs and outputs of the cortical areas that impinge on the hippocampus – the subicular complex and entorhinal cortex – together with some of the interconnections of these respective regions. The dorsolateral prefrontal cortex sends inputs to the presubiculum or parasubiculum, depending on the species; the subiculum in turn projects to the ventral prefrontal cortex (Cavado and Reinoso-Suárez, 1988). The subiculum also projects to the hypothalamus, septum, anterior thalamus, cingulate cortex, and entorhinal cortex (Brodal, 1981), as well as the medial frontal cortex, parahippocampal region, amygdala, nucleus accumbens, and lateral dorsal thalamic nuclei (Rosene and Van Hoesen, 1977). There are inputs to the entorhinal cortex from the orbitofrontal cortex, temporal pole, perirhinal cortex, superior temporal gyrus, parahippocampal gyrus, and retrosplenial cortex (Insausti and Amaral, 1988). Brodal (1981) lists as inputs to the EC the following: olfactory bulb, prepyriform and periamygdaloid cortex, amygdala, medial septum, dorsal raphe nucleus, locus ceruleus, the CA3 region of the hippocampus, and parts of the thalamus. Most of the output from the EC is sent to the hippocampus, via the lateral and medial perforant paths. Seltzer and Pandya (1976), in studies of the rhesus monkey, found that the rostroventral temporal lobe, peristriate cortex, and caudal inferior parietal lobule (association areas for hearing, vision, and touch, respectively) projected to regions of the parahippocampal gyrus that in turn are known to project to the EC. The existence of these pathways implies that the EC receives multimodal "highly processed" information from several cortical regions (Lopes da Silva et al., 1985). In addition to exciting the hippocampus, the EC sends fibers to the septum (Crutcher, Madison, and Davis, 1981), as does the hippocampus, as discussed later. The subiculum receives inputs from CA1, the EC, and "virtually all areas along the base of the temporal lobe" (Van Hoesen, Rosene, and Mesulam, 1979). It projects back to many of these same regions (Berger et al., 1980; Finch et al., 1986; Rosene and Van Hoesen, 1977).

The cingulate cortex is another part of the "limbic system."[2] In addition to receiving afferents from the hippocampus, the cingulate is also excited by the anterior thalamus, subiculum, lateral septum, and areas of pareital, temporal, and prefrontal cortex (Brodal, 1981). The cingulate likewise projects to the hippocampus, but also to the amygdala, septum, thalamus, prefrontal cortex, parietal association cortex, superior colliculus, pretectal area, periaqueductal gray, midbrain tegmentum, and locus ceruleus (Brodal, 1981). (The reader will have noticed how the same regions are multiply interconnected with one another.)

We shall now briefly consider the subcortical inputs to the hippocampus. Many, perhaps all, of the transmitters released by these inputs act via intracellular second messengers (Nicoll, 1988). Most fibers from the septum release acetylcholine, whereas others release GABA; substance P is another possible transmitter (Vincent and McGeer, 1981). Acetylcholine has a number of actions, most of which have a slow onset and long duration (minutes). It decreases transmitter release from both excitatory and inhibitory presynaptic terminals (Haas, 1982; Segal, 1982, 1983, 1985; Valentino and Dingledine, 1981), blocks a slow calcium-dependent potassium conductance, $g_{K[Ca]}$ (Benardo and Prince, 1982; Cole and Nicoll, 1984), and blocks a voltage-dependent potassium current called the M current (Halliwell and Adams, 1982), with possible cellular depolarization and an increase in input resistance. Acetylcholine also seems to excite inhibitory cells (McCormick and Prince, 1985, 1986; Reece and Schwartzkroin, 1988; Strowbridge and Shepherd, 1988). The effects of acetylcholine have a latency of onset of tens of milliseconds to minutes and tend to last for minutes. Most of the GABA fibers from the septum appear to synapse onto inhibitory cells in the hippocampus (Freund and Antal, 1988); it is not known if $GABA_A$ or $GABA_B$ receptors are involved (Alger and Nicoll, 1982b). The latter case would be interesting, because the effects of activation of $GABA_B$ receptors are mediated by a second messenger and tend to be relatively long-lasting (Andrade, Malenka, and Nicoll, 1988). Further details of the septum-to-hippocampus pathway will be discussed later in the section on theta rhythm.

The locus ceruleus of the pons uses norepinephrine as transmitter. This compound decreases $g_{K[Ca]}$ and also hyperpolarizes pyramidal cells (Madison and Nicoll, 1982, 1986a,b). The raphe nuclei use serotonin, a transmitter that hyperpolarizes many CA1 cells (Andrade et al., 1986; Segal, 1980), and may directly excite inhibitory neurons (Guy and Ropert, 1990). Occasionally, serotonin depolarizes CA1 cells in association with a decreased input resistance (Jahnsen, 1980). Variable effects of serotonin may derive from the existence of multiple receptor types, which may lead to activation of one potassium conductance while others are suppressed (Andrade and Nicoll, 1987; Colino and Halliwell, 1987). Some serotonin receptors are coupled via a second messenger to the same potassium channels that are activated by $GABA_B$ receptors (Andrade et al., 1986). Cells in the mesencephalic reticular formation release histamine into the hippocampus (Garbarg et al., 1974). Peptides that are found in the hippocampus or that exert effects on hippocampal neurons include cholecystokinin (CCK), vasoactive intestinal peptide (VIP), substance P, neurotensin, met-enkephalin, leu-enkephalin (Tielen, van Leeuwen, and Lopes da Silva, 1982), vasopressin (Mühlethaler, Dreifuss, and Gähwiler, 1982), and somatostatin (Roberts et al., 1984). The latter compound may act presynaptically to diminish GABA release (Scharfman and Schwartzkroin, 1988a). Similarly, neuropeptide Y (NPY) is a peptide transmitter found in the hippocampus that appears to diminish, by a presynaptic mechanism, the action-potential-evoked release of excitatory transmitter (Colmers, Lukowiak, and Pittman, 1987). The cells of origin for NPY are not known with certainty; they may be intrinsic to the hippocampus, perhaps with NPY co-released with another transmitter.

Having reviewed some of the anatomical organization of the hippo-campus, we shall devote the remainder of this introductory chapter to four manifestations, normal and pathological, that have been associated with the hippocampus: memory disorders, spatial performance, certain types of EEG findings, and epilepsy.

Amnestic syndromes and the hippocampus

We shall now consider some behavioral syndromes wherein there is either definite or suggestive evidence of hippocampal dysfunction. In general, these clinical and experimental observations suggest that the hippocampus is essential for conceptual or declarative (Squire, Shima-mura, and Amaral, 1989) memory (particularly for memory of events to which one is exposed only once), but not for procedural memory (the kind of memory involved in learning a skill with practice) (Squire, 1986).

A remarkable clinical syndrome called transient global amnesia was vividly described by Fisher and Adams (1964); see also Shuping, Rol-linson, and Toole (1980a). In this syndrome, there is a sudden onset of altered behavior, but with preservation of consciousness and personal identity. The patient appears bewildered and repeats certain questions over and over. He or she is not able to record new information for more than a few minutes. This state persists for some hours, and there is permanent amnesia for the period of involvement; but the patient can record new memories once the transient amnesic period is over (Krit-chevsky, Squire, and Zouzounis, 1988). There is some suggestive evi-dence that this syndrome involves the hippocampus. For example, it has been reported in association with a glioma in the left (dominant) hippo-campus (Shuping, Toole, and Alexander, 1980b), but it has also been reported with a thalamic lesion (Goldenberg, Wimmer, and Maly, 1983). The underlying pathogenesis is not known. One interesting hypothesis is that the hippocampus becomes transiently nonfunctional because of spreading depression (Olesen and Jurgensen, 1986), a phenomenon to which this brain region is known to be susceptible in vitro (Snow, Taylor, and Dudek, 1983). In this regard, transient global amnesia has been triggered by mild trauma (Haas and Ross, 1986), a procedure that can initiate spreading depression in the hippocampal slice. Complex partial seizure activity in the hippocampus also disrupts the registration of ongo-ing events, as described later (Halgren and Wilson, 1985). It is interest-ing that transient global amnesia can be triggered by orgasm (Mayeux, 1979). During orgasm there is intense electrical activity in the septum (Heath, 1972) that presumably would strongly drive the hippocampus.

Surgical lesions of the hippocampus bilaterally, in humans and in subhuman primates, also produce an amnestic syndrome in which "single-exposure" memory is particularly involved (Squire, 1986). In humans, the temporal stem, an area of subcortical white matter in the temporal lobe, was thought to represent a critical region for memory (Horel, 1978), but this idea has not been confirmed by primate experiments (Zola-Morgan, Squire, and Amaral, 1989a,b). The work with lesions dates back to the nineteenth century (Brown and Schäfer, 1888), but is now identified particularly with the Klüver-Bucy syndrome, seen in monkeys after a bilateral surgical lesion of the medial temporal region (including amygdala and hippocampus) (Klüver, 1951). The lesion also leads to secondary degenerative changes elsewhere, including changes in the anterior commissure, frontotemporal white matter, and connections to the cingulate cortex (Klüver, 1951). It may be relevant that the amygdala and hippocampus are interconnected structures; specifically, in primates, the amygdala projects to CA1, to the subiculum, and to entorhinal cortex (Amaral, 1986). The operated animals show a failure of visual recognition and lose their fear of creatures that would normally frighten them (snakes, for example). They are compulsively hypersexual; they will put everything graspable into their mouths. Two recent abstracts suggest that in a temporal-lobe lesion of this sort, the amygdala lesion contributes to the "emotional" component, while damage to the perirhinal, parahippocampal, and perhaps hippocampal areas contributes to the memory deficit (Alvarez-Royo et al., 1988; Zola-Morgan, Squire, and Amaral 1988).

Further insight into the role of the hippocampus in memory has come from clinical observations of patients with more restricted lesions, as well as from animal experiments with controlled lesions. Thus, the famous patient HM had more restricted bilateral amygdala/hippocampal lesions produced in a neurosurgical procedure aimed at relieving his severe epileptic seizure disorder (Scoville and Milner, 1957). Postoperatively, he had severe anterograde amnesia (inability to form new memories) that has persisted; there was loss of some memories from a few years prior to surgery. HM remains unable to learn the meanings of new words (Gabrieli, Cohen, and Corkin, 1988).

Patients who recover from anoxic encephalopathy, such as that following cardiac arrest, may well have dementia, including a severe disorder of memory.[3] The underlying neuropathology may be diffuse in these cases, however. One patient had dementia with more limited pathology: bilateral lesions involving CA1, the subiculum, and the amygdala (Volpe and Petito, 1985). Of particular interest is a patient with an amnestic syndrome in whom the lesion was confined to the hippocampi: There was bilateral destruction of CA1 (Zola-Morgan, Squire, and Amaral, 1986) (Figure 1.3). In this patient, immediate memory was relatively preserved, but material to be recalled was irrevocably lost over some minutes.

Patient HM was more amnesic than was the patient of Zola-Morgan et

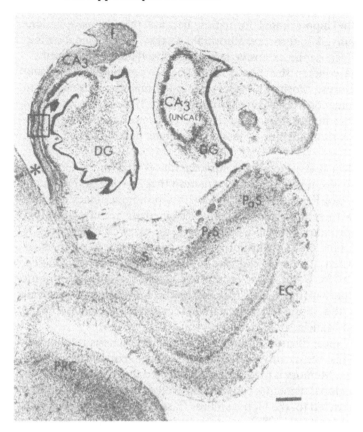

Figure 1.3. Dropout of CA1 cells in a patient with memory loss. The area of cell loss is the region between the two arrows. Calibration: 2 mm. (From Zola-Morgan, Squire, and Amaral, 1986, with permission.)

al. (1986). Presumably, this was due to his more extensive medial-temporal-lobe damage, such as to the amygdala. In the view of Mishkin (1978), removing both amygdala and hippocampus is more detrimental (in primates) to mnemonic function than is removing the hippocampus alone; Mishkin believed that the cooperative functions of the amygdala and hippocampus could be attributed to the overlap in inputs and outputs of the respective structures, together with their interconnections with each other. On the other hand, Zola-Morgan and Squire (1986) have documented amnestic problems in monkeys with bilateral hippocampal lesions sparing the amygdala (but the monkeys did have variable destruction in the EC and parahippocampal gyrus). The data of Zola-Morgan et al. (1989b) suggest that extensive medial-temporal-lobe lesions are more disruptive of mnemonic function than are lesions restricted to the hippocampal formation because the extensive lesions involve periamygdaloid cortex, entorhinal cortex, and perirhinal cortex, rather than because the extensive lesions involve the amygdala itself. These data concern the effects of damage to the hippocampus and related structures. "Positive" evidence that the hippocampus is used in mnemonic behavioral tasks comes from studies of 2-deoxyglucose utilization. Thus, the hippocampus and dentate gyrus are metabolically activated by "working-memory" tasks (Friedman and Goldman-Rakic, 1988).

It seems clear that although the hippocampus is vital for the formation of new memories, it is not the only structure that is required. For example, in Wernicke-Korsakoff syndrome with a profound amnestic deficit (but again with relative preservation of immediate recall), pathology may not be prominent in the hippocampus, as reviewed by Victor, Adams, and Collins (1973). Furthermore, lesions restricted to the thalamus, even when unilateral, can cause an amnestic syndrome (Goldenberg et al., 1983). Note, however, that the medial dorsal nucleus of the thalamus is part of the same "system" as the hippocampus, receiving inputs from the septum, amygdala, and mammillary bodies (Gritti, Mariotti, and Mancia, 1987).

Another clinical disorder that involves the hippocampus is limbic encephalitis. This occurs in association with cancer, particularly oat-cell cancer of lung. Memory is predominantly affected, but behavioral abnormalities and global dementia can occur as well. The pathology involves, but is not restricted to, the hippocampus (Case Records of the Massachusetts General Hospital, 1988). Areas affected include the hippocampus proper, the parahippocampal gyrus, uncal cortex, and amygdala. Lesions have also been described in the orbitofrontal cortex and the cingulate gyrus (Henson, Hoffman, and Urich, 1965). Corsellis, Goldberg, and Norton (1968) describe the pathology as either degenerative or inflammatory. Because paraneoplastic syndromes such as limbic encephalitis may be mediated immunologically, it is intriguing that there is a particular antigen found throughout the limbic system (although in other brain areas, too) (Horton and Levitt, 1986; Levitt, 1984).

Thus, certain types of memory appear to be stored somehow in the hippocampus and/or connected regions for periods upward of several minutes. The types of memory involved are "single-exposure" memory and perhaps verbal and spatial memory as well, as discussed later. Memory of the more distant past is less sensitive to hippocampal damage than is memory of the very recent past. A relevant time scale for analysis of population activities in the hippocampus would thus appear to be tens of seconds to minutes. This is what we must aim for in our experimental and modeling work. At the moment, however, most of our simulations deal with events on the time scale of milliseconds to hundreds of milliseconds.

The hippocampus and spatial performance in rodents

The hippocampus is also critical for rats to navigate a maze or to perform in the Morris milky-water test (Morris et al., 1982). In the latter test, the animal must repeatedly find a platform submerged in a tank of milky water. The animal cannot see the platform, but may be able to locate it by using spatial cues in the environment. Surgical lesions of the hippocampus or of the fimbria/fornix (Nilsson et al., 1987) impair performance of such tasks. Ischemic lesions destroying only half of the CA1 region in rats are sufficient to impair performance of spatial tasks (Auer, Jensen, and Whishaw, 1989). A tetanus-induced transient epileptic encephalopathy can be produced in rats by injection of tetanus toxin into the hippocampus; this syndrome is also followed by reduced performance in a maze (Brace, Jefferys, and Mellanby, 1985; Jeffreys and Williams, 1987). In at least one study, administration of AP5 (a blocker of the NMDA receptor) impaired the learning of a spatial task (Morris et al., 1986). This is of interest because the hippocampus has a particularly high concentration of NMDA receptors (Greenamyre et al., 1985; Monaghan and Cotman, 1985) and because NMDA-receptor activation is required for long-term potentiation (LTP) at many (but not all) synapses in the hippocampus. LTP, however, is normal in rats with tetanus encephalopathy, even though these rats still perform poorly in a maze (Jefferys and Williams, 1987).

The hippocampus in rodents is remarkable also for the existence of place cells (O'Keefe and Nadel, 1978). These cells increase their rate of firing when the animal is in a particular part of a certain locale: the place field of the respective cell; see Eichenbaum and Cohen (1988) for a review. Muller, Kubie, and Ranck (1987) have performed elegant quantitative experiments on these cells in rats. The relative increase in firing of a place cell is particularly noticeable during theta rhythm, an EEG activity that appears in the hippocampus during walking (as described later) and that tends to be associated with a low overall rate of firing of pyramidal cells in the hippocampus proper. However, place specificity persists for CA1 cells after theta is abolished by septal microinjection of the local anesthetic tetracaine (Mizumori et al., 1989). Muller et al. (1987) found that more than 60% of CA3 cells were place cells. Spatial coordinates in the environment were not clearly correlated with the location of place cells in the hippocampus; that is, nearby cells could have place fields that were far apart; see, however, Eichenbaum et al. (1989). Although multiple sensory modalities (visual, olfactory, and auditory) can contribute to the definition of a place field for a given cell, visual cues appear to be primary (O'Keefe, 1979). The place field of a cell may be altered by tampering with distant visual cues (Muller et al., 1987). There is recent evidence that the place field for hippocampal neurons is modifiable by experience, as, for example, by putting drinking water (Breese, Hampson, and Deadwyler, 1989) or transparent Plexiglas (Muller and Kubie, 1987) into particular spots in the environment. It is of interest that the hippocampus in monkeys is used not only for memory of new experience, but particularly for memory of where objects are in space (Parkinson, Murray, and Mishkin, 1988), and neurons have been found in monkey hippocampus that increase their firing rate in response to the spatial location of a visual stimulus (Rolls et al., 1989). These observations in rats may have correlates in the hippocampal function of primates and humans.

Synchronization and EEG in the hippocampus

We shall now consider several types of neuronal population behaviors in the hippocampus. The most obvious population behaviors are those in which neuronal firing is synchronized. Such synchronous activities include rhythmical EEG waves, sharp waves and other EEG transients (both normal and pathological), and seizures. Synchronization, like many fundamental concepts, is difficult to define precisely. The concept involves three ideas: a time scale Δt, a spatial scale ΔV, and a distinguishable state S of the neurons. Synchrony depends on how many neurons within ΔV during Δt are in state S. For the model, Δt is 1 ms, ΔV is either the whole model or $\frac{1}{15}$ of it, and state S is "soma depolarized more than 20 mV," this being the criterion for sending an axonal output. Synchrony is calculated every millisecond, defining the *synchronization curve*. The characteristics of this curve (amplitudes of peaks, silent intervals, Fourier spectrum, and so on) can then be analyzed. It would not be easy experimentally to measure synchrony, because we would need to record from all of the cells. The character of the synchronization curve must be inferred either from dual intracellular recordings or from field-potential recordings. The correspondence between experimental observation and a simulated synchronization curve is straightforward only when all of the cells are firing together, as during epileptiform events.

Because observation of all of the cells is possible only in computer simulations, we must briefly consider what measurements are actually practical in vivo. The behavioral state of an animal is associated with different behaviors of the hippocampal neuronal population. One therefore needs to observe the brain during different behavioral states, and this effectively makes intracellular recording impossible. Most in vivo neurophysiological experiments are done with electrodes that record either (i) the potential in the extracellular space between neurons or (ii) the potential some distance from the brain substance (e.g., on the brain surface, the dura, or the scalp), but with the assumption that the recorded potentials indirectly reflect neuronal activity. The relation between neuronal activity and extracellular potentials is complex; see

Pedley and Traub (1990) and the references therein for a review. Very concisely, action-potential currents produce brief extracellular-potential fluctuations, which can be recorded with a nearby electrode. In addition, propagated action potentials cause synaptic currents to flow across the membranes of target cells (which may be local or at a distance from the firing cell); the synaptic currents may be either excitatory or inhibitory and will have a spatial distribution that will depend on the transmitter and receptor types, as well as the membrane locations of the synapses. Extracellular currents produced by summed synaptic currents constitute the major "source" of the EEG, except at very low frequencies. Slow potential shifts in the EEG can be produced by activity-induced changes in the extracellular milieu, for example, in potassium-ion concentration. Clearly, measurement of EEG signals does not define neuronal activities precisely, but rather provides a set of constraints on what the neurons might be doing (see also Chapter 7).

We shall consider only a few of the many types of hippocampal EEG patterns. These are theta rhythm or rhythmic slow activity (RSA) and EEG sharp waves and spikes and ictal or seizure events. EEG sharp waves form a spectrum between normal and abnormal degrees of cellular synchronization. In each case, there are three general issues to discuss: What are the behavioral correlates of the EEG pattern? [We emphasize again that the behavioral state is inseparable from the collective neuronal behaviors (and in turn the EEG patterns) that are expressed in any given brain region; the behavioral state is even correlated with the transmission of action potentials through hippocampal circuitry (Buzsáki, 1989; Buzsáki et al., 1981; Winson and Abzug, 1978).] What parts of the brain generate the EEG pattern, and are the individual EEG waves in these different parts in phase, or at least phase-locked? What is known about the cellular physiology underlying the EEG pattern?

Throughout, we must consider two alternative mechanisms underlying the collective neuronal behavior and EEG pattern in a brain region. Is population activity imposed by some corresponding collective behavior in an input structure, possibly one or more subcortical nuclei? Or, on the other hand, does the EEG pattern result from some autonomous collective behavior in the observed structure, with the effect of inputs from other structures being to set "system parameters" (e.g., the maximum values of membrane conductances such as $g_{K[Ca]}$), and so emphasize or bring out different collective modes of activity? This latter idea has been explored in invertebrate central pattern-generating networks (Heinzel, 1988b; Heinzel and Selverston, 1988). If population behaviors are generated within relatively small neuronal networks, we can, in principle, gain understanding of the EEG from observing collective neuronal behaviors in brain slices. Such behaviors cannot be directly imposed by inputs from other brain structures, because these structures are disconnected in the

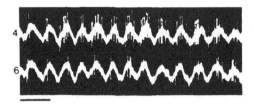

Figure 1.4. Hippocampal theta in the rat during walking. Simultaneously recorded unit activity from interneurons in CA1 stratum oriens. Electrodes are 500 μ apart. Calibration: 250 ms. (From Buzsáki et al., 1989a, with permission.)

slice preparation. And furthermore, we can manipulate pharmacologically various system parameters in the slice and observe which collective modes are thereby expressed.[4]

Theta rhythm (Figure 1.4) is an EEG signal recorded from the hippocampus in the approximate frequency range 4–12 Hz; for a review, see Buzsáki (1985) and Buzsáki, Leung, and Vanderwolf (1983).[5] Theta rhythm is easier to detect in rodents and rabbits than in cats and primates (including humans), and its cellular mechanisms have been better characterized in rodents and rabbits than in other species. Its behavioral correlates in cats are also more complex than in rodents (Wilson, Motter, and Lindsley, 1976). We shall therefore be discussing rodents and/or rabbits, unless specified otherwise. Theta occurs during locomotion, sensory stimulation (such as stroking the fur), rapid-eye-movement (REM) sleep, and urethane or ether anesthesia. Even with urethane present, sensory stimulation can increase the amplitude and frequency of theta. Theta rhythm can be elicited in anesthetized animals by stimulation of the mesencephalic reticular formation (Vertes, 1982, 1985). Theta can also be induced by repetitive stimulation of the septum at theta frequencies. High-frequency stimulation (at greater than 100 Hz) leads to desynchronization of the hippocampal EEG (Vertes, 1985). Stimulation of the lateral hypothalamus tends to suppress theta (Grastyán et al., 1965; Wilson et al., 1976), perhaps via concurrent stimulation of the median forebrain bundle (Vertes, 1985). Theta rhythm in waking animals has been classified into types 1 and 2 (Kramis, Vanderwolf, and Bland, 1975; Sainsbury, 1985). Type-1 theta, of frequency 6–12 Hz, occurs during walking and running and is resistant to muscarinic blockade, such as that produced by atropine. Type-2 theta, of frequency 4–9 Hz, occurs during immobility and is sensitive to atropine. Type 2 is rarely observed as a spontaneous event in rats, but is common in rabbits. Lesions such as disconnection of the septum or the entorhinal cortex from the hippocampus suggest that both types of theta can occur simultaneously in the awake rat. Frequency doubling of theta can occur during running (Buzsáki, Rappelsberger, and Kellényi, 1985). The extracellular potentials recorded during theta rhythm, using electrodes at different tissue depths, suggest that the potentials reflect synaptic currents produced by excitatory and inhibitory inputs to different membrane locations of pyramidal and dentate granule cells (Buzsáki et al., 1986). This does not explain how the synaptic inputs themselves are generated by cells firing within and outside the hippocampus; this issue will become critical in our consideration of EEG-like activity generated autonomously in hippocampal slices (Chapter 7). Although theta has been most often studied in CA1 and in the dentate, it can also be recorded in CA3 and in the hilus (Buzsáki et al., 1986).

In exploring rats, theta waves are phase-locked to sniffs and to motion of the vibrissae (whiskers), although the precise phase relations can drift with time (Komisaruk, 1970). Theta waves can be correlated with other types of motor activity such as limb movements (Semba and Komisaruk, 1978) or the onset of bar pressing in rats that press a bar in order to stimulate the lateral hypothalamus (Buño and Velluti, 1977). Theta waves can also be phase-locked to a sensory stimulus, such as a tone presented durĩng conditioning experiments (Buzsáki et al., 1979).

Theta rhythm occurs in multiple limbic-system locations, not just in the hippocampus. [These limbic areas are all reciprocally connected with the septum, as well as with each other; see Alonso and Köhler (1984), as well as the references cited later.] The occurrence of theta in the *subiculum* (Buzsáki et al., 1986) is expected, because the subiculum receives a major input from CA1 (Buzsáki, 1985). In the entorhinal cortex, theta rhythm occurs in both deep and superficial layers, 180° out of phase with each other; the rhythm is at the same frequency as CA1 theta and is phase-locked to CA1 theta (Alonso and Garcia-Austt, 1987a,b; Mitchell and Ranck, 1980). Interestingly, different layers of the entorhinal cortex project to CA1, as compared with the dentate gyrus (Lopes da Silva et al., 1985; Steward and Scoville, 1976): CA1 theta and dentate theta are also out of phase with each other. Like the hippocampus, the medial septum/diagonal band is reciprocally interconnected with the entorhinal cortex, and the input from the septum is both cholinergic and noncholinergic (Alonso and Köhler, 1984).

An intriguing aspect of theta rhythm is that entorhinal-cortex cells tend to fire in a manner phase-locked to the rhythmical theta waves, even when the cells themselves do not fire rhythmically (Alonso and Garcia-Austt, 1987a,b) (Figure 1.5). Rhythmic cells fire more than one action potential per theta wave, on average. Whether these cells are interneurons or bursting excitatory neurons is not known. This feature of theta raises an interesting question: How does a neuronal population generate a rhythm that is not clearly evident in the firing of any single neuron? A similar phenomenon occurs in hippocampal slices. We shall return to this question in Chapter 7.

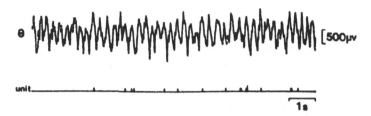

Figure 1.5. Simultaneous recording of theta activity and a single unit (neuron) in the rat entorhinal cortex. Note the apparently irregular firing of thc unit. (From Alonso and Garcia-Austt, 1987b, with permission.)

Theta rhythm in the septal nuclei is believed somehow to drive hippocampal theta. One can record theta rhythm in the septum before it has begun in the hippocampus, as, for example, after a seizure (Alonso et al., 1987; Petsche, Stumpf, and Gogolak, 1962). Cooling the fimbria/ fornix eliminates theta in the hippocampus while septal theta continues (Stewart and Fox, 1989). Certain lesions also suggest that the septum is critical for hippocampal theta: Medial septal lesions abolish theta in the hippocampus and entorhinal cortex (Vanderwolf and Leung, 1983). Although subcortically denervated (i.e., disconnected from the septum) hippocampus does not exhibit theta, theta can be restored by a transplant (into the fimbria/fornix) that includes fetal septal neurons (Buzsáki et al., 1987b).

Rhythmic firing can occur in septal neurons in vitro with no connected hippocampus (Vinogradova, Zhadina, and Brazhnik, 1987). More commonly, in vivo, septal theta and hippocampal theta occur together, at the same frequency and phase-locked. When cells fire (including nonrhythmic cells), they tend to do so at a particular phase of theta, although the phase involved depends on the individual cell (Alonso et al., 1987). Most rhythmically firing cells in the septum continue their rhythmic firing even in the presence of muscarinic cholinergic blockade (Stewart and Fox, 1989).

It is appropriate to review here the reciprocal septal-hippocampal connections and the physiology of the septal region. The rat septal region is large relative to total brain size. The medial-septum/diagonal-band projection extends all over the hippocampus. The septum-to-hippocampus connection has been studied using horseradish peroxidase (HRP) injections (Crutcher et al., 1981). This connection is dense to the dentate hilus and stratum oriens of CA3, "modest" to the dentate molecular layer and stratum radiatum of CA3, and "sparse" to the strata oriens and lacunosum/moleculare of CA1 (Meibach and Siegel, 1977b; Raisman, 1966). Reciprocally, CA1 projects to the medial septum (Raisman, 1966) and to the lateral septum (Knowles and Schwartzkroin,

1981b). Areas CA3 and CA4 also project to the lateral septum. Nonpyramidal neurons have been observed sending axons into the medial septum/diagonal band (Alonso and Köhler, 1982; Chronister and DeFrance, 1979).

The septum exerts influences on the hippocampus via cholinergic, GABAergic, and perhaps other pathways. The details of the different pathways are important for understanding the mechanisms underlying theta generation, as well as for interpreting the results of pharmacological manipulations, particularly the fact that theta rhythm is (sometimes) abolished by agents that block muscarinic acetylcholine synapses, as described later. A large fraction of septal neurons are cholinergic, although one group has estimated that the fraction of cholinergic cells in the medial septum/diagonal band is less than 50% (Baisden, Woodruff, and Hoover, 1984). Cholinergic terminals ramify throughout the hippocampus. Most of the terminals originate in the septum/diagonal band, but some conceivably may originate from intrinsic hippocampal cells (Amaral and Kurz, 1985; Matthews et al., 1987). Explants of septal nuclei also make cholinergic synapses with cocultured hippocampal explants (Gähwiler and Brown, 1985a), providing an interesting experimental model for studying the cellular physiology of septal-hippocampal relations.

Cholinergic agents such as carbachol or eserine (physostigmine) can elicit rhythmic activity both in vivo (Bland and Bland, 1986; Malisch and Ott, 1982; Vanderwolf and Leung, 1983) and in vitro (Konopacki et al., 1987; Leung and Yim, 1988; MacVicar and Tse, 1989). It is not clear whether or not the in vitro rhythmic activity should be called "theta," because pyramidal-cell firing is much more prominent in vitro than in vivo. These data suggest that acetylcholine released by septal neurons into the hippocampus might elicit or facilitate theta rhythm through a tonic action rather than through a phasic action. The long duration of effects (minutes) of iontophoretically applied acetylcholine supports this hypothesis. One view (G. Buzsáki, personal communication) suggests that a slow septal cholinergic input is permissive for the septal GABAergic input to induce or facilitate theta generation in hippocampal, subicular, and entorhinal circuitry. However, acetylcholine applied to neocortical slices can elicit phasic inhibitory effects (Strowbridge and Shepherd, 1988); such an action conceivably may exist in the hippocampus, because hippocampal GABAergic cells probably receive cholinergic input from the septum (Freund and Antal, 1988).

The mutual interrelations of the septum, hippocampus, and entorhinal cortex appear to be rather complicated. Vanderwolf and Leung (1983) studied the effects of bilateral (but incomplete) entorhinal-cortex lesions in rats. The animals were jumpy. Theta disappeared in CA1, but was found in the dentate during walking. The lesions favored the occur-

rence of hippocampal sharp waves, as discussed later. Eserine (physostigmine) injections elicited theta in both normal and entorhinal-lesioned
rats, suggesting that the septal cholinergic input to the hippocampus –
suitably amplified by the acetylcholinesterase inhibitor eserine – can
elicit hippocampal theta, without requiring an entorhinal input. On the
other hand, atropine abolished theta in lesioned animals (but not in
normal animals), as though the entorhinal cortex supplied some noncholinergic input to the hippocampus sufficient to elicit theta there even
with septal cholinergic influences blocked.

In addition to the cholinergic input, there is a GABAergic input to the
hippocampal formation from the septum (Freund and Antal, 1988).
These fibers predominantly inhibit GABAergic cells within the hippocampus. This connection may be relevant to the genesis of both theta
rhythm and sharp waves, as discussed later. Septal inhibition of hippocampal inhibitory neurons could produce an oscillatory phasic or a tonic
disinhibition in the hippocampus. Phasic disinhibition at the right frequency might contribute to theta, whereas tonic disinhibition would be
expected to lead to sharp waves. The firing patterns of septal GABA-
ergic cells during different behavioral states remain, however, to be
determined. Septal afferents onto GABAergic cells in the dentate gyrus
have been demonstrated (Schwerdtfeger, 1986), but it is not known if
these afferents are themselves GABAergic.

Cellular physiology of septal neurons

Some in vitro septal neurons exhibit spontaneous rhythmicity at 2–10 Hz
that depends, at least in part, on intrinsic membrane properties, because
it disappears when the cell is hyperpolarized (Segal, 1986). These neurons appear to be generating intrinsic bursts, with fast action potentials,
slower calcium spikes, and a long-lasting (up to about 500 ms) afterhyperpolarization (AHP) (Lopez-Barneo, Alvarez de Toledo, and
Yarom, 1985) (see Chapter 2). Griffith (1988) distinguishes three classes
of septal cells: bursting cells (7%); cells with a slow AHP, lasting about
600 ms (40%); and cells with a fast (5–50 ms) AHP (53%). The bursting
cells develop a rebound burst after a long hyperpolarizing current is
released, in a manner reminiscent of thalamic neurons. Similarly, a
fimbria shock causes an inhibitory postsynaptic potential (IPSP) that is
followed by an 80–250-ms depolarization that may reach firing threshold
(Dutar, Lamour, and Jobert, 1985). This property could well be relevant
to theta generation in the septum, just as it appears to be for EEG
spindle-rhythm generation by cells in the nucleus reticularis thalami and
connected thalamic nuclei (Steriade and Llinás, 1988). Cells with a slow
AHP do not exhibit rebound bursting (Griffith and Matthews, 1986).
Interestingly, cells with a slow AHP appear to be cholinergic, based on

acetylcholinesterase staining, whereas fast-AHP cells do not appear to be cholinergic (Griffith and Matthews, 1986). Perhaps the latter cells will prove to be GABAergic. Acetylcholine depolarizes septal neurons, while increasing cellular input resistance (Segal, 1986), an effect similar to that produced by acetylcholine on hippocampal pyramidal cells (Halliwell and Adams, 1982).

Theta rhythm has also been recorded in rat cingulate cortex during walking. The waves recorded in the cingulate seem to be locally generated rather than being volume-conducted (Leung and Borst, 1987). The occurrence of theta in the cingulate is interesting, because this structure receives input from the subiculum. Because theta is not recorded in most six-layer cortex, it is useful to examine what is distinctive about the cingulate cortex. The cingulate cortex receives cholinergic inputs from the nucleus of the diagonal band of Broca, from the ventral globus pallidus, and from the substantia innominata (Borst, Leung, and Mac-Fabe, 1987). The cingulate cortex is distinguished from other six-layer neocortex in anatomical and electroencephalographic ways: Its major thalamic input is from the anterior nuclear group. In cats, the anterior nuclear group of the thalamus does not generate EEG spindles (apparently because it receives no input from the "spindle pacemaker," the nucleus reticularis thalami), and, in turn, the cingulate does not produce EEG spindles (Mulle, Steriade, and Deschênes, 1985). In contrast, other parts of the cortex, reciprocally connected with spindling regions of the thalamus, themselves generate spindles. Spindles are rhythmic EEG waves of 8–13 Hz, seen in slow-wave sleep and under barbiturate anesthesia, conditions not associated with limbic theta in rodents or cats. For a review of spindles and thalamic physiology, see Steriade and Llinás (1988). Spindles are rarely observed in rat cingulate cortex (Leung and Borst, 1987).

Brain-stem influences on theta rhythm

Influences of the brain stem on theta probably are mediated through the septum. The most potent positive effect on theta generation occurs after stimulation of the nucleus pontis oralis in the rostral pontine reticular formation (Vertes, 1985). Cells in this nucleus do not fire in rhythmic bursts, but rather tonically at high rates. The connection from this nucleus to the septum is apparently indirect, through the supramammillary nucleus. At least some cells in the nucleus pontis oralis appear to be cholinergic, because there is choline acetyltransferase and acetylcholinesterase staining there (Mizukawa et al., 1986). Interestingly, stimulation of this nucleus during active sleep (REM sleep) leads to hyperpolarization of motoneurons (Fung et al., 1982); thus, the nucleus pontis oralis may contribute to the muscular atony characteristic of REM sleep as well as to theta rhythm. Stimulation of the median raphe nucleus (containing serotoninergic cells) leads to desynchronization of theta, an effect apparently mediated by serotonin (Vertes, 1982, 1985). Desynchronization is seen in both the septum and the hippocampus itself. There is a direct projection from the median raphe to the medial septum through the median forebrain bundle. Median raphe cells also provide direct input to the hippocampus.

Cellular physiology of theta

In discussing the physiology of theta rhythm, one must always consider whether or not and how the animal is anesthetized. Thus, walking theta and urethane theta have different phase relations and depth profiles (Winson, 1974, 1976a,b). Here, we shall be interested not so much in laminar depth profiles (Buzsáki et al., 1985, 1986) as in the correlations of cellular firing with theta waves, with intracellular recordings, and with comparisons of behavior between different hippocampal regions. The results from different laboratories are sometimes conflicting.

Bland et al. (1980) found in urethane-anesthetized rabbits that CA1 pyramidal cells fired during the (locally) negative phase of theta waves.[6] The cells could fire during most theta waves (exceptions will be discussed later). Increased theta amplitude was correlated with increased theta frequency. The correlation of inhibitory cell firing with theta waves was less than was the correlation for pyramidal cells. Pyramidal-cell bursting is rare during in vivo theta rhythm (G. Buzsáki, personal communication). Bland, Seto, and Rowntree (1983), in studying awake rabbits, also found that increased theta frequency correlated with increased unit firing rates in the dentate gyrus.

Buzsáki and Eidelberg (1983), in studying rats under urethane anesthesia, likewise found that CA1 pyramidal cells fired during the locally negative theta phase, whereas CA1 interneurons fired mainly during the positive phase. Dentate interneurons could fire during either phase, depending on the cell. During theta rhythm, interneurons increased their firing, but pyramidal cells decreased their firing. Buzsáki et al. (1983) observed that interneuron firing was more likely during theta than was pyramidal-cell firing. They also showed that CA3 cells and dentate granule cells fired during the same theta phase; see, in addition, Fox, Wolfson, and Ranck (1986). The mean firing rate for granule cells, like that for interneurons, is increased during theta.

Leung and Yim (1986), with intracellular recordings from CA1 cells in rats under urethane anesthesia, found cyclic 10-mV membrane-potential fluctuations that were phase-locked to extracellular theta waves (up to 0.5 mV in amplitude). Maximum cellular hyperpolarization occurred during local theta positivity. This is consistent with the observations noted earlier that cell firing should be most probable during local theta negativity. Measurements of reversal potentials suggest that the intracellular waves represented IPSPs. Leung and Yim also observed synchrony in theta between the two hippocampi, provided recordings were taken at homologous locations.

Nuñez, Garcia-Austt, and Buño (1987) performed intracellular recordings in CA1 and CA3 neurons in rats under urethane anesthesia. They found that there was a sustained depolarization during theta, with superimposed membrane-potential oscillations. The oscillations could be either 5–10-mV subthreshold sine waves or slow spikes up to 60 mV in amplitude (presumably calcium spikes). The sine-wave oscillations behaved like EPSPs when the membrane potential was altered by current injection, in contrast to the findings of Leung and Yim (1986). Bursts of action potentials occurred in phase with theta waves. The bursts were periodic in some cells and random in other cells, even though the bursts still occurred in phase with theta waves. When the amplitude of extracellular theta waves was increased by stroking the fur, a nonperiodic cell could become periodic. Firing tended to occur on the depolarizing part of intracellular theta waves. Figure 2 of Nuñez et al. (1987) illustrates a cell bursting with each theta wave, at intervals of 250 ms. This high interburst frequency resembles the activity seen in hippocampal slices that have been bathed in cholinergic agents (Leung and Yim, 1988; MacVicar and Tse, 1989). Such high interburst frequency is not seen during theta in walking rats. Indeed, complex spikes, which correspond to cellular bursts, are rarely observed during walking theta.

Leung (1984) found that depth records of CA1 theta could be best explained by assuming cyclical excitatory and inhibitory inputs to CA1 pyramidal cells, with excitation leading inhibition. Excitatory synaptic inputs seem to be critical for theta generation, because Destrade and Ott (1980) could abolish theta rhythm after local injection of a glutamate blocker. On the other hand, the source of the relevant glutamatergic inputs is not clear. Whishaw and Sutherland (1982) observed theta after the CA3 and CA4 regions were lesioned with kainic acid. One might guess, then, that excitatory inputs from the entorhinal cortex are essential for theta generation. This notion receives some support from the disappearance of CA1 theta after entorhinal-cortex lesions (Vanderwolf and Leung, 1983).

Bullock, McClune, and Buzsáki (1988) have recorded theta with 16 separated electrodes (Figure 1.6). The waves are synchronized along the entire length of the hippocampus (G. Buzsáki, personal communication). Intrinsic factors within the hippocampus that could regulate the spatiotemporal characteristics of theta waves are discussed in the context of our model in Chapter 7.

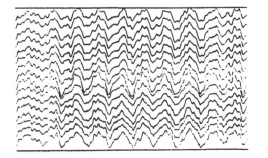

Figure 1.6. Theta rhythm recorded in an awake, exploring rat with 16 simultaneous extracellular electrodes in CA1 stratum radiatum. When the electrodes are aligned in the same architectonic layers (as in the present case), synchrony of waves occurs along the entire length of the hippocampus. Calibration: 125 ms, 1 mV. (Figure kindly supplied by Dr. G. Buzsáki.)

Theta rhythm in primates and humans

The behavioral correlates of hippocampal EEG appear to be different in humans and in rodents. Thus, hippocampal EEG desynchronization has been reported in humans during movement (Halgren, Babb, and Crandall, 1978). Arnolds et al. (1980) observed no change in hippocampal EEG when their patient went from walking to sitting, although changes were seen during different verbal behaviors. Isokawa-Akesson, Wilson, and Babb (1987) recorded hippocampal units in awake, resting epileptic patients; the hippocampus under study did not itself exhibit recognized epileptic activity. Cells were observed that fired rhythmically, sometimes in doublets or bursts, but no particular frequency stood out. Unfortunately, no correlation with the local field potential was reported. Hippocampal theta has been recorded in some human epileptic patients during REM sleep (P. Rutecki, personal communication).

Some conclusions about theta

1. Multiple interconnected areas of the limbic system generate theta during characteristic behaviors, including walking, running, and REM sleep. Areas generating theta include the septum, hippocampus, subiculum, entorhinal cortex, and cingulate cortex. Of these regions, the septum is the only one that seems able to generate theta rhythm in vivo when isolated from the other regions. We can hypothesize that large neuronal populations have preferred "resonant frequencies" that they can express under either tonic or phasic input conditions from connected regions. Acetylcholine may be permissive for a population oscillation through a tonic influence; this would be analogous to some invertebrate

pattern-generating circuits that exhibit different oscillatory modes under the influence of different neuromodulatory substances (Getting and Dekin, 1985a,b; Heinzel and Selverston, 1988). Alternatively, the predominant theta-generating influence of the septum may be mediated via phasic inputs onto inhibitory interneurons, as suggested by Buzsáki and Eidelberg (1983). Such influences could be mediated either by acetylcholine (which excites inhibitory cells in the neocortex and hippocampus) (McCormick and Prince, 1985, 1986; Reece and Schwartzkroin, 1988; Stewart and Fox, 1988; Strowbridge and Shepherd, 1988) or by GABA. Septal neurons have been observed to form both types of connections onto hippocampal inhibitory cells (Freund and Antal, 1988).

2. Whereas some cells fire rhythmically in phase with theta waves, other cells fire nonrhythmically; yet, when these latter cells do fire, their firing is still correlated with theta. The general question of how a population of neurons can generate rhythmic oscillations not apparent in individual neurons may be amenable to in vitro studies (see Chapter 7).

3. Because theta rhythm is not present during all behavioral states in awake rodents, nor is it readily apparent in humans, we wonder if theta is really critical for hippocampal function. Perhaps rhythmic hippocampal activity is difficult to detect in primates with field-potential recordings because relatively few neurons are involved or because the lamination of cells in the primate hippocampus is not as "tight" as in rodents and rabbits.

EEG spikes and sharp waves

We shall now discuss certain EEG transients, both normal and pathological: EEG (interictal) *spikes* and *sharp waves*. Both phenomena result from brief, synchronized discharge of a population of neurons, although the necessary degree of synchrony is not clear.

EEG spikes are defined as events lasting less than 70 ms that exceed the amplitude of background activity (Daly, 1979). They are usually negative at the brain surface and may be followed by a surface negative slow wave. Spikes can be biphasic or polyphasic. Sharp waves probably represent a similar cellular phenomenon, but are longer in duration (70–200 ms). Spikes may be inhibited by alerting or by sensory stimuli. In a series of 6,497 individuals without epilepsy, EEG spikes or sharp waves were found in only 2.2%, and seizures developed in 15% of those cases (Zivin and Ajmone-Marsan, 1968). Patients with focal epilepsy are much more likely to have EEGs containing spike foci. Currie et al. (1971) studied 666 patients with complex partial seizures; there were focal temporal abnormalities in 92%, including spikes or sharp waves in more than half of these. Trojaborg (1968) studied 242 children with EEG spike foci; 82% had seizures, and 13% had structural abnormalities of the brain without (recognized) epilepsy. In 10–20% of patients with complex partial seizures, spikes occur only during sleep, whereas in 1–7%, spikes disappear during sleep (Daly, 1979). This is another example wherein subcortical influences appear to regulate the extent of neuronal synchronization.

In some patients with myoclonus, afferent stimulation can evoke giant somatosensory potentials that resemble EEG spikes (Rothwell, Obeso, and Marsden, 1986). Spike/wave complexes evoked by a verbal memory task have been recorded in the human hippocampus (Altafullah and Halgren, 1988). Clinical seizures evoked by specific activities (eating, mental arithmetic) are well known, albeit rare.

The link between interictal spikes and synchronized neuronal firing has been demonstrated in humans (Wyler, Ojemann, and Ward, 1982). That result was expected after a number of studies of cellular electrophysiology of experimentally induced EEG spikes. These events (possibly leading into sustained seizures) can be produced in vivo by electrical stimulation (Sawa, Kaji, and Usuki, 1965; Sawa, Maruyama, and Kaji, 1963), by freezing the cortex (Goldensohn and Purpura, 1963), or by local application of $GABA_A$-blocking compounds like penicillin (Dingledine and Gjerstad, 1979, 1980; Wong and Prince, 1979), bicuculline (Curtis et al., 1971), or picrotoxin (Yakushiji et al., 1987). GABA blockade may be induced in either the neocortex (Matsumoto and Ajmone-Marsan, 1964a; Prince, 1968) or the hippocampus (Dichter and Spencer, 1969a,b). In each case, the cells demonstrate synchronized synaptic potentials and cellular firing. Generally, large EPSPs that initiate action potentials (the "paroxysmal depolarization shift") are observed in cells within the "focus"; more distant cells can demonstrate prolonged hyperpolarizations after the paroxysmal discharge (Dichter and Spencer, 1969b; Prince and Wilder, 1967). These hyperpolarizations may underlie the slow wave that often follows an EEG spike. The cellular mechanisms that underlie in vitro analogues of these in vivo events will be considered in detail in Chapter 6.

There is a normal EEG phenomenon called the small sharp spike (SSS). Although the cellular basis of the SSS has not been demonstrated directly, SSSs probably result from a limited degree of synchronous cell firing over a relatively large region of cortex or hippocampus. White, Langston, and Pedley (1977a) found that 24% of normal subjects have one or more SSSs after 24 hr of sleep deprivation, usually during stage-1 or stage-2 sleep. They occur at low frequency (less than one per 7 s) and can be bilaterally synchronous. Each SSS has a wide spatial distribution, but the boundaries of the distribution change from event to event. The SSS is followed by a slow wave. White et al. (1977a) never saw SSSs when a patient was awake (but note that human EEGs usually are taken with the patient at rest, not walking, drinking, etc.). In patients known

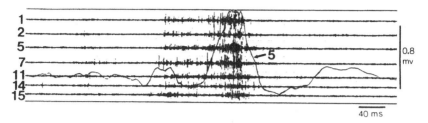

Figure 1.7. Synchronized firing during a physiological sharp wave in an intact rat during awake immobility. Recordings made with an array of 16 extracellular electrodes aligned along the longitudinal extent of the hippocampus in the stratum pyramidale of CA1. A filtered signal is also shown from electrode 5. Note the widespread synchrony. (From Buzsáki, 1989, with permission.)

to have complex partial seizures, EEG spikes occurred (at least on occasion) during the waking state; spikes could occur in runs, and sharp waves as well as spikes were recorded. None of these features is associated with the normal EEG.

Sharp waves detected in EEG recordings from animals

A possible animal correlate of the SSS is the sharp wave observed in rat hippocampus under physiological conditions. Sharp waves (SPWs) occur during "consummatory" behaviors, such as drinking and grooming, and during slow-wave sleep and awake immobility, but not normally during other behaviors such as walking (Buzsáki, 1986; Buzsáki et al., 1983; Suzuki and Smith, 1985, 1987, 1988a–d) (Figure 1.7). Moreover, they are suppressed by sensory stimulation. SPWs can be up to 3.5 mV in amplitude and can occur at rates of 0.2 to 5 per second (Suzuki and Smith, 1987). Although maximum SPW frequencies overlap the frequency range of theta rhythm, theta waves are much more regular than are SPWs. Clearly, though, a detailed comparison of the cellular mechanisms of an SPW with a single theta wave would be most interesting. SPW extracellular potentials are positive in layers 2–4 of the subiculum and in the strata oriens and pyramidale of CA1 and CA3, but are negative in the stratum radiatum of CA1. This laminar distribution is consistent with the occurrence of synaptic excitation into the stratum radiatum during an SPW. A similar laminar distribution is recorded in CA1 after stimulation of the Schaffer collaterals, suggesting that the partially synchronized burst recorded in CA1 is induced by partially synchronized firing in CA3 (Buzsáki et al., 1983; Suzuki and Smith, 1988b). A similar pattern of CA3-to-CA1 spread of synchronized firing is seen in hippocampal slices exposed to convulsant agents (Wong and Traub, 1983).

Extracellular-potential gradients during SPWs are 8–12 mV/mm; such gradients are large enough to influence cellular activity, at least in the dentate gyrus (Jefferys, 1981).

During an SPW, there is increased firing of pyramidal cells, interneurons, and granule cells (Buzsáki et al., 1983; Suzuki and Smith, 1988a) (Figure 1.7). The occurrence of an SPW is also associated with an increased response to an afferent volley. Blocking $GABA_A$ inhibition can further increase the amplitude of the SPW (Buzsáki, 1986; Suzuki and Smith, 1988d). This suggests that during an SPW inhibition is not completely blocked and that synchronization is incomplete. Buzsáki (1986) has directly shown that a single pyramidal cell does not fire during each SPW. SPWs are followed by EEG silence lasting 100 to 500 ms, and the larger the SPW the longer the silence (Buzsáki, 1986). The amplitude and frequency of SPWs are increased by high-frequency stimulation of the commissural/Schaffer system (Buzsáki, 1984), which should enhance the efficacy of excitatory synapses and which might suppress recurrent inhibition. Of special interest is the observation that SPWs are widely synchronized throughout both hippocampi (Figure 1.7). Buzsáki's criteria for the epileptiform (as opposed to normal physiological) nature of SPWs are these: Epileptiform SPWs can be rhythmic, of amplitude greater than 4 mV, or can occur during theta-associated behaviors. [Theta rhythm suppresses not only physiological SPWs but also epileptiform activity induced by local penicillin application (Lerma et al., 1985).] Epileptiform events tend to be of shorter duration than physiological SPWs (Buzsáki, 1986). The medial septum and entorhinal cortex are not essential for the generation of SPWs, although these inputs may modulate the rate (Buzsáki et al., 1983; Suzuki and Smith, 1988c).

Because CA1 SPWs appear to result from Schaffer-collateral input and commissural synaptic input, and because the septum and entorhinal cortex are not essential for SPW generation, these data suggest that the CA3 region in vivo can autonomously generate synchronized bursts, at least under certain conditions (Buzsáki et al., 1983). This again underscores the relevance of understanding how synchronization can be regulated within the CA3 region itself, an issue most readily studied in vitro.

SPWs have also been observed in the cingulate cortex in normal rats during drinking, grooming, and eating. In the cingulate cortex, unlike the hippocampus, SPWs occasionally occur interspersed with walking-associated theta (Leung and Borst, 1987).

Could SSSs be the human analogues of physiological SPWs in rats? Both events have wide spatial distributions. Further knowledge of the behavioral concomitants of SSSs and of their cellular mechanisms could help to answer this question.

The hippocampus and epilepsy

Interictal EEG spikes and sharp waves do not indicate seizures. EEG spikes and sharp waves have no observable clinical concomitant, whereas seizures usually do. EEG spikes and sharp waves last less than 200 ms, whereas seizures last seconds and longer (a precise minimum duration is not clear). EEG spikes and sharp waves appear to result from excitatory synaptic interactions, as discussed later. For seizures, the situation is more complex. Thus, many different types of collective neuronal behaviors qualify as "seizures." These behaviors include the following: (i) Absence seizures and their related experimental syndromes produced by systemic administration of penicillin (Avoli et al., 1983; Fisher and Prince, 1977a,b). This type of epilepsy may result from a global, but incomplete, blockade of certain types of IPSP in the cortex. (ii) The series of synchronized bursts that sometimes occur in the presence of $GABA_A$ blockers (see Chapter 6) (Hablitz, 1984; Miles, Wong, and Traub, 1984; Swann and Brady, 1984). Such events may be analogous to the so-called epileptic recruiting rhythm (Brenner and Atkinson, 1982) and/or to the clonic phase of grand mal seizures. Picrotoxin-induced seizures are dependent on excitatory synapses (Miles et al., 1984). (iii) The series of synchronized action potentials, associated with very large extracellular-potential transients, that occur in low-calcium media and sometimes in high-potassium media (Jefferys and Haas, 1982; Jensen and Yaari, 1988; Konnerth, Heinemann, and Yaari, 1984, 1986a; Taylor and Dudek, 1982, 1984a, 1984b; Traynelis and Dingledine, 1988a,b). These events appear not to require synaptic transmission at all. They may represent what the cortex is doing during the tonic phase of a grand mal seizure. (iv) Seizures occurring in hippocampal slices bathed in a low-magnesium solution (Swartzwelder et al., 1987). These events may depend on unblocking of the NMDA-activated channels. Mg^{2+} normally closes the NMDA-activated channel, unless the membrane is depolarized (Mayer, Westbrook, and Guthrie, 1984), but other factors, such as increased membrane excitability, could also be essential. No doubt, other types of seizures occur,[7] and such types may be relevant in poorly understood clinical seizure syndromes, including infantile spasms, atonic seizures, and myoclonic seizures. In summary, numerous physiological types of seizures occur, apparently involving different mechanisms, and some of the mechanisms are nonsynaptic (see Chapter 8).

The hippocampus is regarded as having a particularly low seizure threshold. Although this concept is not simple to quantify, we can cite two observations that support it. First, in epileptic patients whose seizures originate focally (Gastaut, 1970) (this being the majority of epileptic patients), the seizure focus is more commonly in the medial temporal lobe than in other cortical areas. Second, spontaneous epileptiform events are much more readily observed in hippocampal in vitro slices than in neocortical in vitro slices. Two issues must be considered to explain the low hippocampal seizure threshold: (i) What properties of the normal hippocampus (intrinsic cell properties, synaptic connectivity, subcortical inputs, and so on) render it susceptible to seizures? We suggest that recurrent excitatory synapses and a low pyramidal-cell firing threshold may be critical in this regard. (ii) Is the hippocampus especially prone to alter its structure or cellular properties after injury (head trauma, anoxia, prior seizures) so as to render it even more epileptogenic? If this is the case, what are the mechanisms?

Several factors may provide a link between injury and susceptibility to seizures. First, the subcortically deafferented hippocampus is extremely seizure-prone (Buzsáki et al., 1989b). Second, following an injury, some brain regions, including the dentate gyrus and hippocampus proper, develop aberrant recurrent excitatory connections, which would be expected to be epileptogenic (Cook and Crutcher, 1985; Frotscher and Zimmer, 1983; Sutula et al., 1988; Tauck and Nadler, 1985). Finally, the CA1 area is susceptible to cell loss after strong excitation (Sloviter, 1983), perhaps because of the rich abundance of NMDA receptors in CA1 (Monaghan and Cotman, 1985). Loss of target CA1 cells could lead to reactive sprouting of CA3 cell axons and so to the formation of new recurrent CA3-CA3 connections, although this has not been directly shown. Excitotoxic damage might explain several other features of hippocampal pathology and epileptogenesis: the loss of CA1 cells after sustained stimulation of the perforant path (Sloviter, 1983); the susceptibility of the hippocampus to ischemic damage (Brierley and Cooper, 1962; Kass and Lipton, 1982; Levine, 1960); and the neuropathological lesion called hippocampal sclerosis often found in patients with partial complex seizures of hippocampal origin.[8]

The clinical phenomenology of partial complex seizures is interesting in its own right, as well as for the hints it may provide as to hippocampal function. With respect to understanding hippocampal function, however, we must always remember that the expression of a clinical seizure depends not just on the site of origin but also on those brain structures involved in abnormal behavior as the seizure progresses and spreads. This defines yet another problem for cellular electrophysiology and modeling: Not only must we study how the seizure is initiated under special conditions (Delgado-Escueta et al., 1986) and what the involved neurons do during the seizure, but we must study how seizures spread from one brain region to another.

Using simultaneous videotape and EEG recording, Theodore, Porter, and Penry (1983) studied a series of patients with medically intractable seizures (such a series may not be representative of complex-seizure patients as a group). In this series, the focus of seizure onset was always in the temporal lobe, although complex partial seizures originating from other cortical lobes have been described (White et al., 1977a). Automatisms occurred in almost all seizures, usually involving the face and arms, and consisting of purposeless, repetitive movements. The patient could appear angry, or might vocalize or blink. An aura was unusual. Examples of auras included a characteristic smell or the experience of déjà vu [the best description we know of déjà vu, presumably not ictal, however, is by Proust (1927)]. Other auras were fear, a rising feeling in the stomach, blurred vision, and a feeling of helplessness. Many other examples of auras of complex partial seizures have been described; see, for example, the list of seizure experiences reported by Shorvon (1986). The seizure itself lasted about a minute, and the postictal state about a minute and a half. The initial seizure manifestation was staring, followed by automatisms (e.g., lip smacking, sucking, chewing, swallowing, and so on), stereotyped movements, and vocalizations. The latter might or might not be formed speech (Maldonado et al., 1988).

The interictal (i.e., "between seizure") EEG at the scalp in the Theodore et al. (1983) series could be normal or diffusely slow or could contain EEG spikes (unilateral, bilateral, or multifocal). The ictal (i.e., during the seizure) EEG could be unchanged, could contain bilateral sharp waves and slowing, or could show spikes; or there might be a transition from unilateral interictal spikes to bilateral ictal spikes. In nonmotor simple seizures (i.e., without alterations of consciousness) the EEG may show temporal theta[9] (Devinsky et al., 1988). Seizure phenomena associated with temporal theta included "dizziness," déjà vu, speaking, distortions of visual perception, and anxiety.

Halgren (1982) suggested that the hippocampus was involved in déjà vu, because he found that electrical stimulation of the medial temporal lobe could elicit the experience. Care was taken to use stimuli that were below threshold for seizure initiation. The hippocampus also seems to be somehow concerned with the sense of familiarity, because different potentials are evoked in the human hippocampus after exposure to familiar words as compared with unfamiliar words (Halgren, Smith, and Stapleton, 1985). The reader should be experiencing a sense of familiarity at this point, too, because place cells in rodents also register a recognition of familiarity for parts of the environment.

What is the relation between complex-seizure phenomenology and amnestic syndromes? In general, seizures that alter consciousness also alter memory for the seizure episode. (This is difficult to interpret in itself, however, because a seizure that begins, say, in the hippocampus may end up involving diverse brain structures.) Halgren and Wilson (1985) stimulated the amygdala, hippocampus, and parahippocampal gyrus in epileptic patients. They observed that impairment of delayed recall correlated with the occurrence of an evoked afterdischarge. Even though an evoked afterdischarge involved a more limited brain area than did a clinical seizure, the afterdischarge could still produce functional impairment of memory, possibly requiring specific tests for the recognition of the impairment. Interestingly, immediate recall and mental arithmetic were not affected by the afterdischarge. Bridgman et al. (1989) likewise observed acute impairment of memory tasks during subclinical electrographic seizures confined to a single hippocampus. Thus, we would guess that a functional disruption of hippocampal activity (as well as bilateral structural destruction of the hippocampi) can disrupt long-term memory.

The two-stage memory model. Buzsáki (1989) has developed a theory that ties together many of the observations we have been discussing. He supposes that during exploration, associated with hippocampal theta and with increased firing rates of (at least some) dentate granule cells, particular groups of entorhinal-cortex cells excite particular groups of dentate granule cells. These latter, in turn, excite particular groups of CA3 pyramidal cells. The selected CA3 cells, while not firing excessively during exploration,[10] are assumed to be altered, so that these same CA3 cells initiate the sharp waves that occur after exploratory behavior. LTP of Schaffer-collateral synapses probably occurs during the sharp waves, owing to the synchronized repetitive firing of a large group of CA3 cells. Likewise, the synapses formed by CA1 pyramidal cells, subicular cells, and dentate granule cells, which all participate in sharp waves, may well be potentiated during sharp waves. One can imagine the formation of complex loops involving cellular subsets of CA3, CA1, subiculum, entorhinal cortex, dentate, and back to CA3. Physiological studies – in which a shock is given to the perforant path, leading to both immediate and delayed responses throughout the hippocampus – suggest that loops such as this are possible (Buzsáki, 1989). It is an open question, however, how the divergence and convergence of the different connecting pathways might affect such loops (Amaral and Witter, 1989).

In summary, we have discussed the hippocampus and connected structures in vivo, emphasizing clinical, behavioral, and EEG issues. These issues suggest three broad types of scientific questions that have been explored in physiological experiments in vitro and in simulations: (i) cellular mechanisms of epilepsy; (ii) the nature of the EEG; (iii) memory (or at least synaptic plasticity; behavioral memory, as it is usually understood, is not even defined in vitro). These three issues are, in fact, intricately interrelated. For example, epileptiform EEG spikes are an extreme form of partially synchronous firing that characterizes an EEG wave. Likewise, repetitive afferent synaptic stimulation that induces synaptic plasticity can, if continued long enough, lead to epileptiform discharges.

It may be helpful to expand on these three main themes. With respect to epilepsy, we wish to know what types of electrographic seizures can be elicited in vitro (again, behavioral seizures are not defined in vitro). How can we account for such seizures? Historically, this was one of the first issues to be studied in hippocampal slices (Schwartzkroin and Prince, 1977). With respect to EEG, do slices exhibit rhythmic potential waves analogous to the in vivo EEG? Again, what are the mechanisms? If in vitro rhythmic activity is different from EEG, what can it tell us about the functional properties of the hippocampus? Historically, this question was studied after epilepsy, but the motivation for it came from interest in low concentration of epileptogenic agents (Miles and Wong, 1987a; Schneiderman, 1986; Schneiderman et al., 1989; Traub, Miles, and Wong, 1989) and from a search for characteristic behaviors in brain slices taken surgically from epileptic patients (Schwartzkroin and Knowles, 1984). The physiology of EEG-like waves is more subtle and difficult to understand than epileptiform behavior, but is important because it is closer to normal brain physiology. The common issue for epilepsy and EEG is this: How is synchronization of neuronal activity regulated? Two questions have provided the basis for the many studies on synaptic plasticity: How is it induced? How is it expressed? We might also ask another: What are the consequences for population activity of altering a given synapse or set of synapses? This question requires modeling in addition to experiments.

A more elusive set of questions with biological and theoretical components concerns the computational role of the hippocampus.[11] From a biological point of view, we would ask this: What mathematical computations are performed in the hippocampus? This is extremely difficult to address experimentally, either in vivo or in vitro. First, it is not known how information is encoded either in the input pathways to the hippocampus or in the output pathways from the hippocampus. Second, the hippocampus in vitro, and probably also in vivo, can generate its own spontaneous activity in the absence of outside stimulation. This means that the hippocampus cannot simply be an input–output device. We have also asked a different type of question: Given a model of hippocampal circuitry that reproduces known physiology, does a basis emerge for views of computation that differ from existing models such as the Turing machine, the Hopfield model, and layered neural networks? (See Chapter 9.)

The next two chapters will review the physiology of hippocampal neurons and of the synaptic connections. We shall then discuss how we model hippocampal neurons and networks. Finally, we shall consider the collective behavior of hippocampal neuronal populations, from experimental and theoretical points of view.

2 Physiology of single neurons: voltage- and ligand-gated ionic channels

In this chapter we ask how hippocampal neurons translate their synaptic inputs into an output signal sent toward other neurons. This basic question has two aspects. First, what are the firing patterns for pyramidal cells and interneurons? Neuronal firing patterns determine both how cells respond to synaptic inputs and the timing of synaptic events that they elicit in other cells. Second, what are the detailed physiological mechanisms, such as electrotonic properties or ionic-channel density and kinetics, that determine how and why a neuron responds as it does? We wish to know how a neuron functions as a device that processes its inputs that are distributed in space and time. A model of a neuron (Chapter 4) must capture the phenomenology correctly; preferably, the model will accurately represent underlying mechanisms to achieve that objective.

Before expanding on these themes, let us first consider the preparations that are used for cellular neurophysiology, with some of their advantages and disadvantages. In vivo studies are the sine qua non for understanding the normal repertoire of neuronal firing patterns and synaptic inputs and how these are correlated with behavioral states. However, stable intracellular recording is very difficult when animals are moving, such as during exploration-associated theta rhythm. Voltage-clamping cells in vivo is likely to be extraordinarily difficult. In vitro slices possess the advantages that much of the circuitry is retained from the intact brain, the ionic and chemical environment of the cells can be conveniently manipulated, and stable intracellular recordings can readily be obtained, even from two cells at once. Single-electrode voltage-clamping can be performed (Brown and Griffith, 1983a,b; Brown and Johnston, 1983; Johnston and Brown, 1983; Johnston, Hablitz, and Wilson 1980), as can intradendritic recording (Benardo, Masukawa, and Prince, 1982; Wong, Prince, and Basbaum, 1979). Drugs can be iontophoresed to portions of the cell membrane (Newberry and Nicoll, 1984, 1985), as well as globally, and groups of cells can be stimulated electrically or chemically, with hypertonic KCl (Wong and Traub, 1983), 4-aminopyridine (4-AP) (Segal, 1987), or glutamate (Christian and Dudek, 1988a,b), as well as other agents. Optical recording of neuronal populations can be achieved (Grinvald, Manker, and Segal, 1982). Recently, patch-clamp techniques have been applied to neurons in slices, promising new data on basic synaptic mechanisms, with an improved signal/noise ratio (Konnerth et al., 1988). Obviously, neurophysiology cannot be correlated with behavior in a brain slice. The cells may not be in a completely normal state, because they are, to some extent at least, deafferented; many cells will have had parts of their dendrites and some of their axonal branches sheared off. Voltage-clamping of neurons in slices suffers from problems of incomplete spatial control of the membrane potential, because of the dendrites (see the Appendix to Chapter 4 for some review of voltage-clamp concepts). Because of the high resistance of the intracellular electrodes used for switching the clamp, together with their limited current-carrying capacity, it is difficult to voltage-clamp currents that are rapidly varying in time or are large.

Cultured neurons offer many of the advantages of slices, particularly the ability to control the chemical milieu. With the ability to visualize single neurons, it is possible to iontophorese drugs to selected portions of the membrane and to insert two microelectrodes into a given cell (Segal and Barker, 1984a–c, 1986). The latter is an advantage for voltage-clamp studies, although problems of incomplete spatial control remain. Optical recording is readily done on cells in culture, with simultaneous measurements of membrane potentials in multiple dendritic and somatic locations (Grinvald, Ross, and Farber, 1981) and intracellular calcium transients (Ross, Arechiga, and Nicholls, 1987). Cells in culture may not be normally differentiated, however, nor is the synaptic connectivity normal (see Chapter 3). A recently developed technique involves the slice culture, in which a hippocampal slice is maintained in culture conditions for weeks, long enough for the cells to redistribute into a monolayer, yet with retention of much of the normal synaptic organization (Frotscher and Gähwiler, 1988; Gähwiler, 1981; Llano et al., 1988; Thompson and Gähwiler, 1989a–c).

Isolated pyramidal neurons are particularly favorable for biophysical and biochemical studies (Kay and Wong, 1986). Cells are readily visualized and can be patched under different modes (whole cell, isolated patch, etc.). Voltage-clamp studies can then be undertaken with low-resistance electrodes (Kay and Wong, 1987; Numann, Wadman, and Wong, 1987; Stelzer, Kay, and Wong, 1988). Remarkably, the internal chemical environment can now be modified during the course of an experiment (Chen et al., 1990; Kostyuk, Krishtal, and Pidoplichko, 1981). Unfortunately (or perhaps fortunately for voltage-clamping), isolated cells lose most of their dendrites, so that an important contribution to cell function is lost. Likewise, there are no normal physiological synaptic inputs to these cells.

Data deriving from all of these techniques, and others yet to be devel-

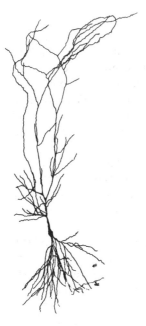

Figure 2.1. CA3 pyramidal cell, horseradish peroxidase (HRP) injection. Note apical dendrites (above) and basilar dendrites (below). (Drawing by Dr. A. I. Basbaum.)

oped, are important to achieve an integrated understanding of the physiology of the hippocampus.

Types of cells. About 90% of the cells in the CA3 region are pyramidal cells (Figure 2.1), the principal output neurons, whose synapses are excitatory (Misgeld and Frotscher, 1986). Most of the remainder of the cells probably are inhibitory and use GABA as their transmitter. The inhibitory cells have a number of different locations within CA3, as well as different axonal arborization patterns, firing behaviors, and postsynaptic actions. A complete classification does not yet exist, but many data are available (Gamrani et al., 1986; Lacaille and Schwartzkrain, 1988a; Lacaille et al., 1987; Ribak, Vaughn, and Saito, 1978; Sloviter and Nilaver, 1987). The taxonomy of cell types may prove complicated, because cells of pyramidal morphology may take up GABA (Hoch and Dingledine, 1986) or react with anti-GABA antibodies (Gamrani et al., 1986). The presence in some cells of different peptides, which may be released from terminals, and of different calcium-binding proteins may help to define further subsets of hippocampal inhibitory neurons. The physiology of inhibitory cells is considered briefly at the end of this chapter and in the next chapter. We shall mainly be concerned with pyramidal cells; there are far more data for pyramidal cells than for inhibitory cells.

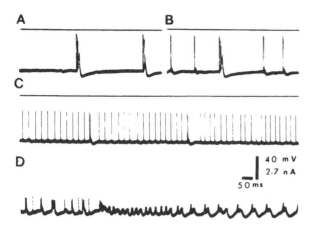

Figure 2.2. Some of the repertoire of firing behaviors of a CA3 pyramidal cell in the slice. A: Intrinsic bursts, each followed by an AHP, at a small injected depolarizing current. B: At a larger current, bursts are interspersed with spike doublets. C: At a still larger current, bursts do not occur, but rather single spikes and spike doublets (followed by a brief AHP). D: At a larger current still, the membrane develops ~20-Hz oscillations. (From Wong and Prince, 1981, with permission.)

General observations on pyramidal cells: phenomenology of their behavior. The input resistance of CA3 pyramidal cells in the slice ranges from 20 to over 50 MΩ, and the membrane time constant is typically from 30 to 50 ms.[1] CA3 pyramidal cells contain a variety of voltage- and calcium-dependent currents, as reviewed later. These currents allow pyramidal cells to fire not only single action potentials but also intrinsic bursts of up to eight spikes at intervals of 5–10 ms (Figure 2.2). Bursts occur both in vivo (Kandel and Spencer, 1961b; Spencer and Kandel, 1961b,c) and in vitro (Wong and Prince, 1978). A burst consists of a series of action potentials, riding on a depolarizing wave, with one or more slow, calcium-mediated action potentials. It lasts from 30 to 50 ms. The burst is followed by a long AHP (Hotson and Prince, 1980) that may last about 1 s. A burst can be triggered as an all-or-none event, analogous to a single action potential, by a brief excitatory stimulus (i.e., lasting only a few milliseconds) (Wong and Prince, 1981; Wong et al., 1979). Thus, a burst represents a form of amplification, both in terms of total membrane current and in terms of duration.

According to the data of Masukawa, Benardo, and Prince (1982), obtained from guinea pig slices, not all CA3 stratum pyramidale cells (presumed to be pyramidal cells by virtue of action-potential morphology) are burst-firing; some of the cells respond to either brief or sustained depolarizing currents with one or a few action potentials. These authors found burst generation to be more common in CA3a cells (near CA2) than in CA3b cells.

The burst depends on at least one calcium current (Wong and Prince, 1981). The existence of such a calcium current can be demonstrated when sodium channels are blocked with tetrodotoxin (TTX). A slow, calcium-dependent action potential can then be elicited (Schwartzkroin and Slawsky, 1977; Wong and Prince, 1981). It takes rather large currents to elicit this slow action potential, and even then it has a latency delayed for tens of milliseconds. The calcium spike is more readily shown when (at least some) outward currents are blocked, as, for example, with tetraethylammonium (TEA) (Segal and Barker, 1986), a property shared with many other types of neurons [e.g., dentate granule cells (Fricke and Prince, 1984)]. The relevance of a calcium current to intrinsic bursting is known because blockers of calcium current prevent typical bursting while allowing individual action potentials to occur (Wong and Prince, 1981). Specifically, what disappears from the burst in the presence of calcium blockers are spike-depolarizing afterpotentials (DAPs),[2] as well as the single or multiple slow spikes that often occur toward the end of a burst. Apparently, summation of DAPs leads eventually to generation of one or more calcium spikes. The long latency of calcium spikes could reflect a high threshold or slow activation kinetics of the responsible current, or dendritic [perhaps in multiple sites (Wong and Prince, 1978)] location of the channels, or both. However, not all calcium channels are located in the dendrites. Calcium currents are detectable in isolated cells deprived of distal dendrites (Kay and Wong, 1987), and calcium channels have been demonstrated on the somata of cultured neurons (Jones, Kunze, and Angelides, 1989). The detailed mechanisms by which one or more calcium currents, and perhaps other inward currents, contribute to bursting are yet to be fully elucidated.

Dendritic electrogenesis. The varying shapes and latencies of calcium spikes suggest that they are initiated at diverse dendritic locations (Wong and Prince, 1978). Direct intradendritic recordings suggest that calcium spikes can indeed be generated in apical dendrites of hippocampal pyramidal cells (Benardo et al., 1982; Masukawa and Prince, 1984; Wong et al., 1979) and in basilar dendrites (Lacaille et al., 1987). The presence of possibly multiple dendritic sites, each capable of generating sodium or calcium spikes, or both, is intriguing; such sites would vastly increase the complexity of the cell as a "logical device."[3]

It appears that both the soma and the dendrites of CA3 pyramidal cells are able to generate bursts. In contrast, CA1 pyramidal cells have somewhat different properties: Dendritic burst generation occurs in response to a brief injected current (Wong et al., 1979) or after orthodromic stimulation with inhibition blocked. But steady current injected into the soma usually leads to accommodating repetitive firing, rather than a burst (Lanthorn, Storm, and Anderson, 1984; Madison and

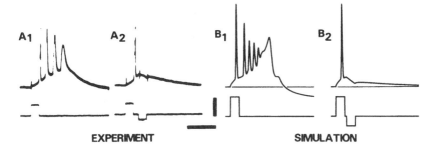

Figure 2.3. An intrinsic burst can be triggered by a brief current pulse in a CA3 pyramidal cell; a properly timed hyperpolarizing pulse can prevent the burst from developing, while leaving a depolarizing afterpotential. For details of the simulation, see Chapter 4. This particular model used multiple dendritic bursting sites, but that is not critical for the behavior illustrated. Note the slow Ca^{2+}-mediated action potentials. Calibrations: 15 ms, 20 mV, 1.3 nA for A, and 1 nA for B. (From Wong and Prince, 1981, and Pedley and Traub, 1985, with permission.)

Nicoll, 1984; Schwartzkroin, 1978). Nevertheless, bursting can be seen in the somata of CA1 pyramidal cells when inhibition is blocked and the cells are driven maximally by synchronized firing in CA3 (Schwartzkroin and Prince, 1978; Wong and Traub, 1983). CA1 cells in different subregions tend to have different firing properties (Masukawa et al., 1982).

A burst is terminated by a slow, intrinsic hyperpolarizing afterpotential (AHP) mediated by one or more calcium-dependent K^+ currents (Hotson and Prince, 1980) that increase the input conductance of the cell by 25–40% (Alger and Nicoll, 1980a; Hotson and Prince, 1980). The ionic basis of this AHP is rather complex; the AHP has two or three distinguishable components mediated by different calcium-dependent K^+ currents (Lancaster and Adams, 1986; Lancaster and Nicoll, 1987; Numann et al., 1987; Storm, 1989). Furthermore, if the cell bursts as part of a synchronized population burst, still another K^+-dependent (but not calcium-activated) afterpotential is present (Domann, Dorn, and Witte, 1989; Schwartzkroin and Stafstrom, 1980).

Bursting is truly intrinsic to the individual cell, and not an emergent property of hippocampal circuitry. It is particularly noteworthy that a burst can be elicited by injection of a brief current pulse. Additional support for the intrinsic character of bursting comes from the observation that spontaneous burst frequency is modulated by currents injected into an individual cell, with burst frequency increasing as the cell is depolarized (Hablitz and Johnston, 1981; Wong and Prince, 1981). Even more definitive is the observation that bursts (without, however, clearly evident calcium spikes) can be elicited in isolated hippocampal neurons not synaptically connected to anything at all (Figure 2.4).

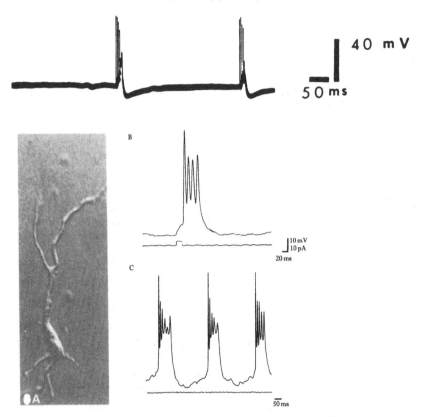

Figure 2.4. Intrinsic bursts in pyramidal cells in a slice (above) and in isolated pyramidal cells sheared of many of their dendrites (A–C). Note that the isolated cell can produce a burst after a brief current pulse (B), or it can produce a series of bursts during a sustained current injection (C), but Ca^{2+} spikes are not apparent. (Top from Wong and Prince, 1981; A–C from Wong, Traub, and Miles, 1986, with permission.)

Not only does steady depolarization of a CA3 hippocampal neuron lead to increasing burst frequency, but further depolarizations lead to a characteristic sequence of behaviors: repetitive bursts separated by trains of single action potentials, then action potentials only without bursts, and finally membrane oscillations (at about 20 Hz) without somatic action potentials (Wong and Prince, 1981). On the other hand, hyperpolarization of the membrane tends to suppress spontaneous bursting; Hablitz (1984) found a highest rate of spontaneous bursts (about 1 Hz) at a holding potential of about −55 mV. [His slices were bathed in picrotoxin, however, but that ought not to affect spontaneous burst frequency; a similar dependence of burst frequency on membrane potential was found in normal media by Hablitz and Johnston (1981), with depolarization (from about -59 mV to about -51 mV) tending to increase burst frequency. These authors observed spontaneous bursts at frequencies from 0.28 to 1.0 Hz.]

Some of the important functional consequences of the ability of CA3 pyramidal cells to burst are as follows: (i) Pyramidal cells do not readily fire sustained high-frequency trains of action potentials, but rather tend to fire groups of closely spaced (5–10 ms apart) action potentials, separated by long intervals with reduced firing, or else single or paired action potentials. (ii) A given sequence of excitatory inputs may evoke, in a postsynaptic neuron, a burst, one or two action potentials, or only a subthreshold depolarization; the response will depend on whether or not the postsynaptic cell is hyperpolarized and on the concurrence of appropriately timed and located inhibitory inputs. The probabilistic nature of synaptic transmission (see Chapter 3) may also be relevant in determining how the postsynaptic neuron responds. (iii) Calcium entry during the burst, in addition to opening potassium channels, may serve a variety of second-messenger functions, as described later. Calcium entry into a postsynaptic cell seems to be crucial in initiating long-term potentiation (Gustafsson and Wigström, 1988; Malenka et al., 1988). Excessive calcium entry may mediate excitotoxic cell death (because during ischemia with impaired energy metabolism there could be problems in pumping calcium out of the cell and/or in sequestering calcium). (iv) The effect of a bursting neuron on postsynaptic connected neurons will consist of a sequence of EPSPs. Because the time constant for pyramidal cells (30–40 ms or more) is much longer than the interspike interval during a burst (5–10 ms), these EPSPs will summate. As a consequence, even if individual EPSPs are subthreshold for spike triggering, a burst-evoked sequence of EPSPs can (and often does, see Figure 3.9) elicit a burst in a connected neuron. This concept turns out to be important for understanding the CA3 region (see Chapters 3, 6, and 7).

When the process of DAP summation is diminished by injection of a suitably timed pulse of hyperpolarizing current, a developing burst can be terminated, to yield only one or two action potentials followed by a DAP (Figure 2.3). This property of hippocampal neurons is critical for their role in network behavior. It may be appropriate to jump ahead a bit and comment on why this is so. If a bundle of hippocampal afferents is stimulated by a brief shock, pyramidal cells typically respond with a single spike or an EPSP, followed by a fast, Cl^--mediated IPSP and then by a slower K^+ IPSP; see, for example, Newberry and Nicoll (1984), Knowles et al. (1984), Thalmann (1984), and Gähwiler and Brown (1985a,b). The fast IPSP plays a functional role analogous to the brief hyperpolarizing potential in Figure 2.3; if this IPSP is blocked, the same afferent stimulus can evoke a dendritic burst (Wong et al., 1979), which may, in turn, elicit a somatic burst. Consider now another, more physio-

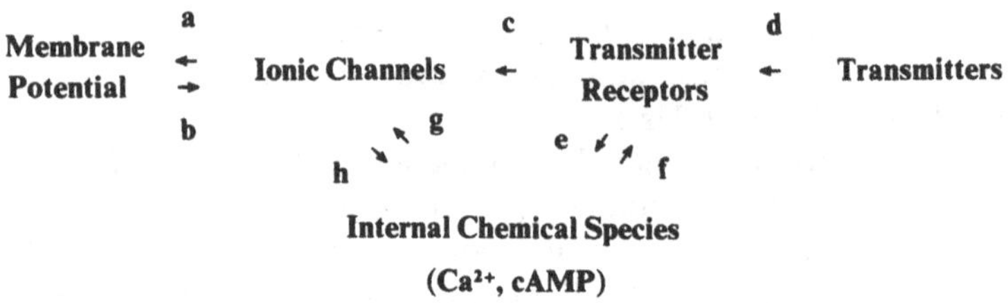

```
          a                      c                    d
Membrane  ←                   Transmitter  ←
Potential    Ionic Channels  ←  Receptors     Transmitters
          b              g
                    h  ↖ ↖      e ↙ ↗
                                     f
```

Internal Chemical Species

(Ca²⁺, cAMP)

Figure 2.5. The essential elements that regulate the behavior of neurons on a time scale of milliseconds to seconds. Some of the interactions between these elements are shown.

logical, situation. Suppose that there is a group of CA3 cells that are firing synchronously. Synaptically connected neurons, either in CA3 or in CA1, will receive in consequence a mixture of excitatory and inhibitory inputs, the relative timing and amplitude of which will determine whether or not and how the postsynaptic cells will fire, and in particular whether or not they will burst (Mesher and Schwartzkroin, 1980). Because CA3 cells are interconnected through divergent connections, the effects of one neuron not firing, firing a single action potential, or firing a burst will be amplified "downstream"; that is, differing firing behaviors in any given cell will be "experienced" by all of the cells to which that cell sends outputs, and a single input to any of these cells may in turn critically influence its behavior. (These concepts will be expanded in Chapter 6.)

Ideally, we would have a complete description of the currents generating bursts and afterpotentials based on voltage-clamp data. Unfortunately, quantitative data, though increasing rapidly, are still incomplete. Furthermore, in neurons, not only are there many types of ionic channels, but these channels are gated by multiple factors besides the membrane potential (Figure 2.5). Thus, an understanding of how the cell functions as a device requires (i) an understanding of how localized ionic currents result in a spatial and temporal distribution of membrane potential (this is the domain of cable theory, see Chapter 4) and (ii) an understanding of how membrane potential itself, transmitter-receptor complexes, and the internal milieu of the cell interact to determine the states of the different ionic channels; these channel states, in turn, determine (along with the distribution of ionic species across the membrane) what the various ionic currents will be. This vast subject ultimately requires a sophisticated understanding of the structure, function, and regulation of neuronal membrane proteins, something we can only attempt to summarize very briefly. Membrane channel physiology has been reviewed by Adams and Galvan (1986) and by Llinás (1988); receptor–channel interactions mediated through the interior of the cell have been reviewed by

Nicoll (1988); see also McCormick and Williamson (1989). Table 2.1 lists some of the interactions known to occur in hippocampal neurons, referring to Figure 2.5. The list is not comprehensive.

Inhibitory cells. Inhibitory cells have widely different shapes (Lorente de Nó, 1934; Tömböl, Babosa, and Somogyi, 1979; Tömböl, Somogyi, and Hajdu, 1978), axonal distributions, locations (Sloviter and Nilaver, 1987), and firing patterns, with some inhibitory cells resembling pyramidal cells in their firing patterns (Kawaguchi and Hama, 1988; Traub, Miles, and Wong, 1987b). Interneurons also differ in the presence or absence of different calcium-binding proteins (Sloviter, 1989). Many interneurons fire trains of brief action potentials, without succeeding long-duration AHPs, and with the frequency of firing continuously controllable by synaptic input (Kawaguchi and Hama, 1988; Lacaille and Schwartzkroin, 1988a,b; Lacaille et al., 1987). Other inhibitory neurons fire broader action potentials, a series of which may be followed by an AHP (Kawaguchi and Hama, 1988; Figure 1 of Traub et al., 1987b). These latter cells tend to accommodate; that is, a high frequency of firing cannot be sustained. GABA staining or GAD staining of cells reveals that putative inhibitory cells occur in all layers of the hippocampus, with diverse morphology and axonal branching patterns, and with synapses onto the soma, dendrites, or axon initial segments of target cells (Schlander and Frotscher, 1986; Sloviter and Nilaver, 1987; Somogyi et al., 1983b,c).

Examples of inhibitory cells include basket cells (located in or near the stratum pyramidale, and with perisomatic synapses), oriens/alveus interneurons (Lacaille et al., 1987), moleculare/lacunosum interneurons (Lacaille and Schwartzkroin, 1988a,b), and chandelier cells, forming synapses onto axon initial segments (Somogyi et al., 1983b). (See Chapter 3 for more details about these cells.)

The input resistance of CA3 inhibitory cells is 50–60 MΩ (Miles, 1990), and the membrane time constant is 8–12 ms. Some inhibitory cells in CA3 show adaptation during sustained depolarizing-current injection, but others do not. Compared to pyramidal cells, CA3 inhibitory cells exhibit narrower action potentials, each of which is followed by a spike AHP. These findings are similar to those for many types of inhibitory cells in CA1. It is possible that CA1 stratum lacunosum/moleculare cells possess a low-threshold calcium current, because they exhibit rebound depolarizations (sometimes with firing) after hyperpolarization (Lacaille and Schwartzkroin, 1988a). Some CA3 inhibitory cells also exhibit this property (Miles, 1990).

Two types of synaptic inhibition. One type of synaptic inhibition is mediated by the action of GABA on the GABA$_A$ receptor, with resulting flow

Table 2.1

Ionic channels → membrane potential
This is the subject of cable theory (Chapter 4)

Membrane potential → ionic channels (i.e., voltage-dependent channels)
g_{Na}, action potential (Sah, Gibb, and Gage, 1988)
g_{Na}, slowly inactivating (French and Gage, 1985)
g_{Ca}, high threshold, slowly inactivating (in isolated cells) (Kay and Wong, 1987; Meyers and Barker, 1989)
g_K, transient or A type (Gustafsson et al., 1982; Numann, et al., 1987; Segal, Rogawski, and Barker, 1984)
g_K, delayed rectifier (Numann et al., 1987)
$g_{K[Ca]}$, C current (Storm, 1987)
$g_{K[Ca]}$, type 1 (Numann et al., 1987)
$g_{K[Ca]}$, type 2 (Numann et al., 1987)
g_K, M-type, voltage-dependent conductance decreased by acetylcholine (Halliwell and Adams, 1982)
g_{AR}, anomalous rectifier (Hotson, Prince, and Schwartzkroin, 1979)
g_L, leakage conductance, involves several cations
NMDA-activated channels (ligand, Mg^{2+}, and voltage-sensitive) (Mayer et al., 1984; Nowak et al., 1984)
GABA-activated Cl^- channels (both ligand and voltage-sensitive) (Gray and Johnston, 1985)

Transmitter → receptor → ionic channel
Glutamate binds to NMDA, quisqualate, or kainate receptor types, coupled to Na- and/or Ca-permeable channels.
GABA (A-type receptor) coupled to Cl^- channels.
NMDA-activated channels (see above)

Transmitter → receptor other than "normal" one (cross-modulation)
Glycine modification of NMDA receptor (Johnson and Ascher, 1987)
Glutamate modification of $GABA_A$ receptor (Stelzer and Wong, 1989)

Ionic channel → internal milieu
Ca^{2+} entry through voltage-dependent and NMDA-gated channels.

Internal milieu → receptor
Phosphorylation-step regulation of $GABA_A$ receptor function (Stelzer et al., 1988; Chen et al., 1990)

Transmitter → receptor → internal milieu → ionic channel (i.e., second-messenger effects) (Nicoll, 1988)
GABA → B receptor → G protein → K channel
Serotonin → receptor →G protein → K channel
Adenosine → receptor → G protein → K channel
Acetylcholine → phosphatidylinositol breakdown → M-type K channel
Acetylcholine → receptor → protein kinase C activation → reduction of
$g_{K[Ca]}$

Table 2.1 *(cont.)*

Norepinephrine → β receptor → cAMP → reduction of $g_{K[Ca]}$
Norepinephrine → ? steps → modulation of voltage-dependent Ca channel (Gray and Johnston, 1987)
(Histamine and corticotrophin-releasing factor similar to norepinephrine β receptor (Haas and Konnerth, 1983))
Internal milieu → direct (?) modification of ionic channels
Ca^{2+} inactivation of Ca^{2+} channels (Kay and Wong, 1987)
Ca^{2+} activation of K current $(g_{K[Ca]})$ (Numann et al., 1987)

of cl⁻. There is another type of inhibition, with "delayed" or "slow" IPSPs mediated by GABA$_B$ receptors (perhaps on dendrites) that are coupled to K⁺ channels (Kehl and McLennan, 1985a,b; Knowles et al., 1984; Newberry and Nicoll, 1984, 1985; Thalmann, 1984).

An interesting question concerns the existence of a special class of interneurons mediating delayed or slow IPSPs, and whether such a class of cells is excited by both feedforward and feedback (recurrent) pathways. Lacaille and Schwartzkroin (1988a,b) suggest that stratum lacunosum interneurons in the CA1 region might generate slow IPSPs. Several lines of evidence suggest indirectly that separate inhibitory cells mediating slow IPSPs exist in the CA3 region and are activated by recurrent circuitry: (i) Prolonged stimulation of individual cells mediating fast IPSPs has never been observed to produce as well a delayed IPSP (R. Miles, unpublished data). (ii) Spontaneous slow IPSPs are observed that are not preceded by large fast IPSPs. (iii) Small drops of 4-AP cause both repetitive firing in selected interneurons and the appearance of long-duration K-dependent hyperpolarizations (not affected by picrotoxin) in pyramidal cells, suggesting that 4-AP excites a subpopulation of inhibitory cells (Segal, 1987). (iv) Synchronized bursts in CA3 in the presence of GABA$_A$ blockers are followed by hyperpolarizing potentials that are not blocked by intracellular EGTA (i.e., that do not seem to be calcium-dependent) (Schwartzkroin and Stafstrom, 1980); one of these hyperpolarizing afterpotentials is blocked by phaclofen, a GABA$_B$ antagonist (Domann et al., 1989; Kerr et al., 1987). Inhibitory cells generating these potentials presumably are excited by pyramidal-cell activity in feedback fashion. On the other hand, in the CA1 region, slow IPSPs are not activated by antidromic stimulation (Newberry and Nicoll, 1984), suggesting that in this part of the hippocampus there is little recurrent activation of cells mediating slow inhibition. Dual intracellular recordings also suggest that the CA1 stratum lacunosum/moleculare interneurons that may mediate slow IPSPs within CA1 are not excited by pyramidal cells (Lacaille and Schwartzkroin, 1988a,b).

3 Synaptic function and organization of the CA3 region

In this chapter we review data on unitary synaptic interactions between hippocampal neurons necessary to construct a model of the CA3 neuronal network. First, the properties of excitatory and inhibitory synapses between hippocampal neurons are described. We then show that the properties of single synapses allow certain details of the operation of simple recurrent circuits to be deduced. Finally, we consider how activity occurring in multiple parallel circuits is integrated into the summed activity of a large neuronal network. These matters will be further expanded in later chapters.

Our current knowledge of synaptic function has been derived from only a few synapses, such as neuromuscular junctions in frog (Katz, 1969) and crayfish (Atwood and Wojtowicz, 1986), the giant synapse of the squid stellate ganglion (Llinás and Nicholson, 1975), synapses on goldfish Mauthner cells (Korn and Faber, 1987), and Ia afferents terminating on spinal motoneurons (Rall, 1967; Redman and Walmsley, 1983). Are these synapses useful models for understanding connections between cortical cells? Clearly, cortical synapses must be studied directly to provide appropriate information. Such studies have proliferated with the increasing use of isolated preparations. From these studies, values are emerging for several critical parameters of cortical synaptic function. We shall give current estimates from connections between hippocampal neurons.

First, what is the amplitude of postsynaptic potentials evoked by a single presynaptic excitatory or inhibitory neuron? The operation of cortical neuronal networks depends crucially on these units of cellular interaction. Second, can we use fluctuations in amplitudes of synaptic events to estimate two factors that determine PSP amplitude – the number of transmitter release sites at a synapse and the number of channels activated by transmitter released from one site?

Next, we begin to consider a central question for mammalian neurobiology: What is the use of so many cells? Obviously, large numbers of motoneurons can optimally time and weight the activation of many muscle groups and so generate sophisticated movements. Similarly, the parallel processing of multiple aspects of visual information requires large numbers of cells in primary visual cortical areas. But what are the millions of CA3 pyramidal cells in one human hippocampus doing? We first consider anatomical and physiological techniques to measure connectivity in a large neuronal population. Next, we examine the probabilistic operation of synaptic circuits built on this anatomical substrate. Finally, we ask whether or not neuronal population behaviors can be synthesized and understood from the operation of simple synaptic circuits.

Unitary synaptic events

Electrical stimulation of afferent pathways elicits similar sequences of synaptic potentials in most hippocampal neurons. In granule cells from the dentate gyrus, and in CA1 or CA3 pyramidal cells, a small, short depolarization is succeeded by a larger and often biphasic hyperpolarization. This complex waveform lasts for several hundred milliseconds and is a superimposition of events generated at many excitatory and inhibitory synapses (Barrionuevo et al., 1986). The basic paradigm of recording complex synaptic events initiated by simultaneously activating many afferent fibers (Adrian, 1936) has been extremely productive, especially for pharmacological studies. However, massive, coherent presynaptic discharge seems likely to occur only in pathological situations, such as when cells receive inputs from an epileptic focus. For a deeper understanding, events generated at individual synapses must be examined. Several techniques have been used to generate unitary events at single hippocampal synapses:

1. Weak, carefully placed stimuli may activate a few similar cells or fibers (McNaughton, Barnes, and Anderson, 1981; Turner, 1988). Pharmacological antagonists that selectively block receptors at excitatory or inhibitory synapses may enhance the value of this approach.

2. Focal glutamate application can activate spatially restricted cell groups, while passing axons are not excited (Christian and Dudek, 1988a,b). Correlating postsynaptic events with extracellular spikes from a single neuron in the region of glutamate application (Jankowska and Roberts, 1972; Yamamoto, 1982) is helpful, but it is difficult to show that only one cell fires.

3. Spontaneous synaptic events impinging on single neurons can provide useful data on aspects of transmitter release and receptor pharmacology (Brown, Wong, and Prince, 1979; Collingridge, Gage, and Robertson, 1984; Cotman et al., 1986). However, synaptic events may result from activity in more than one group of presynaptic cells.

4. Presynaptic and postsynaptic cells can be recorded simultaneously (MacVicar and Dudek, 1980a). Synaptic events can then be unambiguously attributed to a single cell whose activity can be controlled. However, the success rate will be low unless neuronal connectivity is high.

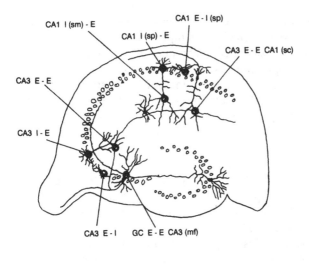

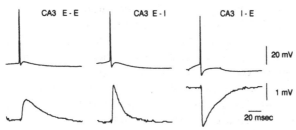

Figure 3.1. Schematic diagram showing hippocampal cell types and the synapses between them. Averaged presynaptic and postsynaptic records from three types of synapses between CA3 neurons: E–E, recurrent excitatory synapse between pyramidal cells; E–I, excitation of an inhibitory cell by a pyramidal cell; I–E, inhibition of a pyramidal cell by an inhibitory cell.

One or more of these techniques have been used to examine synapses between cells in hippocampal slices, as shown in Figure 3.1. Work on synapses between cultured hippocampal neurons has provided valuable insights into mechanisms of transmitter action, but neuronal identity and spatial context are lost in dissociated-cell culture. Abnormal connectivities may develop, possibly because of reduced competition of presynaptic terminals for postsynaptic sites. For instance, the proportion of inhibitory cells that survive in culture seems to be larger than in situ (Hoch and Dingledine, 1986; Segal and Barker, 1984c). In addition, the number of terminals made at a connection between neurons in culture (Pun et al., 1986) may be abnormally high. This can result in unusually high values for the conductance of single synaptic events (Forsythe and Westbrook, 1988; Segal and Barker, 1984c). It remains unclear whether or not culture conditions influence the number of receptors inserted in the matrix facing a single release site. However, synapses between cultured cells possess several advantages. Receptor agonists and antagonists may be applied rapidly to specific visualized sites (Bekkers and Stevens, 1989). In addition, the membranes of cultured cells are accessible for recordings with low-resistance patch electrodes. In contrast, penetration of neurons in slices with sharp, high-resistance electrodes may result in significant leak conductances and thus may affect synaptic events (Clements and Redman, 1989). The developments of explant slice culture (Gähwiler, 1981), where some spatial organization is retained in a single cell layer, and of patch-electrode recording from slices may combine some advantages of both techniques (Edwards et al., 1989; Llano et al. 1988; Sakmann et al., 1989).

We next review some properties of unitary synaptic actions at hippocampal synapses.

EPSP from dentate granule cell to CA3 cell (mossy fiber)

By means of glutamate microapplication to excite granule cells, mossy-fiber EPSPs of 2–12 mV amplitude were recorded in CA3 pyramidal cells (Yamamoto, 1982; Yamamoto, Higashima, and Sawada, 1987). EPSPs with an amplitude of several millivolts and fast rise times occur spontaneously in many CA3b and CA3c cells (Brown et al., 1979; Cotman et al., 1986). These events are presumed to result from activity in mossy-fiber terminals that are electrotonically close to the CA3 pyramidal-cell soma.

Recurrent EPSP from CA3 pyramidal cell to CA3 pyramidal cell

In recordings from pairs of CA3 pyramidal cells, we have found that recurrent EPSPs initiated by single presynaptic action potentials have mean amplitudes ranging between 0.6 and 1.3 mV (Miles and Wong, 1986). The time to peak for averaged events varies between 5 and 12 ms. Figure 3.1 shows records from a presynaptic cell and postsynaptic cell at a recurrent excitatory synapse between CA3 neurons. In immature rat hippocampus, larger recurrent EPSPs, up to 3 mV in amplitude, have been recorded in the same way (Smith, Turner, and Swann, 1988).

EPSP from CA3 pyramidal cell to CA1 pyramidal cell (Schaffer collateral)

Sayer, Friedlander, and Redman (1990) recorded EPSPs of mean amplitude 0.13 mV in CA1 cells following CA3 cell spikes. This value compares with amplitudes of 0.4 mV for minimal EPSPs elicited in CA1 cells by weak afferent stimulation (Turner, 1988). This low amplitude agrees with the observation that spontaneous EPSPs are difficult to resolve in CA1 neurons, in contrast to the large EPSPs apparent in CA3 cells.

EPSP from pyramidal cell to inhibitory cell (CA1 and CA3)

EPSPs initiated by CA1 and CA3 pyramidal-cell firing have been recorded in neurons identified as inhibitory by their firing patterns or by showing that they inhibited another cell (Lacaille and Schwartzkroin, 1988a,b; Miles, 1990). These events have amplitudes in the range 2–3 mV, as shown in Figure 3.1. Large, fast-rising EPSPs occur spontaneously at high frequency in many inhibitory cells. Their rise time is 2–4 ms, considerably faster than recurrent EPSPs that impinge on pyramidal cells, possibly because of different electrotonic locations of the synapses, as well as the different time constants between pyramidal and inhibitory cells.

IPSP from CA1 inhibitory cell (stratum pyramidale) to CA1 pyramidal cell

Schwartzkroin and associates recorded inhibitory potentials in CA1 pyramidal cells when inhibitory cells were made to fire repetitively (Knowles and Schwartzkroin, 1981a; Lacaille et al., 1987). The summed IPSPs resulting from 50–100-Hz presynaptic firing were 2–4 mV in amplitude, suggesting that the unitary IPSPs probably were less than 0.5 mV in amplitude. It is difficult to observe spontaneous IPSPs in CA1 pyramidal cells unless the driving force for Cl^- is enhanced by intracellular Cl^- injection (Alger and Nicoll, 1980b). In voltage-clamped Cl^--loaded CA1 cells, the conductance of spontaneous IPSPs was in the range 3–10 nS (Collingridge et al., 1984).

IPSP from CA1 inhibitory cell (stratum lacunosum/moleculare) to CA1 pyramidal cell

These inhibitory cells differ from those located close to the stratum pyramidale in regard to firing pattern and source of excitatory input (Lacaille and Schwartzkroin, 1988a,b). They may mediate the late K^+-dependent phase of the afferent evoked synaptic inhibition, rather than the Cl^--dependent phase that inhibitory cells in the strata oriens and pyramidale are assumed to generate. Single action potentials in these inhibitory cells do not evoke a measurable event, but repetitive firing can elicit a summed IPSP of peak amplitude about 1 mV.

IPSP from CA3 inhibitory cell (stratum pyramidale) to CA3 pyramidal cell

Interactions between inhibitory cells located within or close to the CA3 stratum pyramidale and CA3 pyramidal cells seem to be more diverse than in CA1 (Miles and Wong, 1984). We have found that inhibitory cells possess different firing patterns: Some exhibit the pronounced spike AHPs characteristic of CA1 basket cells, whereas other inhibitory cells have much less pronounced AHPs (Figure 3.2). Unitary IPSPs were always resolved on averaging responses to single action potentials. However, IPSP amplitudes vary over an eightfold range between different connections. Synaptic transmission fails at weak inhibitory synapses (Figure 3.2B), but failures do not occur at strong synapses (Figure 3.2A). This points to a presynaptic source for the differences in efficacy, possibly a difference in the number of inhibitory terminals. Peak conductance changes for averaged IPSPs vary between 2 and 10 nS. The time to peak for IPSPs is in the range 3–10 ms.

Electrotonic interactions between CA3 cells and between dentate cells

Dual impalements have shown that some dentate granule cells and some CA3 pyramidal cells are electrically coupled (MacVicar and Dudek, 1980b, 1981, 1982; MacVicar, Ropert, and Krnjevic, 1982; R. Miles, unpublished data). The junctions do not appear to rectify: Hyperpolarizations and depolarizations are transmitted equally well between coupled cells. Coupling ratios typically are 0.05 to 0.15, and potential changes transmitted to the postsynaptic cell are attenuated at high frequencies.

In summary, most unitary synaptic events recorded in the hippocampus are quite large. Peak somatic conductances are in the range 0.1–3 nS for unitary EPSPs and 0.8–10 nS for unitary IPSPs. EPSPs are sufficiently large that single presynaptic cells can initiate postsynaptic firing. Spike-to-spike transmission occurs readily at excitatory synapses made onto inhibitory cells. At recurrent excitatory synapses between CA3 pyramidal cells, presynaptic bursts of action potentials often are needed to elicit a postsynaptic burst.

Fluctuations in transmiter release

Synaptic events fluctuate in amplitude at all hippocampal synapses that have been examined (Lacaille and Schwartzkroin, 1988a,b; Miles and Wong, 1984, 1986; Sayer et al., 1988, 1990; Smith et al., 1988). Figure 3.3 shows six responses: five EPSPs and one transmission failure, generated at a recurrent synapse between CA3 pyramidal cells. Analysis of these fluctuations, assuming that transmitter is released in quantal fash-

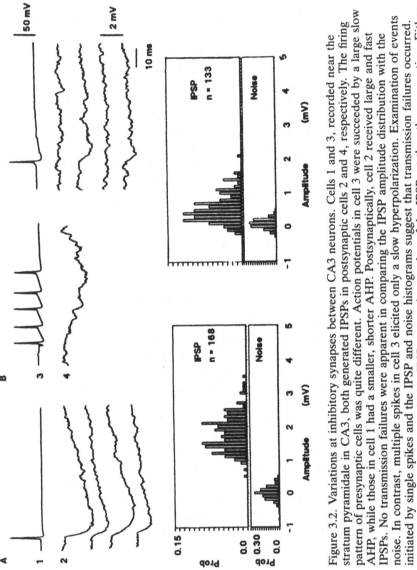

Figure 3.2. Variations at inhibitory synapses between CA3 neurons. Cells 1 and 3, recorded near the stratum pyramidale in CA3, both generated IPSPs in postsynaptic cells 2 and 4, respectively. The firing pattern of presynaptic cells was quite different. Action potentials in cell 3 were succeeded by a large slow AHP, while those in cell 1 had a smaller, shorter AHP. Postsynaptically, cell 2 received large and fast IPSPs. No transmission failures were apparent in comparing the IPSP amplitude distribution with the noise. In contrast, multiple spikes in cell 3 elicited only a slow hyperpolarization. Examination of events initiated by single spikes and the IPSP and noise histograms suggest that transmission failures occurred. However, the shape of recognizable IPSPs approximates that of the IPSPs at the other connection. Either different numbers of transmitter release sites or different probabilities of release could account for the difference.

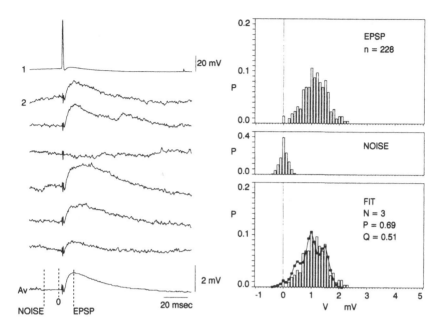

Figure 3.3. EPSP amplitude fluctuations at an excitatory synapse between two CA3 pyramidal cells. Six responses in cell 2 to single action potentials in cell 1 are shown. Transmission failed on one occasion. An EPSP averaged from 228 responses is shown below them. Distributions of EPSP amplitudes and noise, from cellular and recording-system sources, are plotted on the right. EPSPs were measured for each response between the points marked 0 and EPSP, which was the peak of the averaged response. Noise was measured from 0 to a previous point with the same time difference, marked NOISE. The lower panel shows a fit to the EPSP distribution assuming simple binomial statistics. Values were $n = 3$, $p = 0.69$, and q was distributed normally with mean 0.51 and standard deviation 0.05 mV. The distribution derived from these parameters was then convolved with the experimental noise distribution to yield the curve shown.

ion (del Castillo and Katz, 1954), allows estimation of two important parameters: (i) How many transmitter release sites exist at a single connection? (ii) How many postsynaptic channels are activated by transmitter released from a single site?

A simple view of transmitter release is that one unit, or quantum, of transmitter corresponds to the contents of a single presynaptic vesicle. One transmitter quantum has a postsynaptic action q (in units of potential, conductance, or change transfer). The probability that one quantum will be released from a single release site after an action potential is p. If n sites release transmitter independently, the number of quanta released follows a binomial distribution. The mean amplitude of the postsynaptic event is then npq. Statistical methods must be used to extract values for n, p, and q from fluctuations in amplitude of synaptic events. This simple model clearly provides a useful framework to describe synaptic function and plasticity, although at cortical synapses it is hard to demonstrate directly some of its assumptions.

How many release sites (n)? With the simple model described earlier, values for n derived from fluctuations in synaptic events should correspond to the anatomical number of release sites (Korn et al., 1982; Grantyn, Shapovalov, and Shiriaev, 1984a,b; Redman and Walmsley, 1983). Morphological estimates of terminal number provide an independent measure of n. Values for n from statistical analysis and from counting release sites defined at the electron-microscopic level have not always agreed. However, one fact emerges when values for n from morphology and statistical analysis are examined (Table 3.1). At most vertebrate synapses, n is in the range 3–30, much lower than values from neuromuscular junctions and the squid giant synapse (McLachlan, 1978).

Anatomical work at cortical synapses where PSP fluctuations have not been analyzed also suggests that there may be only a few release sites (Table 3.1). With a small n and a moderate p, few quanta will be released, and statistically transmission should sometimes fail. Transmission failures do occur at excitatory synapses between CA3 pyramidal cells, at excitatory synapses from pyramidal cells onto CA3 inhibitory cells, and at some inhibitory synapses onto CA3 pyramidal cells. A statistical analysis of fluctuations at a recurrent excitatory synapse between CA3 pyramidal cells is shown in Figure 3.3. Synaptic transmission at this particular synapse can be described with a binomial model with $n = 3$, $p = 0.69$, and $q = 0.51$ mV. The probability of a transmission failure at this synapse was $(1 - 0.69)^3 = 0.03$.

How many receptors at each postsynaptic site (q)? Values for quantal amplitude can be obtained in two ways: from analysis of PSP fluctuations and also from measurements of miniature synaptic events. These small synaptic potentials recorded in cortical cells, when sodium currents are blocked, are presumed to reflect exocytosis of single transmitter quanta independent of presynaptic action potentials (Brown et al., 1979; Cotman et al., 1986; Konnerth et al., 1988; Ropert, Miles, and Korn, 1990).

Single quanta recorded in cortical neurons cannot be attributed to one particular presynaptic cell as they can at neuromuscular junctions. However, miniature inhibitory events can be shown to result from activation of GABA receptors at synapses that often are located somatically. In the presence of TTX, miniature IPSCs (inhibitory postsynaptic currents)

Table 3.1. *Values for n from morphology and from PSP fluctuations*

***

Inhibitory cell "commissural" → *Mauthner cell of goldfish*
Morphology: 3–42 terminals
Quantal: binomial n = morphology
(Korn et al., 1982; Korn, Faber, and Triller, 1986)

Sensory afferent → *frog spinal motoneuron*
Morphology: 5–23 terminals, 1–12 release sites each
Quantal: binomial n close to morphology
(Grantyn et al., 1984a,b)

Spinal-cord group-Ia afferent → *spinal motoneuron*
Morphology: 3–8 terminals
Quantal: n = 1–3, 2–6, less than morphology
(Clements, Forsythe, and Redman, 1987; Redman and Walmsley, 1983)

Group-I muscle afferent → *dorsal-spinocerebellar-tract neurons*
Morphology: 1:18 terminals, 1–4 release sites each
Quantal: n = 3–30, less than morphology
(Tracey and Walmsley, 1984; Walmsley, Edwards, and Tracey, 1988)

Pyramidal cell → *pyramidal cell, visual-cortex layers III and V*
Morphology: 1 terminal; 1–4 terminals, 1 release site each
(Gabbott, Martin, and Whitteridge, 1987; Kisvarday et al., 1986; Martin, 1988)

Inhibitory cells (axo-axonal, clutch, basket) → *pyramidal cell, visual-cortex layers IV and V*
Morphology: 6–14 terminals (axo-axonal cell); 3–34 terminals (basket cell)
(Kisvarday et al., 1985, 1987; Somogyi, Freund, and Cowey, 1982; Somogyi et al., 1983a)

Inhibitory cell → *hippocampal pyramidal cell*
Morphology: 8–30 terminals (axo-axonal cell); 5–12 terminals (basket cell)
(Nunzi et al., 1985; Somogyi et al., 1983b,c)

***

recorded from CA1 cells and dentate granule cells have a mean conductance of about 0.4 nS (Konnerth et al., 1988; Ropert et al., 1990). If GABA opens Cl⁻ channels each having a conductance of about 20 pS, a single quantum of transmitter opens about 20 GABA channels. Quantal inhibitory events in spinal motoneurons also seem to open 20–40 glycine channels. In contrast, a single quantum of acetylcholine opens 2,000–4,000 nicotinic channels at the frog neuromuscular junction. Quantal events recorded in TTX can be compared with spontaneous inhibitory events in the absence of TTX, thus giving an estimate for the mean number of quanta released by presynaptic action potentials. A quantal event of conductance 0.4 nS (Ropert et al., 1990) and a mean conduc-

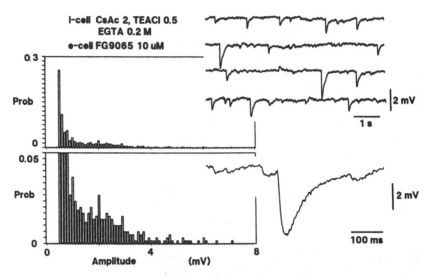

Figure 3.4. Spontaneous inhibitory synaptic events impinging on a CA3 pyramidal neuron fluctuate in amplitude over a 10-fold range. Potassium-current antagonists in the intracellular solution allowed membrane depolarization to a potential about 60 mV positive to the IPSP reversal potential. The excitatory amino acid antagonist CNQX suppressed most spontaneous excitatory synaptic events. IPSP amplitude distributions are plotted, at two magnifications, on the left. On the right, IPSPs are shown at two different time scales.

tance of 5 nS for spontaneous events (Collingridge et al., 1984) suggests that single action potentials in CA1 inhibitory cells release on average about 12 quanta.

Analysis of miniature excitatory events is more difficult than analysis of inhibitory events, because several groups of presynaptic cells that form synapses at varying dendritic loci may be involved. The largest miniature EPSPs resolved in CA3 neurons, with amplitudes up to 2–3 mV, have been assumed to derive from the electrotonically close mossy-fiber terminals (Cotman et al., 1986; Brown et al., 1979). It seems to be difficult to resolve miniature EPSPs in CA1 cells. Miniature EPSCs (excitatory postsynaptic currents) in cultured hippocampal cells may consist of fast and/or slow current components, which correspond to the activation of quisqualate-kainate and NMDA receptors, respectively (Bekkers and Stevens, 1989). Comparison of single-NMDA-channel conductance (about 50 pS) with the amplitude of miniature currents suggests that 5–10 NMDA channels are opened in extracellular media without Mg^{2+}. The estimated number of quisqualate-kainate channels opened by transmitter released from a single site can vary between 20 and 100, depending on the conductance of single quisqualate-kainate channels. Single-channel conductances between 10 and 50 pS have been reported, and the receptor may have multiple conductance states (Ascher and Nowak, 1988; Cull-Candy and Usowicz, 1987; Tang, Dichter, and Morad, 1989).

Probability of transmitter release (p). The simple binomial model assumes that transmitter will be released with equal probabilities from all sites at a connection between two cells. Suggestions that p is not uniform at all sites have been made on statistical grounds from analysis of EPSP fluctuations at the Ia synapses onto spinal motoneurons and neuromuscular junctions in crayfish (Redman and Walmsley, 1983; Wojtowicz and Atwood, 1986). In both cases, some sites were thought to release transmitter with probabilities close to 1, but other sites were not functional ($p = 0$). At amphibian neuromuscular junctions, the probability of release appears to decay systematically along the junction beween the presynaptic terminal and the muscle (Bennett, Jones, and Lavidis, 1986). Surprisingly, it appears that p may, under normal conditions, be zero at all contacts between two cells. Synaptic transmission from club endings onto goldfish Mauthner cells has both electrotonic and chemical excitatory components (Lin and Faber, 1988). At some connections, only electrotonic coupling has been apparent, but latent chemically mediated monosynaptic EPSPs have been revealed following presynaptic injection of 4-AP.

In summary, cortical synapses involve few release sites, with inhibitory synapses perhaps having more than excitatory synapses. Quantal content is low, and consequently postsynaptic responses fluctuate widely in amplitude, and transmission failure is not uncommon. In other words, cortical synapses, especially excitatory ones, are not reliable. The number of receptor channels activated by one quantum of transmitter may represent a fundamental unit. For inhibitory synapses in the hippocampus, about 20 GABA channels may be opened. Less than 100 quisqualate-kainate channels may be opened by a single quantum at an excitatory synapse. The number of transmitter release sites is also small, possibly 1–5 at excitatory synapses and 3–30 at inhibitory connections. The role of this synaptic uncertainty in cortical information processing remains to be clarified.

Neuronal connectivity

Specificity of neuronal connections presumably is crucial to the operation of the nervous system. In the hippocampus, long-range pathways are clearly specific: dentate granule cells connect to CA3 cells, which connect to CA1 cells. However, it is not clear whether or not specific arrangements exist for the shorter-range collateral synapses or how such arrangements may be quantitated. In order to explore synaptic connec-

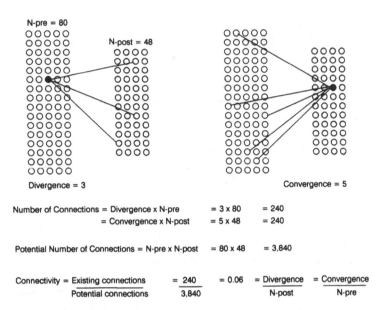

Figure 3.5. A simple treatment of synaptic connectivity between two cell populations; there are 80 presynaptic cells and 48 postsynaptic cells. Each presynaptic cell makes three divergent synapses, and five synapses converge onto a postsynaptic cell. Connectivity, the probability that a presynaptic cell is connected to a postsynaptic cell, is calculated as 0.06. Connectivity can be determined knowing either the divergence and the number of postsynaptic cells or the convergence and the number of presynaptic cells.

tivity in greater detail, several questions may be posed. How many cell classes really exist? What is synaptic divergence – how many synapses does one cell make? What is convergence – how many synapses does one cell receive? What is the probability that two cells are connected, and how does it vary with the distance between them? Finally, is synaptic connectivity uniform for apparently similar cells?

Some of these questions can be examined using sets of presynaptic and postsynaptic cells, as in Figure 3.5. In this treatment, convergence and divergence are given as average parameters for cells of a population. Statistical differences between cells seem certain. That is, it seems unlikely that each cell sends precisely the same number of outputs, or receives the same number of inputs, as every other cell. Figure 3.5 shows that average neuronal connectivity may be estimated if convergence, divergence, and the sizes of neuronal populations are known. For recurrent connections between neurons of the same population, such as excitatory synapses between CA3 pyramidal cells, the presynaptic and postsynaptic populations are identical, so that convergence is equal to divergence. We now turn from an abstract treatment to estimates, from anatomy and physiology, for synaptic divergence, convergence, and neuronal connectivity.

Divergence. The number of cells receiving synapses from one neuron may be estimated both anatomically and physiologically. Anatomically, the axonal tree of one cell must be fully visualized (Tamamaki, Watanabe, and Nojyo, 1984) and the number of terminals counted. With an estimate for the number of terminals per connection, a value for divergence may be obtained. Preferably, electron-micrographic evidence that presumed terminals do possess ultrastructural features of release sites should be obtained.

The mean distance between presumed release sites on axon collaterals of cortical pyramidal cells is close to 10 μ (Martin and Whitteridge, 1984; Schüz and Munster, 1985). With a total axon collateral length of about 10,000 μ, a single cell may possess approximately 1,000 terminals (Braitenberg, 1978). And if there are 1–5 terminals per connection, a cortical pyramidal cell may contact 200–1,000 postsynaptic cells. Cortical pyramidal cells innervate both pyramidal and inhibitory cells, in a ratio of about 5:1 (Gabbott et al., 1987; Kisvarday et al., 1986). It may be important to remember that anatomical connections may not be functional (Pun et al., 1986; Wojtowicz and Atwood, 1986).

To estimate divergence physiologically, one cell should be activated while potential postsynaptic neurons are examined for PSPs that are evoked. Connections made by single preganglionic axons in small clusters of rat submandibular ganglion cells have been mapped in this way (Lichtman, 1980). Similarly, spike-triggered averaging has been used to detect connections between Ia sensory fibers from muscles and motoneurons (Mendell and Henneman, 1971; Scott and Mendell, 1976). Each sensory afferent fiber diverges widely, connecting with about 90% of the 300 motoneurons innervating the muscle from which it originates. Divergence onto synergist motoneurons (not in the pool innervating the muscle of origin) is somewhat less, with each fiber making synapses with about 200 motoneurons.

For hippocampal neurons, the following data are pertinent. Inhibitory cells may contact 100–300 neighboring pyramidal cells (Somogyi et al., 1983b). This is probably a small fraction of the potential target cells within the volume of the inhibitory cells' axonal arborization. Contacts between dentate granule cells and target CA3 pyramidal cells seem to be even more selective. Claiborne et al. (1986) showed that a single mossy fiber arose from each granule cell and formed 12–15 terminals, spaced at roughly equal intervals of about 150 μ, in the CA3 region. Even if the large mossy terminals form functional synapses with several neurons, each granule cell can contact only a very small fraction of the CA3 cell population. CA3 pyramidal-cell axons have synaptic terminals, on averaging, every 7 μ; the total axonal extent within a 400-μ-thick transverse slice ranges from 2.6 mm to 12.5 mm, implying a total of 370–1,785 release sites within the slice (Ishizuka et al., 1990). Transmitter released from these sites will excite other CA3 pyramidal cells, interneurons, and CA1 pyramidal cells.

Quantitation of synaptic divergence in the hippocampus with electrical recordings is difficult because there are so many cells. It is probably impossible to keep a recording from one cell and test for connections in all possible postsynaptic neurons. However, both excitatory and inhibitory cells make divergent connections. Single CA3 cells can elicit polysynaptic recurrent EPSPs in two simultaneously recorded CA3 pyramidal cells (Miles and Wong, 1987a). Spontaneous IPSPs occur simultaneously in most pairs of neighboring CA3 pyramidal cells (Miles and Wong, 1984), consistent with anatomical evidence that inhibitory-cell axons diverge widely.

Convergence. The number of synapses a cell receives can also be estimated both anatomically and physiologically. Anatomically, the number of synaptic contacts (excitatory or inhibitory) that a cell receives must be estimated and divided by the number of terminals per connection. So, for instance, CA3 pyramidal cells receive inhibitory inputs on the initial segments of their axons from the chandelier type of inhibitory cells. The number of symmetric terminals located on CA3 pyramidal-cell initial segments is about 50–100 (Kosaka, 1980), and the number of terminals that an axo-axonal cell makes on a particular cell is 15–30 (Somogyi et al., 1983c). This suggests that 2–6 chandelier cells make axo-axonal inhibitory contacts with a single pyramidal cell.

Convergence can be estimated electrically by comparing a unitary PSP with the PSP evoked when all similar presynaptic cells are activated simultaneously (Hume and Purves, 1983). Thus, Figure 3.6 shows that a unitary IPSP generated in a CA3 pyramidal cell by a single inhibitory cell reverses polarity at a potential similar to the apparent reversal of the fast component of the maximal IPSP generated by afferent stimulation. The conductances of these two events can then be compared to give the number of inhibitory cells that generate the afferent event. The conductance of IPSPs evoked by single inhibitory cells is in the range 4–10 nS (Figure 3.6). The conductance of the maximal synaptic inhibition evoked by afferent-fiber stimulation is about 80–160 nS, suggesting that 8–40 inhibitory cells converge onto each pyramidal cell (Figure 3.6). To make this estimate, all inhibitory cells must be assumed to fire only once, and contamination by EPSPs of the maximal evoked IPSP must be ignored.

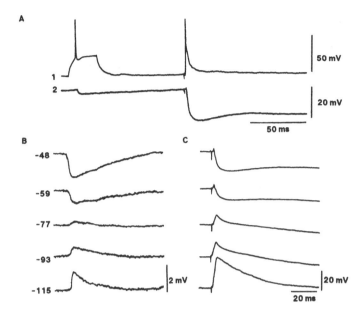

Figure 3.6. Convergence of inhibitory synapses on a pyramidal cell estimated by comparing a unitary IPSP with the maximal afferent IPSP. Action potentials in cell 1 evoked monosynaptic IPSPs in pyramidal cell 2. Maximal mossy-fiber stimuli evoked a single spike in the inhibitory cell and a small EPSP succeeded by a large IPSP in the pyramidal cell. Varying the membrane potential of cell 2 showed that the unitary IPSP reversed at a potential (about −75 mV) similar to that of the early Cl⁻-dependent phase of the afferent IPSP. Comparing conductance changes induced by unitary (6-nS) and afferent (114-nS) IPSPs suggested that about 20 similar inhibitory cells might converge onto pyramidal cell 2. It is conceivable that cell 2 receives IPSPs from inhibitory cells that are not themselves excited by an afferent stimulus.

Connectivity. Connectivity, or the probability that one cell is connected to another cell, depends on convergence, divergence, and the size of the neuronal population (Figure 3.5). Connectivity can also be estimated by counting the number of interactions seen in many recordings from presynaptic- and postsynaptic-cell pairs. In our work in the CA3 region, two cells typically are recorded within about 400 μ of each other. So, for a given presynaptic cell, postsynaptic cells are selected from a population of about 2,000–3,000 pyramidal cells, assuming that slices are about 400 μ thick, that the diameter of the CA3 cell soma is about 20 μ, and that there are three cells at each point in the pyramidal-cell layer. With a ratio of 1:10 for inhibitory cells to pyramidal cells, 200–300 inhibitory cells may be associated with these pyramidal cells. With this in mind, estimates for connectivity of different cell types from our work and that

Table 3.2. *Probabilities that synapses exist between cells of different types within the hippocampus*

Connection	Region	Probability	Conditions	References
E → E	CA3	0.02		MacVicar and Dudek (1980a)
E → E	CA3	0.02		Miles and Wong (1986, unpublished data)
E → E	CA3	0.05	Young rats	Smith et al. (1988)
E → E → E	CA3	0.04		MacVicar and Dudek (1980a)
(polysyn.)	CA3	0.10	In PTX	Miles and Wong (1987a, unpublished data)
	CA3	0.55	Young rats	Smith et al. (1988)
I → E (s.p.)	CA3	0.60		Miles and Wong (1989, unpublished data)
E → I (s.p.)	CA3	0.10		R. Miles (unpublished data)
E → I → E	CA3	0.30		Miles and Wong (1984, unpublished data)
E → E	CA3 → CA1	0.06		Sayer et al. (1988)
E → I (s.p.)	CA1	0.28		Knowles and Schwartzkroin (1981a)
I → E (s.p.)	CA1	0.30		Knowles and Schwartzkroin (1981a)
E → I (s.o.)	CA1	0.64		Lacaille et al. (1987)
I → E (s.o.)	CA1	0.07		Lacaille et al. 1987)
I → E (s.m.)	CA1	0.24		Lacaille and Schwartzkroin (1988a,b)

Abbreviations: E, excitatory; I, inhibitory, PTX, picrotoxin; s.p., stratum pyramidale; s.o., stratum oriens; s.m., stratum moleculare.

of others are presented in Table 3.2. Based on the data, a CA3 pyramidal cell in an adult slice may contact at least 40–60 other nearby pyramidal cells and 20–30 nearby inhibitory cells. An inhibitory cell in CA3 would be expected to contact several hundred pyramidal cells.

Patterns of connectivity. A modular arrangement of neurons is well established for some areas of the brain. Cells in vertical columns of the visual cortex tend to respond in a similar way to visual stimuli. This organization depends in part on a segregation of thalamic inputs to particular columns. In addition, intracortical connections may support the columnar organization. Axon collaterals of single pyramidal cells ramify both

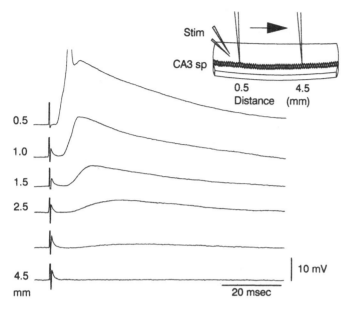

Figure 3.7. Spatial distribution of excitatory synapses activated by stimulation at one point. Averaged EPSPs recorded from cells penetrated sequentially at different distances from a fixed stimulus in a longitudinal slice from the CA3 region. Picrotoxin (50 μM) in the external solution blocked synaptic inhibition, and elevating $[Ca^{2+}]_o$ to 10 mM suppressed firing and thereby reduced polysynaptic EPSPs. EPSPs were likely mediated by recurrent connections of the longitudinal association pathway between CA3 cells. They were detected over distances up to 4 mm from the stimulus, but not throughout the whole slice.

locally and in isolated columnar regions some distance away (Gilbert and Wiesel, 1983; Kisvarday et al., 1986).

A modular arrangement of the hippocampus in parallel lamellae, similar to transverse slices, has been postulated (Andersen et al., 1971). Although modalities of cellular response seem not to be organized according to hippocampal lamellae, some axonal projections are constrained to lie within a single transverse plane. The mossy-fiber axons of dentate granule cells do lie in a single transverse slice, and the longitudinal extent of their hilar collaterals is also limited (Claiborne et al., 1986). However, the axon collaterals of CA3 pyramidal cells, both those that make synapses with other CA3 cells and those that form the Schaffer-collateral projection to CA1 pyramidal cells, are much less constrained. Anatomically, these axon collaterals can ramify through at least half of the longitudinal extent of the hippocampus (Ishizuka et al., 1990; Swanson, Wyss, and Cowan, 1978; Tamamaki et al., 1984). Figure 3.7 shows a physiological mapping of the organization of these collaterals in a longitudinal slice from the CA3 area (Miles, Traub, and Wong, 1988). The spatial distribution of synapses activated by a fixed stimulus was examined by recording EPSPs in cells at various distances from the stimulus. IPSPs were blocked with picrotoxin, and polysynaptic EPSPs were suppressed with elevated concentrations of divalent cations. In all cases, monosynaptic EPSPs were largest close to the stimulation site and declined monotonically over distances of 3–5 mm. This suggests that the probability that one CA3 pyramidal cell innervates another declines with distance between them. In simulations, connections between pyramidal cells were assumed to be random locally and to have a probability density that declined exponentially with distance from the presynaptic cell (see Chapter 6).

It is not clear whether there is a microorganization for inhibitory and excitatory connections in the hippocampus or whether connections are made at random. Focal stimulation of small groups of CA3 cells with glutamate suggests that recurrent excitatory synapses are most dense between nearby pyramidal cells, with an asymmetric distribution weighted toward the hilar → CA2 direction (Christian and Dudek, 1988a). The same technique shows that excitatory connections exist between CA1 pyramidal cells at a lower density than that between CA3 cells (Christian and Dudek, 1988b). A different insight into the structure of excitatory connections within the CA3 region came from stimulation of single CA3 pyramidal cells in the presence of blockers of synaptic inhibition. Single CA3 cells can influence – entrain or initiate – the synchronous burst firing of the entire CA3 pyramidal-cell population that occurs under these conditions. The extent of this influence measures physiologically the efficacy of synaptic pathways from one cell to the rest of the CA3 cell population. Some neurons have a very strong effect, others have a moderate action, and many cells appear to have no influence (Miles and Wong, 1983; Neuman, Cherubini, and Ben-Ari, 1987). These differences could reflect a true microorganization, with some cells making more numerous or more effective local synaptic contacts. Alternatively, this may reflect the extent to which axons are cut during preparation of the slice.

Clearly, more work is needed to define quantitatively the neuronal connectivity in the hippocampus. However, for excitatory connections, including the mossy-fiber and Schaffer-collateral pathways and the recurrent connections between CA3 pyramidal cells, connectivity appears to be 0.01–0.1. This is much lower than the value of 0.9 for Ia afferent connectivity with (a specific pool of) spinal motoneurons. Inhibitory connectivity onto pyramidal cells is much higher than for excitatory connectivity. However, the axonal arborization pattern of the inhibitory cells is more restricted than that of pyramidal cells.

Synaptic circuits

We now move from anatomical connectivity to the operation of simple synaptic circuits in the hippocampus. Synaptic circuits are built from anatomical connections between cells. However, anatomical circuits translate into functional synaptic circuits only when intercalated cells fire. So, for a disynaptic circuit to work, one cell must excite another cell sufficiently that it will fire and thus induce a PSP in a third cell. Both unitary EPSP amplitude and the difference in potential between rest and firing threshold in an intercalated cell are critical in determining whether or not single cells can initiate polysynaptic events. If single presynaptic cells cannot initiate polysynaptic events, attention must focus on mechanisms available to synchronize groups of cells so that the resulting summed EPSPs will cause intercalated cells to fire. We shall now show that the properties of transmission in disynaptic circuits can be predicted from probabilities and latencies for spike-to-spike transmission at monosynaptic excitatory and inhibitory connections. Disynaptic transmission can occur only if an intercalated cell fires. Therefore, disynaptic events usually are transmitted with lower probabilities than are monosynaptic EPSPs.

Disynaptic IPSPs in the CA3 region. Inhibitory cells of the stratum pyramidale have a low firing threshold. CA3 pyramidal cells elicit large, fast unitary EPSPs that frequently cause inhibitory cells to fire (Miles, 1990). The interval between presynaptic and postsynaptic spikes may be as short as 2–3 ms (Figure 3.8, upper portion), and the probability that spikes will be transmitted as high as 0.6. This strong excitation of inhibitory cells allows single pyramidal-cell spikes to initiate disynaptic IPSPs in other pyramidal cells with latencies of 3–5 ms (Figure 3.8, lower portion). The amplitude of unitary EPSPs in CA1 inhibitory cells also facilitates disynaptic inhibitory interactions (Knowles and Schwartzkroin, 1981a; Lacaille and Schwartzkroin, 1988a,b). In CA3, disynaptic inhibitory interactions between pyramidal cells are detected with probability about 0.3. The high divergence of the inhibitory-cell axon collaterals may largely account for the high probability of disynaptic interaction. In addition, several disynaptic pathways can exist between a particular pair of pyramidal cells, so the pyramidal-cell excitation of inhibitory cells also seems to be divergent.

Polysynaptic EPSPs. CA3 pyramidal cells can generate polysynaptic EPSPs, involving transmission along chains of neighboring pyramidal (excitatory) cells (Lorente de Nó, 1938; Miles and Wong, 1987a,b). In adult animals, these interactions are most easily detected when synaptic

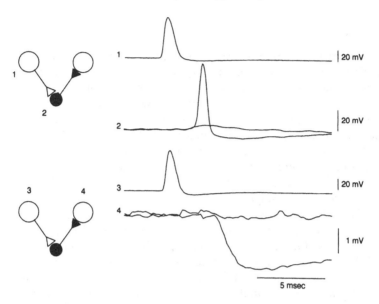

Figure 3.8. Components of the disynaptic inhibitory synaptic circuit. Large, fast EPSPs are generated at excitatory synapses onto inhibitory cells and can make them fire. In this case, single spikes in pyramidal cell 1 caused inhibitory cell 2 to fire with probability about 0.4 and mean latency about 2.5 ms. An EPSP and an action potential are shown. These monosynaptic interactions can account in part for a powerful short-latency disynaptic coupling between pyramidal cells, such as that between cell 3 and cell 4. Firing in an intercalated inhibitory cell would generate the IPSP and no response would occur when the inhibitory cell did not discharge.

inhibition mediated by $GABA_A$ receptors is suppressed. In young animals, polysynaptic EPSPs are observed more frequently (Smith et al., 1988), suggesting that an interesting regulation of recurrent circuitry may occur during development.

The probability that single spikes in pyramidal cells will evoke firing in a monosynaptically coupled pyramidal cell is quite low – about 0.05 (Miles and Wong, 1986). Presynaptic bursts elicit larger, summed EPSPs, and the probability of postsynaptic firing increases to about 0.3–0.5. Thus, presynaptic bursts often can evoke postsynaptic bursts at monosynaptic connections (Figure 3.9). The relatively slow rise time of summed EPSPs initiated by presynaptic bursts, shown in Figure 3.9, results in long intervals, 8–30 ms, between presynaptic and postsynaptic firing. This is significantly longer than that at excitatory synapses made onto inhibitory cells. Latencies for spike-to-spike transmission at monosynaptic connections between pyramidal cells agree closely with the latencies (mean 10–15 ms) observed for polysynaptic EPSPs (Miles and

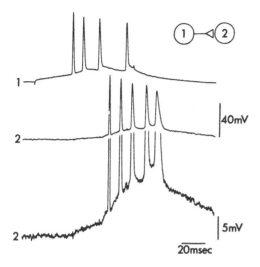

Figure 3.9. Burst transmission between two monosynaptically connected CA3 pyramidal cells. A presynaptic burst in cell 1 evoked a summed EPSP that caused cell 2 to fire a burst. In this case, the probability of burst transmission was about 0.3, at a stimulation rate of 0.5 Hz, and the latencies from first spike to first spike varied between 12 and 30 ms.

Wong, 1987a). That is, if most polysynaptic EPSPs are actually disynaptic, the latency of the EPSP results from the time it takes to recruit a single intercalated pyramidal cell. As expected, transmission of polysynaptic EPSPs is not obligatory: Presynaptic bursts fail to evoke postsynaptic responses with probabilities in the range 0.5–0.7.

Single presynaptic cells may also initiate polysynaptic events via the longer-range intrahippocampal pathways. If the amplitude of unitary mossy-fiber EPSPs is about 5 mV, activity in single granule cells probably will cause individual CA3 pyramidal cells to fire. This could induce a secondary wave of recurrent EPSPs in a cluster of connected CA3 pyramidal cells, depending on the strength of inhibition. (Exactly which of these connected CA3 cells will fire, as a "secondary response" to the mossy input, will depend on complex factors such as afterpotentials caused by recent firing, and feedforward and recurrent inhibition.) In contrast, a small unitary EPSP (Sayer et al., 1990) and relatively higher CA1 cell firing threshold suggest that single CA3 pyramidal cells cannot cause CA1 cells to fire. It appears that unless there is some synchronous firing of CA3 cells, the CA1 region will be functionally amputated from CA3.

Inhibitory control of polysynaptic excitation. Latent excitatory pathways between apparently unconnected CA3 pyramidal cells may be un-

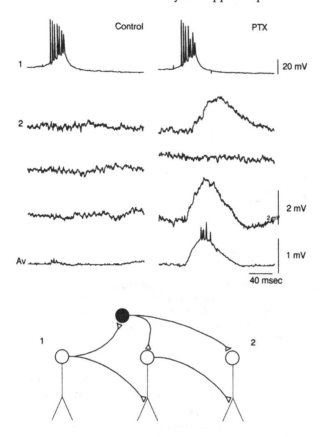

Figure 3.10. Inhibitory control of excitatory transmission via polysynaptic pathways between pyramidal cells. In control conditions, cells 1 and 2 seemed not to communicate in either single or averaged traces. When inhibition was suppressed with picrotoxin (50 μM), bursts in cell 1 evoked EPSPs of variable latency (6–28 ms), which failed sometimes. These events, which otherwise resembled summed EPSPs initiated by presynaptic bursts at monosynaptic connections (Figure 3.8), were presumed to be polysynaptic. Thus, suppressing Cl^--mediated inhibition uncovers latent polysynaptic pathways between CA3 pyramidal cells. Inhibition could act to block burst firing in intercalated pyramidal cells, or it could act to shunt weaker and slower dendritic EPSPs through a postsynaptic action. At a sufficient dose of picrotoxin, cell 2 would itself fire a burst (Figure 3.11).

covered when synaptic inhibition is suppressed. Figure 3.10 shows that bursts in one pyramidal cell elicited no response in another cell under control conditions. In contrast, in the presence of picrotoxin, depolarizing potentials were apparent in individual and in averaged responses; these responses had a shape similar to that of summed EPSPs initiated by presynaptic bursts at monosynaptic connections. The events mediated by this newly functional pathway had latencies and transmission probabilities consistent with those of polysynaptic events (Miles and Wong, 1987a). This "trick" may allow functional synaptic circuitry in the CA3 region to be rapidly rearranged under the influence of transmitters that modulate intrinsic synapses. New synaptic pathways can open to link previously uncoupled pyramidal cells in the CA3 region when synaptic inhibition is suppressed. Furthermore, we shall show that the release of latent excitatory pathways is also associated with the expression of a range of rhythmic neuronal population activities in the CA3 region.

Synaptic inhibition may control the spread of polysynaptic excitation in several ways. First, consider a unitary EPSP and a unitary IPSP converging simultaneously on a pyramidal cell. The EPSP impinges dendritically rather than somatically, causes a smaller change in somatic conductance, and is more likely to fail because of the statistics of transmitter release of the two synapses. Second, a disynaptic IPSP initiated by one pyramidal cell in another is more effective than a disynaptic EPSP generated by a different pathway between the same two cells. As we have discussed, disynaptic IPSPs have shorter latencies than disynaptic EPSPs, because single presynaptic spikes can activate intercalated inhibitory cells, whereas intercalated pyramidal cells are most effectively driven by presynaptic bursts. Furthermore, the connectivity of the inhibitory pathway is higher than that of the excitatory pathway, because inhibitory connections are more divergent than excitatory ones. This is, to some extent, counteracted by the fact that there are fewer inhibitory cells than pyramidal cells, and so a given pyramidal cell may excite fewer inhibitory cells than pyramidal cells. Finally, a disynaptic IPSP can suppress burst firing in a monosynaptically driven pyramidal cell and so block disynaptic excitation at the site of the intercalated cell (Miles and Wong, 1984).

From synaptic circuits to neuronal population behavior

Fully synchronous bursting. As we discussed in Chapter 1, hippocampal neurons in intact animals express multiple collective behaviors. They range from the theta EEG state, where few pyramidal cells fire with the rhythm, to interictal epileptic spikes, where nearly all cells fire with the rhythm. A variety of treatments can induce activity similar to interictal bursting in hippocampal slices. We shall trace the contribution of CA3 synaptic circuits to the synchronous firing induced by blockade of $GABA_A$-mediated inhibition.

On exposure to picrotoxin, synchronous burst firing is generated within the CA3 region (Miles and Wong, 1983) (Figure 3.11). At inter-

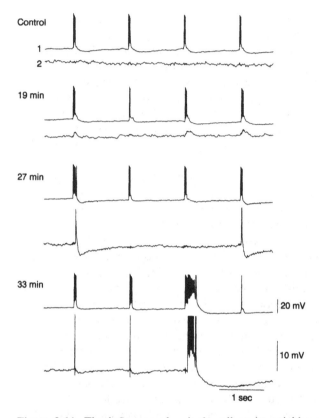

Figure 3.11. The influence of a single cell on its neighbors increases as latent excitatory pathways are uncovered. Cell 1 was stimulated intracellularly at 1.2-s intervals throughout. Initially, it had no discernible influence on cell 2. At 19 minutes after adding picrotoxin, polysynaptic EPSPs were apparent in 3 of 4 trials. At 27 minutes, it triggered (2 times out of 4) larger EPSPs that could induce firing. At 33 minutes, cell 1 initiated firing in cell 2 twice, and on the third trial it triggered the activity of the entire CA3 cell population to form an epileptiform burst. We imagine that polysynaptic pathways from cell 1 eventually involve every cell in the CA3 area. As inhibition is suppressed, activity initiated by cell 1 reaches an increasing number of "nodes," until all postsynaptic cells are involved. See also Miles and Wong (1983).

vals of 2–10 s, all cells recorded have discharged action-potential bursts that have lasted for 50–200 ms and have been correlated with extracellular field potentials (Figure 3.12). This synchronous discharge is synaptic in origin, because it is suppressed by divalent-cation concentrations that do not support synaptic transmission and by antagonists of excitatory amino acid transmitters (Miles, Wong and Traub, 1984). EPSPs underlying burst discharge can be revealed when recording elec-

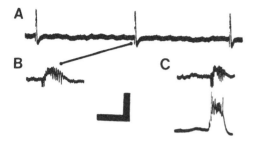

Figure 3.12. Field potentials associated with synchronized bursts. A: Extracellular (field) potential recording of spontaneous events in CA3 in 3.4-mM penicillin, a blocker of GABA$_A$-type IPSPs (Dingledine and Gjerstad, 1979; Wong and Prince, 1979). Note the period of several seconds. These events are analogous to interictal spikes in EEG records. B: A faster sweep shows the characteristic epileptiform field potential: a slow positive envelope (when recorded in the stratum pyramidale) and multiple fast transients. C: During the epileptiform field potential, any pyramidal cell (e.g., lower trace in C) generates a burst with a large depolarizing envelope, the PDS (paroxysmal depolarization shift) (Prince, 1968). Not only are cellular bursts synchronized with the field potential on a time scale of tens of milliseconds, but individual action potentials tend to correlate with the fast (1-ms) field transients (Snow and Dudek, 1984b) (see Chapter 8). Calibration: 1 s in A, 80 ms in B, 120 ms in C; 5 mV in A, 10 mV for fields in B and C, 50 mV for intracellular record in C. (From Traub and Pedley, 1981, with permission. This figure was originally prepared by Dr. Robert K. S. Wong.)

trodes contain agents such as Cs$^+$ that suppress outward membrane currents (Johnston and Brown, 1981; Kay, Miles, and Wong. 1986).

Synchronous firing is also generated in small segments of tissue prepared from the CA3 region (Miles et al., 1984). This observation suggests that synapses between CA3 cells may provide the drive for burst firing in the absence of afferent inputs. If these synapses should prove divergent and firing could spread across them from presynaptic to postsynaptic cell, firing in one cell might spread to other cells in several steps until the whole CA3 population was firing synchronously (Traub and Wong, 1982). As we have shown, recurrent excitatory pathways are divergent, and burst firing can be transmitted transsynaptically. Furthermore, single CA3 cells can entrain or reset spontaneous population bursting (Figure 3.1). We have found that cells that affect the population rhythm often initiate polysynaptic EPSPs in other neurons. This is a rare instance in which one single mammalian cell has a detectable influence on a much larger neuronal population.

Partial synchrony. Figure 3.10 showed that recurrent inhibition controls the spread of activity in polysynaptic recurrent excitatory pathways. When inhibition is completely suppressed, the spread of activity be-

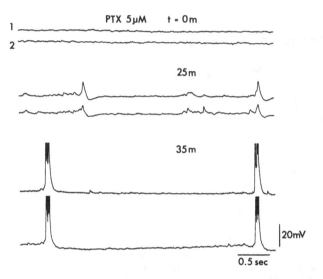

Figure 3.13. A range of rhythmic population activities is expressed as inhibition is reduced: spontaneous membrane-potential fluctuations of cells 1 and 2 at various times after exposure to 5-μM picrotoxin. In control solution ($t = 0$ min), no synchronous activity was apparent. At 25 min, simultaneous EPSPs occurred in both cells. They were much larger than unitary EPSPs, suggesting that small groups of cells presynaptic to both recorded neurons were firing rhythmically and synchronously. (But it is impossible to say that the group of presynaptic firing neurons causing one set of EPSPs is the same as, or even overlaps, the group of neurons causing the next set of EPSPs.) At 35 min, epileptiform bursts, resulting from simultaneous rhythmic discharge of the entire CA3 neuronal population, were apparent in both recorded cells. See also Miles and Wong (1987a).

tween pyramidal cells is unchecked, and population firing is fully synchronous (Figures 3.11 and 3.12). However, when the efficacy of inhibitory circuits is only partly reduced, activity from a single cell might spread to a smaller group of monosynaptically and polysynaptically connected cells and then be extinguished by residual synaptic inhibition. Figures 3.10 and 3.11 show that as inhibition was gradually suppressed, one cell initiated a growing polysynaptic EPSP in another cell. Presumably, the growth of the EPSP reflected firing in an increasing number of intercalated neuronal pathways. A similar growth of partly synchronous CA3 cell firing may be inferred from the growth in rhythmic spontaneous EPSPs that often precedes the onset of fully synchronous discharges (Figure 3.13). This suggests that fully synchronous firing is one extreme of a range of partly synchronous activities that the CA3 neuronal population can generate. Related issues that must be considered include not only what synchronizes the firing of groups of neurons but also (i) what determines the intervals between synchronized events and (ii) what initiates a synchronized event.

The ideas outlined in the preceding section are central to this book. We shall return to them at length in Chapters 6 and 7. First, we must consider in the next two chapters the technical issues involved respectively in modeling individual neurons and in modeling networks of neurons.

4   The single-cell model

There are three general issues to consider in developing an electro-physiological model of a neuron. First, how should one describe the passive electrical features, independent of synaptic inputs and voltage-dependent channels? This issue is addressed by anatomical study of detailed neuronal architecture, by examining the theoretical and experimental responses of neurons to injection of subthreshold currents, and by applying certain of the methods of mathematical physics. Second, how should one describe synaptic inputs? Third, how should one simulate voltage-dependent and calcium-dependent currents? We shall discuss each of these general issues in turn, and then present the particular computer model that we use for a pyramidal cell. The behavior of the model will be compared to the behavior of actual hippocampal pyramidal cells. We shall then present a critique of the model. In the Appendix, we review Hodgkin-Huxley theory, the foundation for our simulation of voltage-dependent currents.[1]

Passive properties, cable theory

Approach to modeling the passive properties of neurons. The goal here is to obtain a quantitative description of membrane potential in a single cell as a function of space and time. This is a necessary step for an understanding of the subthreshold behavior of a neuron and the integration of different synaptic inputs that impinge onto various membrane locations. First we divide the cell into its component pieces: the axon, cell body, and the dendrites. Because of the small diameter of most axons (high input impedance), the effect of the axon on subthreshold membrane behavior is usually ignored. We must thus deal with the soma and dendrites. The soma is generally approximated as a membrane sphere or cylinder to which one or more dendrites are attached. The difficulty comes, then, with the dendrites. How is one to cope with the complex branching?

Let us recall some characteristics of biological membranes. They con-

74

sist of a lipid bilayer with interposed channel proteins. Some of the proteins will pass ions in a relatively nonselective and voltage-independent manner, and they are responsible for the "leak" conductance, usually assumed to be ohmic and described by a membrane parameter R_m (units Ω-cm^2). Other membrane proteins are responsible for (relatively) ion-selective conductances that are gated by one or more of the following: membrane potential, transmitters, Ca^{2+}, and other intracellular messengers. For the passive properties of neurons, we consider only R_m and C_m, the latter describing the membrane capacitance per unit area associated with the lipid bilayer. Neither R_m nor C_m is assumed to be voltage-dependent.

The intracellular medium of cells consists of a complex solution of electrolytes, small, medium, and large molecules (the latter including insoluble cytoskeletal protein structures), and subcellular organelles. We treat the intracellular medium, for modeling purposes, as simply consisting of an electrolyte solution, behaving ohmically, characterized by a parameter R_i (units Ω-cm).

It has been shown that the three-dimensional distribution of potential within a dendrite can be ignored, and that potential can be regarded as a function of (one-dimensional) position along the dendrite (Rall, 1962a). In effect, the diameter of a dendritic branch is small relative to its length. It is also helpful to ignore extracellular potential gradients (i.e., to assume, for purposes of electrotonic analysis, that the extracellular medium is isopotential). Extracellular potentials can be included (Rall, 1962a) (see Chapter 8), but they make the analysis more cumbersome.

Therefore, in analyzing passive properties, we assume that the axon can be ignored and that the only relevant parameters are the geometrical structures of the soma (a cylinder) and dendrites, together with R_m, C_m, and R_i. None of the parameters is voltage-dependent, and all are taken to be constant, that is, not to depend on membrane location or time; see, however, Durand (1984). The main problem is how to describe the passive electrical properties of dendrites.

Passive properties of dendrites. The principles for describing the physics of dendritic trees were set forth by Rall and his colleagues (Rall, 1962a,b, 1967, 1969a,b; Rall and Rinzel, 1973). There are two problems in modeling the passive properties of dendrites: how to map (at least under certain special circumstances) a branching dendrite into a "mathematically equivalent" single cylinder, and how to describe the distribution of potential in such a cylinder. The technique begins by modeling segments of dendrite as leaky coaxial cables. Under appropriate assumptions of symmetry of synaptic inputs,[2] a branching dendrite can be mathematically equivalent to an unbranched dendrite (the "equivalent cylinder"), provided the diameters at branch points satisfy (i) $d^{3/2} = d_1^{3/2} +$

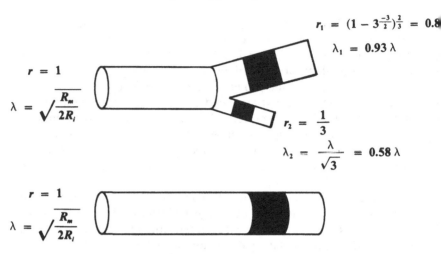

Figure 4.1. A simple branching dendritic structure and its electrotonically equivalent cylinder. At the branch, the $\frac{3}{2}$-power law holds: $d^{3/2} = d_1^{3/2} + d_2^{3/2}$, or, equivalently, $r^{3/2} = r_1^{3/2} + r_2^{3/2}$. Thus, $r_1 + r_2 > r$. Note that the space constants of the branches (λ_1 and λ_2) are smaller than the space constant λ of the parent cylinder, so that a constant electrotonic length is represented by a smaller geometrical length in the branches. The correspondence between the branched structure and the equivalent cylinder identifies the two shaded regions above (areas A_1 and A_2) with the single shaded region below (area A). $A = A_1 + A_2$, so that the identification preserves total membrane area. See also Figure 3B of Rall (1962b).

$d_2^{3/2}$ (d, d_1, and d_2 are the diameters of parent and two daughter branches, respectively) and (ii) the daughter branches have the same "electrotonic length" (i.e., length in membrane space constants) (Figure 4.1). The space constant of a cylindrical cable, in centimeters, is $(rR_m/2R_i)^{1/2}$, where r is the radius in centimeters, R_m is the membrane resistivity in Ω-cm^2, and R_i is the internal resistivity in Ω-cm.

Empirically, hippocampal dendrites approximately satisfy the $\frac{3}{2}$-power branching law (Turner and Schwartzkroin, 1983), although not all dendrites are the same electrotonic length. The latter inhomogeneity may not be of great practical importance, however. The modeler must decide, according to the needs of the problem, how complicated a branching dendritic structure to use for each model neuron. We have tended to use a single branch only in the apical dendrites, or an unbranched structure. In some cases (R. D. Traub, unpublished data), a much more complex dendritic tree has been used, with up to three independent burst sites. We have not attempted to use cell representations with very large numbers of compartments, such as some investigators construct from the detailed anatomy of particular injected neurons; see, for example, Turner (1984a,b) and Turner and Schwartzkroin (1983).

To summarize thus far: The problem of describing potential distribution in a hippocampal dendrite is equivalent to that of describing potential distribution in a cylinder, if we ignore the different electrotonic lengths of some of the branches, and if we consider "radially symmetric" patterns of synaptic input ("Radially symmetric" refers here to electrotonic coordinates). In extending this model to include voltage-dependent membrane channels, we shall have the same symmetry consideration: If such channels are not distributed with radial symmetry, then some degree of branching must be retained to keep the model realistic.

We must now consider the physics of one-dimensional cables, that is, cables whose diameters are small relative to their lengths. The relations among time, potential, and space in such a one-dimensional cable are described by the *cable equation:*

$$\frac{r}{2R_i} \frac{\partial^2 V}{\partial x^2} = I_m = C_m \frac{\partial V}{\partial t} + I_{ionic}$$

a linear partial differential equation. Here, x = length along cable, r = *radius (a constant)*, I_m = total membrane current density, C_m = membrane capacitance per unit area, I_{ionic} = membrane current density carried by ionic charges, t = time, and V is potential across the membrane relative to resting potential. The ionic currents consist of leakage, synaptic, and intrinsic membrane currents. The leakage current is given by $R_m^{-1}V$. The synaptic current (per unit area) is a sum of terms of the form $I_{synaptic} = g_{synaptic}(t)(V - V_{reversal})$, where $V_{reversal}$ is a constant characteristic of the type of synapse. (In fact, many synaptic conductances, including GABA-activated cl⁻ channels and NMDA-activated channels have a more complex dependence on voltage, but we shall assume a simpler linear form for the conductance.) The intrinsic membrane currents, or active currents, are described by equations of the sort $I_{active} = \bar{g}_{active} \times$ (time- and voltage-dependent state variables) $\times (V - V_{reversal})$, where again $V_{reversal}$ is a constant for each type of active current, and $\bar{g}_{active}$ is a constant representing the maximum conductance density for that type of current. Once more, this formalism assumes certain simplifying factors, such as a lack of rectification by the channels (i.e., we assume that the conductance is the same in each direction across the membrane).

In order to solve the cable equation analytically (something that is instructive in simple situations, as where there are no synaptic or active currents), it is helpful to express it in so-called electrotonic coordinates. The cable equation in dimensionless form, using electrotonic coordinates ($X = x/\lambda$, $T = t/\tau_m$, with τ_m, the membrane time constant, equal to $R_m C_m$), and with no ionic currents other than passive leakage current, is

$$\frac{\partial^2 V}{\partial X^2} = V + \frac{\partial V}{\partial T}$$

This equation can be transformed into the classical one-dimensional heat equation by the substitution

$$V(X, T) = U(X, T)e^{-T},$$

yielding

$$\frac{\partial^2 U}{\partial X^2} = \frac{\partial U}{\partial T}$$

(see Carslaw and Jaeger, 1959, p. 144).

We shall now derive analytically some basic results of passive cable theory, with the hope of providing physical insight into the properties of the cable equation. This section includes most of the standard formulas on cable properties that the reader is likely to encounter in the literature. We shall consider only cables with sealed ends, possibly with a defined current injected into the end at $x = 0$, and also infinitely long cables. Problems with one or both ends "leaky" are considered by Rall (1962a). A good understanding of the behavior of single cylinders makes it easier to understand the passive properties of branching dendrites; it is also the "substrate" on which the other currents are superimposed. By "other currents" we mean currents other than the leakage membrane current and internal longitudinal current; examples of these other currents include the synaptic and voltage-dependent currents.

Problem 1

Consider a cable with sealed ends and initial distribution of potential $f(X)$. How does the potential redistribute in time? In electrotonic coordinates, the differential equation is $\partial^2 V/\partial X^2 = V + \partial V/\partial T$. The boundary conditions are $\partial V(0, T)/\partial X = 0$ and $\partial V(L, T)/\partial X = 0$ for all T (L is the electrotonic length of the cable), and $V(X, 0) = f(X)$. We can transform the differential equation into the heat equation $\partial^2 U/\partial X^2 = \partial U/\partial T$ by the substitution $V = Ue^{-T}$ (Carslaw and Jaeger, 1959, p. 101); conveniently, this substitution does not change the boundary conditions. The solution to the heat equation with these boundary conditions is

$$U(X, T) = \bar{f} + \frac{2}{L} \sum_{n=1}^{\infty} a_n e^{-\frac{n^2\pi^2 T}{L^2}} \cos\left(\frac{n\pi X}{L}\right)$$

where $\bar{f}$ and a_n are the Fourier coefficients of f:

$$\bar{f} = \frac{1}{L} \int_0^L f(X')\, dX' \quad \text{and} \quad a_n = \int_0^L f(X')\cos\left(\frac{n\pi X'}{L}\right) dX'$$

It follows immediately that

$$V(X, T) = \tilde{f}e^{-T} + \frac{2}{L} \sum_{n=1}^{\infty} a_n e^{-(1+\frac{n^2\pi^2}{L^2})T} \cos(\frac{n\pi X}{L})$$

To express this solution in physical coordinates (rather than electrotonic coordinates), we recall that $X = x/\lambda$ and $T = t/\tau_m$, where x is the position coordinate along the cable, and t is time. We can write the time-0 initial condition as $g(x) = f(X)$. It is then straightforward to show that

$$V(x,t) = \tilde{f}e^{-t/\tau_m} + \frac{2}{L\lambda} \sum_{n=1}^{\infty} A_n e^{-(1+\frac{n^2\pi^2}{L^2})t/\tau_m} \cos(\frac{n\pi x}{L\lambda})$$

with A_n defined as $\int_0^{L\lambda} g(x)\cos(n\pi x/L\lambda)\, dx$. At the $x = 0$ end of the cable, we thus have

$$V(0, t) = \tilde{f}e^{-t/\tau_m} + \frac{2}{L\lambda} \sum_{n=1}^{\infty} A_n e^{-(1+\frac{n^2\pi^2}{L^2})t/\tau_m}$$

That is, the potential is a sum of terms exponential in time, with the time constants given explicitly in the equation. The slowest (i.e., largest) time constant is τ_m itself. The remaining time constants are $\tau_m/(1 + \pi^2/L^2)$, $\tau_m/(1 + 4\pi^2/L^2)$, and so on. These values rapidly approach zero.

Problem 2

Consider a cable with sealed ends. What is the steady-state input resistance? Because $\partial V/\partial t = 0$, we can write the cable equation as $d^2V/dx^2 = (2R_i/rR_m) V = V/\lambda^2$. Suppose a current I is injected into the end at $x = 0$. If we can determine $V(0)$, we shall know the input resistance: $R_{input} = V(0)/I$. The boundary conditions are $dV/dx = -IR_i/\pi r^2$ at $x = 0$ (drawing a picture will help to convince the reader of this), and $dV/dx = 0$ at $x = L\lambda$. We look for solutions of the form

$$V(x) = a \cosh(\frac{x}{\lambda}) + b \sinh(\frac{x}{\lambda})$$

where a and b are constants to be determined. Note that

$$V'(x) = \frac{a}{\lambda} \sinh(\frac{x}{\lambda}) + \frac{b}{\lambda} \cosh(\frac{x}{\lambda})$$

Using the boundary condition at $x = 0$ and the facts that $\sinh(0) = 0$ and $\cosh(0) = 1$, we see that $b = -\lambda IR_i/\pi r^2$. Now, using the other boundary condition, it follows that $a = (\lambda IR_i/\pi r^2)\coth(L)$. Because $a = V(0)$, it now follows that $R_{input} = (\lambda R_i/\pi r^2)\coth(L)$. This formula is useful in constructing cable models because it relates well-defined physical quantities, some of which can be estimated experimentally (e.g., r and L).

Problem 3

How does the cable, starting at rest [i.e., $V(x, 0) = 0$ for all x] respond to the injection of a constant current I at one end? We must solve the cable equation

$$\frac{r}{2R_i} \frac{\partial^2 V}{\partial x^2} = C_m \frac{\partial V}{\partial t} + \frac{V}{R_m}$$

with the boundary conditions

$$V(x, 0) = 0, \frac{\partial V}{\partial x}(0, t) = J = -\frac{IR_i}{\pi r^2}, \text{ and } \frac{\partial V}{\partial x}(L\lambda, t) = 0$$

for all t. We know already (see Problem 2) that the steady-state solution (i.e., with $\partial V/\partial t = 0$) of these equations is

$$K(x) = \frac{\lambda IR_i}{\pi r^2} \coth(L)\cosh(\frac{x}{\lambda}) - \frac{\lambda IR_i}{\pi r^2} \sinh(\frac{x}{\lambda})$$

Let us define a new function $U(x, t)$ by $U(x, t) = V(x, t) - K(x)$. Then $U(x, t)$ satisfies the differential equation

$$\frac{r}{2R_i} \frac{\partial^2 U}{\partial x^2} = \frac{r}{2R_i} \frac{\partial^2 V}{\partial x^2} - \frac{r}{2R_i} \frac{\partial^2 K}{\partial x^2} = C_m \frac{\partial V}{\partial t} + \frac{V}{R_m} - C_m \frac{\partial K}{\partial t} - \frac{K}{R_m} = C_m \frac{\partial U}{\partial t} + \frac{U}{R_m}$$

That is, U also satisfies the cable equation. The boundary conditions for U are

$$U(x, 0) = -K(x), \frac{\partial U}{\partial x}(0, t) = 0, \text{ and } \frac{\partial U}{\partial x}(L\lambda, t) = 0.$$

Thus, the problem for U is equivalent to Problem 1. Letting $\bar{K}$ be the average of K on the interval $[0, L\lambda]$, we have

$$U(x, t) = -\bar{K}e^{-t/\tau_m} + \frac{2}{L\lambda} \sum_{n=1}^{\infty} A_n e^{-(1+\frac{n^2\pi^2}{L^2})t/\tau_m}\cos(\frac{n\pi x}{L\lambda})$$

with

$$A_n = -\int_0^{L\lambda} K(x)\cos(\frac{n\pi x}{L\lambda}) \, dx.$$

This defines $V(x, t)$. Using the solution for the charging curve, we can then derive the impulse response by piecing together two problems: Inject a large current and obtain the distribution of potential at time δt, and then use the solution to Problem 1 to study the relaxation in time and space of this solution. This procedure indicates that the time constants for the impulse response [i.e., $\tau_m/(1 + n^2\pi^2/L^2)$ for $n = 0, 1, 2, \ldots$] are the same for the impulse problem as for the steady-current problem.

Problem 4

What is the impedance of the cable for a sinusoidal current input $e^{i\omega t}$, $i = \sqrt{-1}$? We need to look at long-term solutions (i.e., ignoring initial transients) of the cable equation

$$\lambda^2 \frac{\partial^2 V}{\partial x^2} = \tau_m \frac{\partial V}{\partial t} + V$$

with $\partial V/\partial x = -R_i e^{i\omega t}/\pi r^2$ at $x = 0$, and $\partial V/\partial x = 0$ at $x = L\lambda$. Because we are looking at long-term solutions, the initial conditions are not relevant. Let us find solutions of the form $V(x, t) = e^{i\omega t}f(x)$. The cable equation implies that f satisfies the differential equation

$$\lambda^2 \frac{d^2f}{dx^2} = f(x)(1 + i\omega\tau_m) = sf(x)$$

where $s = 1 + i\omega\tau_m$. The solutions are then of the form

$$f(x) = a \cosh\left(\frac{x\sqrt{s}}{\lambda}\right) + b \sinh\left(\frac{x\sqrt{s}}{\lambda}\right)$$

for constants a and b to be determined. But f satisfies the differential equation

$$\frac{df}{dx} = \frac{a}{\lambda}\sqrt{s} \sinh\left(\frac{x\sqrt{s}}{\lambda}\right) + \frac{b}{\lambda}\sqrt{s} \cosh\left(\frac{x\sqrt{s}}{\lambda}\right)$$

Using the boundary condition at $x = 0$, we see that $b = -\lambda R_i/\pi r^2\sqrt{s}$. Using the boundary condition at $x = L\lambda$, we see that

$$\frac{a}{\lambda}\sqrt{s} \sinh(L\sqrt{s}) - \frac{R_i}{\pi r^2}\cosh(L\sqrt{s}) = 0$$

Thus, $a = \coth(L\sqrt{s}) \times (\lambda R_i/\pi r^2\sqrt{s})$. Furthermore, the input impedance of the cable is

$$\frac{V(0, t)}{e^{i\omega t}} = \frac{f(0)e^{i\omega t}}{e^{i\omega t}} = a.$$

In the limit $L \to \infty$, $\coth(L\sqrt{s}) \to 1$, so that the input impedance will approach $\lambda R_i/\pi r^2 \sqrt{s}$, a result that, using the definition of λ and some algebra, agrees with Dodge and Cooley (1973):

$$Z_\infty = \frac{\sqrt{R_m R_i}}{\sqrt{2\pi^2 r^3 (1 + i\omega\tau_m)}}$$

Problem 5

What is the frequency-dependent space constant of an infinite cable? See, for example, Katz and Miledi (1968). That is, as we look at the long-term solution $V(x, t)$ for an injected current $e^{i\omega t}$, at what x does the absolute value of $V(x, t)/V(0, t) = e^{-1}$? From Problem 4, we know that

$$V(x, t) = e^{i\omega t}[a \cosh(\frac{x\beta}{\lambda}) + b \sinh(\frac{x\beta}{\lambda})]$$

where $\beta = (1 + i\omega\tau_m)^{1/2}$. Furthermore, $V(0, t) = a$. Also, in the infinite cable $(L = \infty)$, $b = -a$. Thus, the equation we must solve is

$$\text{abs}[\cosh(\frac{x\beta}{\lambda}) - \sinh(\frac{x\beta}{\lambda})] = e^{-1}$$

Using the definitions of cosh and sinh, this equation is the same as $\text{abs}(e^y) = e^{-1}$, where $y = x\beta/\lambda$. Thus, $\text{Re}(y) = -1$. Because x and λ are real, $x = -\lambda/\text{Re}(\beta)$. Writing $\beta = (1 + i\omega\tau_m)^{1/2} = m + in$, m and n real, we find

$$m^2 = 1 + \frac{\sqrt{1 + \omega^2\tau_m^2}}{2} \quad \text{and} \quad \text{Re}(\beta) = m = \pm\sqrt{\frac{1 + \sqrt{1 + \omega^2\tau_m^2}}{2}}$$

(it is the negative root that makes sense physically, because negative values for x are not defined). Thus,

$$x = \frac{\lambda}{\sqrt{\dfrac{1 + \sqrt{1 + \omega^2\tau_m^2}}{2}}}$$

Denoting this x, the frequency-dependent space constant, as λ_ω, we see that $\lambda_\omega/\lambda = m^{-1}$. This result is important because it shows that transient events in a passive cable decrement over smaller distances than do steady-state events, a notion important in understanding some of the physics underlying the EEG (Humphrey, 1968); for a review, see Pedley and Traub (1990).

Even with a single-cable model, one can anticipate the mathematical complexities added when there are synaptic inputs to the middle of the cable: The synaptic conductances will alter the local cable properties, in turn influencing the propagation in space and time of other synaptic currents.

The origin of the $\frac{3}{2}$-power branching rule mentioned earlier is discussed in detail by Rall (1962a), but the physical idea is apparent from considering the input impedance of a cable: The impedance of a cable of electrotonic length L and radius r is $Z_0 = cr^{-3/2}$, where $c = [(R_mR_i)^{1/2}/\sqrt{2}\pi]\coth(L)$. The input impedances of two daughter branches of radius r_1 and r_2 will be $Z_1 = cr_1^{-3/2}$ and $Z_2 = cr_2^{-3/2}$, respectively. For identification of the two parallel branches with the original cable, we must have impedance matching, that is, $1/Z = 1/Z_1 + 1/Z_2$. This relation implies the $\frac{3}{2}$-power rule, $r^{3/2} = r_1^{3/2} + r_2^{3/2}$, provided the electrotonic lengths (L) for the different branches are the same. For this identification to be truly valid, in a neuron with synaptic input and/or active conductances, one must also take care that synaptic inputs and membrane conductances are distributed in a way that is preserved by the mapping between the original single cable and the two branches (Figure 4.1). Two factors are at work here: the relation of membrane areas in the single cable versus the pair of cables, and an appropriate symmetry of conductances. With respect to the latter, one must ensure, for example, that synaptic inputs go to both branches at the same electrotonic location that input goes to the corresponding electrotonic location in the original cable. With respect to the former consideration, we note that the transformation from branching dendrite to single equivalent cylinder preserves area (but not physical length). That is, a portion of dendritic membrane that is $\Delta\lambda$ space constants long, and that includes a branch point, has a physical length less than the corresponding portion (also $\Delta\lambda$ space constants long) in the equivalent cylinder; the total membrane areas are the same, however (Rall, 1962b). To see this, consider the special case of a cylinder of radius r_1 that branches into two equal daughter branches of radius r_2, where, of course, $r_1^{3/2} = 2r_2^{3/2}$. The ratio (space constant parent)/(space constant daughter) $= 2^{1/3} > 1$, from the definition of the space constant and the known relation between the radii. Thus, one λ in the equivalent cylinder corresponds to a greater physical length than one λ in the branched structure. But the ratio (membrane area 1λ equivalent cylinder)/(membrane area 1λ branched structure) is 1. The reason is that the circumference around the parent is $2\pi r_1$, and the total circumference around the two daughters is $4\pi r_2 = \pi r_1 2^{4/3}$. Thus, the ratio of parent circumference to total daughter circumferences is $2^{1-4/3} = 2^{-1/3} < 1$. Thus, the shorter length constant of the daughter branches is exactly balanced by the increase in total circumference, so that one λ of dendrite in each case corresponds to the same total area. This means that in a compartmental model where the compartments have the same electrotonic length, it is best to express conductances in terms of membrane area.

These considerations are also important in modeling field effects, where it is necessary to match the electrotonic coordinates of the cellular model with the physical coordinates that describe the extracellular space in which the cellular model is embedded (Traub et al., 1985a).

Many other cable-theory problems have been treated analytically; see, for example, Rall (1962a,b, 1969a,b), Rall and Rinzel (1973), Rinzel and Rall (1974), and Norman (1972). The last paper illustrates the use of Laplace transform methods.

To apply cable theory to real neurons, there are several considerations. First, in actual neurons, as in much of Rall's analysis, the neuron must be treated not as a single cable but rather as an isopotential "soma" region with several dendritic cables emanating from it. The electrotonic properties (e.g., input resistance, electrotonic length) of the various dendrites need not be all identical. This more complicated configuration makes the mathematics more complex than for a single cable. Much of the experimental literature in this area concerns attempts to estimate the conductance of the soma region relative to the input conductance of the dendrites. Second, measurement of the geometry of real neurons is not straightforward, because of shrinkage artifacts and because of the presence of spines. Spines have the effect of increasing the surface per unit dendritic length (among other things). Different methods of accounting for spines may lead to different estimates of C_m. A review by the Oxford group (Stratford et al., 1989) provides a method of reconfiguring the dimensions of a dendritic cable to compensate for the presence of spines. There is, further, uncertainty as to whether R_m is constant over the entire cell membrane or whether, for example, R_m is different for soma and dendrites (Durand, 1984). In our model, as described later, we follow Turner and Schwartzkroin in not allowing for spines, and therefore we use a value of C_m larger than the usual 1 $\mu F/cm^2$. As previously mentioned, we also assume that R_m is constant.

Passive properties of real neurons are studied physiologically by examination of the charging curve or impulse response,[3] as well as by anatomical reconstruction of cells. The recorded electrical responses can be compared with those expected theoretically, solving boundary-value problems similar to (but usually more complicated than) those described earler. One attempts to determine the basic cable parameters (e.g., R_m) by fitting curves to the observed potentials. Some examples of electrotonic parameters for hippocampal neurons, based on anatomical and/or electrophysiological measurements, have been given by Brown, Fricke, and Perkel (1981b), Turner and Schwartzkroin (1980, 1983), and Johnston (1981). The subject was reviewed by Turner and Schwartzkroin

(1984) and Turner (1984a), who gave a physiological estimate of 0.91 for the electrotonic length of hippocampal pyramidal-cell dendrites. However, those authors pointed out that the equivalent-cylinder model does not really describe pyramidal-cell dendrites because of premature termination of many dendritic branches. Based on anatomical reconstruction from HRP injections and on input-resistance measurements, Turner and Schwartzkroin (1983) estimated 0.69 and 0.32 for the median electrotonic lengths of apical and basilar dendritic branches, respectively. It is not entirely clear how to reconcile this with the estimate of 0.91 for the electrotonic length of the lumped system, but the electrotonically longer branches may be responsible.

Despite its appealing mathematical elegance, electrotonic modeling must be viewed with caution, for reasons outlined by Stratford et al. (1989). These reasons include (i) the unknown size of the shunt at the soma produced by the recording electrode (such a shunt can distort the impulse response), (ii) the need for independent measurements of R_i, (iii) the fact that cells are constantly bombarded by synaptic inputs that may also distort the impulse response, (iv) the existence of voltage-dependent currents active at potentials below threshold for action-potential generation, another source of signal distortion, and (v) most disturbing, the inability to determine uniquely, or sometimes even approximately, the values of the major electrotonic parameters from the available experimental data: cell morphology, steady-state input resistance, impulse response, and so forth.

We conclude that our network models should incorporate reasonable electrotonic parameters for single cells, but also that we should focus on collective phenomena that do not depend on the precise values of these parameters. Indeed, this consideration applies to all of the many types of parameters that enter into our models.

Synaptic inputs

When synaptic inputs are present, it is easier to proceed via simulations than to attempt to use analytical methods. The mathematics are more complicated than for a single cable. In addition, synaptic inputs may terminate on individual dendritic branches, making the expressions still more complex. Analysis is further complicated because many physiological synaptic inputs are not well approximated by an impulse conductance change. Special-purpose simulation programs exist for analysis of these problems; see, for example, Segev et al. (1985).

Certain synaptic events can be described with a time-dependent conductance: $I_{synaptic} = g_{synaptic}(t) \times (V - V_{equilibrium})$, where $V_{equilibrium}$ depends on the type of synapse, and $I_{synaptic}$ is the synaptically induced membrane current at the location of the synapse. The time course of $g_{synaptic}$ produced by a single presynaptic action potential may be determined experimentally (see Chapter 3). Some synaptically gated channels show rectification, that is, the conductance depends on the transmembrane potential, as described by Ashwood et al. (1987), Gray and Johnston (1985), and Barker and Harrison (1988), but we do not consider this effect in our model. Likewise, some transmitters (such as acetylcholine) act not by opening specific ionic channels but by altering the kinetics or conductance of voltage-dependent membrane channels; again, we shall not consider such effects. Finally, as described in Chapter 3, synaptic transmission fluctuates because of quantal effects. We are beginning to incorporate quantal aspects of intercellular communication into our model. For the present, we shall assume that $g_{synaptic}$ (t) has a well-defined time course, fixed for each type of synapse, but perhaps with an amplitude depending on the particular synaptic connection in a network.

   The problem, then, is to glean from the experimental data what form $g_{synaptic}$ should take and where on the postsynaptic cell membrane the appropriate synapses should be located. Some observations that have guided us are as follows. During synchronized epileptiform bursts, which are mediated by recurrent excitatory synapses (Chapter 6), the peak extracellular negativities reflect inward synaptic currents (Johnston and Brown, 1981; Traub et al., 1985a). In the CA3 region, these sinks are in the mid-apical and mid-basilar dendritic regions (Swann et al., 1986a). These data indicate where we should locate, at least approximately, the recurrent excitatory synapses between pyramidal cells.

   Brown and Johnston (1983) voltage-clamped the EPSPs elicited in CA3 cells by weak stimulation of mossy fibers (not a unitary event). They found the synaptic conductance to be proportional to $te^{-t/\tau}$, with t in milliseconds, and $\tau = 2$ ms. (This is a so-called α function. With $\tau = 2$ ms, it will peak at time 2 ms.) In contrast, a unitary recurrent EPSP peaks at about 8–12 ms (Miles and Wong, 1986) (see Chapter 3). To reconcile these observations, and locating recurrent synapses in the mid-dendrites (Figure 4.2), we made the unitary recurrent conductance an α function, but with time constant 3 ms rather than 2 ms. A simulated unitary EPSP then peaks at the soma at about 9.5 ms. [It may be relevant that a high-conductance quisqualate-activated channel in cultured hippocampal neurons produces a current decaying with time constant 3 ms (Tang et al., 1989).]

   Anatomical evidence, as reviewed by Frotscher et al. (1988), indicates that GABAergic terminals are found on the cell bodies, dendritic shafts, and axon initial segments of pyramidal cells. We have therefore located the model's GABA$_A$ synapses on the soma and most proximal dendritic regions. Concerning the kinetics of GABA$_A$-activated channels, the following data are pertinent. Collingridge et al. (1984) found an IPSP current-decay time constant of 8.3 ms at 32°C in CA1 cells. By voltage-clamping cultured hippocampal neurons at room temperature, Segal and Barker (1984b) estimated a mean GABA-activated-channel open time of about 23 ms. If a population of channels were synchronously activated by a short pulse, and the channels were to close with an exponential distribution and mean open time of 23 ms, the macroscopic current would decay with that same time constant, 23 ms.[4] Because we are modeling cells at 37°C, we have used a somewhat faster time constant for decay of the inhibitory conductance (7 ms).

The synapses that mediate $GABA_B$ effects (or slow IPSPs) probably are in the dendrites (Newberry and Nicoll, 1985). Hablitz and Thalmann (1987) found that the slow IPSP was evident within 25 ms, peaked at 120–150 ms, and decayed with a time constant of about 185 ms. Our simulated slow IPSP peaks earlier (30–40 ms) and decays with a time constant 100–200 ms.

Schlander and Frotscher (1986) found excitatory terminals on the soma and dendrites in interneurons, but we have located excitatory synapses only on the soma in inhibitory cells. The unitary EPSP on a (hyperpolarized) inhibitory cell is several millivolts (see Chapter 3). Because a disynaptic IPSP may have a latency as brief as 3–4 ms, it appears that a unitary EPSP onto an inhibitory cell must elicit an action potential with latency as brief as 1–2 ms. In order to achieve such an effect, we were forced to use the unrealistically large unitary conductance of 120 nS. It might be thought that this resulted from our using same electrotonic architecture for inhibitory cells as for pyramidal cells. However, what few data there are on this subject make it unlikely that the electrotonic parameters are the problem. Thus, Turner and Schwartz-kroin (1980) found the following parameters to be similar for interneurons and (CA1) pyramidal cells: R_{input}, C_m, and dendritic electrotonic lengths. Although the membrane time constant was smaller for interneurons (average 3.6 ms), that resulted from a smaller R_m rather than from a smaller C_m; i.e., the membranes of interneurons are leakier than the membranes of pyramidal cells. Experimentally, the threshold for action-potential initiation in inhibitory cells is lower than in pyramidal cells, and inhibitory cells are more likely to fire spontaneously than are pyramidal cells. In models of inhibitory cells with g_{Na} altered to produce a low firing threshold, it is possible to use a unitary EPSP conductance of 8–10 nS (R. Traub, unpublished data), closer to the experimental estimate of 1–2 nS (Miles, 1990).

There are few data concerning the details of IPSPs onto inhibitory cells, although both fast and slow IPSPs are observed in these cells. We therefore made the kinetics and electrotonic location of these IPSPs the same as for the respective IPSP type in pyramidal cells. The unitary IPSP conductance for an inhibitory neuron usually was 0.4 times the corresponding value for a pyramidal cell; this scaling was arbitrary.

Active membrane properties

Our model of a hippocampal neuron is a descendant of the model of Dodge and Cooley (1973) of a motoneuron. The active currents in the Dodge-Cooley model in turn derive from the classical work on the kinetics of the currents underlying the action potential in squid axon (Hodgkin and Huxley, 1952a–d) and frog peripheral node of Ranvier (Frankenhaeuser, 1962). The basic ideas of the Hodgkin-Huxley model are reviewed in the Appendix to this chapter.

Today, investigators record single-channel currents with patch-clamp techniques. They measure membrane gating currents, and they clone and sequence channel and receptor proteins. Why, then, rely on a phenomenological description of membrane currents from the early 1950s? The answer is that whole-cell modelers deal with macroscopic membrane currents, rather than single-channel currents, and Hodgkin and Huxley provide an elegant and useful formulation of the macroscopic currents. Other work in this spirit, which will also prove directly useful for hippocampal cell modeling, includes the voltage-clamp studies of the M current (Halliwell and Adams, 1982), of a slowly inactivating calcium current (Brown and Griffith, 1983b; Johnston et al., 1980; Kay and Wong, 1987), of a rapid sodium current (Sah et al., 1988), and of the calcium-dependent K current (Numann et al., 1987).

In applying the Hodgkin-Huxley formulation to hippocampal neurons, we made numerous modifications, both in the kinetics of the rate functions and in the addition of various ad hoc assumptions suggested by voltage-clamp and other experiments in molluscan neurons. Such modifications were added because the original Hodgkin-Huxley formulation could not generate intrinsic bursts rather than single action potentials. These modifications are discussed next.

The major changes we have made to produce a functional neuron model can be summarized as follows: (i) The model must conform structurally to the neuronal shape and must account for the passive properties of the dendrites. (ii) The Hodgkin-Huxley model has only two types of active channels: sodium and potassium. Neuron models generally need more than two types of active channels. For example, in most neurons there are calcium channels and calcium-dependent potassium channels. (iii) We allow means for modifying channel behavior not present in the original Hodgkin-Huxley model. Examples include the gating of K channels by intracellular calcium, and voltage-dependent inactivation of K channels. (iv) The kinetics and density of Na and K channels are altered. In addition, the densities of these and other voltage-dependent channels are not uniform as in squid axon membrane. Instead, the channels are relatively concentrated at special locations: the soma and probably one or more dendritic sites (Huguenard, Hamill, and Prince, 1989; Wong et al., 1979).

Our model aims to reproduce, reasonably accurately, the intrinsic burst discharges generated by CA3 pyramidal cells in response to injected currents (Traub, 1982). This issue is particularly intricate, given the limited data on the quantitative kinetics of voltage- and calcium-dependent membrane channels and on the spatial distribution of these channels over the soma–dendrite membrane. Some of the experimental features (Chapter 2) that we wish to reproduce are (i) stereotypy of burst morphology for a given cell, (ii) dependence of bursting behavior on the resting potential or the holding potential, (iii) summation of spike afterdepolarizations to produce a depolarizing envelope, (iv) the ability to prevent full burst generation by an appropriately timed hyperpolarizing input, and (v) a long post-burst AHP, intrinsically generated. We shall assume that the multiple conductances necessary to support burst generation are present in localized regions of the cell membrane. There is some evidence in favor of this idea, in that isolated hippocampal neurons, which lose much of the dendritic tree, can generate bursts (see Figure 2.4). Furthermore, dendrites do appear to be capable of generating both Na and Ca spikes (Masukawa and Prince, 1984; Wong et al., 1979). We also assume that patches of cell membrane that contain all the channel species needed to generate bursts are scattered in different somatic and dendritic regions.[5] Note that in CA1 pyramidal cells, apical dendritic regions are capable of generating intrinsic bursts, as, for example, after current injection, whereas the soma membrane is much less likely to do so (Wong et al., 1979). It is not necessary to assume that all the details of burst generation are identical in soma and dendrites; for example, calcium spikes appear to be larger in the apical dendrites than in the soma in CA3 pyramidal cells (Wong et al., 1979).

Because voltage-clamp data were insufficient to permit a full synthesis of cellular membrane behavior, we have developed a model that reproduces qualitatively the essential features of bursting behavior (Traub, 1982). Such a model could serve as a suitable "building block" for network models until a voltage-clamp model is developed. Progress has been made in constructing a model that incorporates voltage-clamp measurements from isolated hippocampal pyramidal cells (Traub, Wong, and Miles, 1990).

The single-cell model used in this book (Traub, 1982) assumes the following: (i) The fast action potential is mediated by a Na^+ current with Hodgkin-Huxley-type kinetics. (ii) Spike repolarization involves a voltage-dependent K^+ current that inactivates with sustained depolarization; such inactivation was found in simulations to allow a growing depolarizing envelope as a burst developed (Aldrich, Getting, and Thompson,

1979). The model spike-repolarizing K^+ current was, in effect, a hybrid of the experimentally observed A and C currents (but without any explicit Ca^{2+} dependence). (iii) The Ca^{2+}-dependent spike-depolarizing afterpotential and the slow Ca^{2+} spike are mediated by the same current. In order to achieve this, a strong Ca^{2+}-dependent inactivation of the Ca^{2+} channel was incorporated into the model; see, for example, Ashcroft and Stanfield (1981), Brehm and Eckert (1978), Brehm, Eckert, and Tillotson (1980), and Brown et al. (1981a). The idea of calcium-dependent inactivation of I_{Ca} was also suggested by the abrupt repolarization of the Ca spike. There is some evidence that I_{Ca} is inactivated by intracellular Ca^{2+} (Meyers and Barker, 1989; Pitler and Landfield, 1987), although whether or not such inactivation occurs rapidly (i.e., within a few milliseconds) after a single calcium spike is not clear. (iv) A single Ca^{2+}-dependent K^+ current is used. This current has some voltage dependence, but is controlled mainly by a threshold-dependent process triggered by an increase in intracellular Ca^{2+} concentration. Once activated, the current is independent of Ca^{2+}. The details of control of the Ca^{2+}-dependent currents remain to be elucidated (Adams et al., 1982; Alger and Williamson, 1988; Lancaster and Adams, 1986; Numann et al., 1987; Storm, 1987).

Details of the hippocampal pyramidal-cell model

The physical structure of the model pyramidal cell is shown in Figure 4.2 (Traub, 1982). The model has a 125-μ-long soma, an equivalent cylinder representing the basilar dendrites (below), and a branched equivalent cylinder representing the apical dendrites (above). The detailed construction of the passive membrane parameters proceeds as follows. First, we specify the membrane parameters, using values concordant with published data: $C_m = 3 \, \mu F/cm^2$ (Kay and Wong, 1987; Turner and Schwartzkroin, 1980), $R_m = 10,000 \, \Omega\text{-}cm^2$ (Turner and Schwartzkroin, 1983), $R_i = 100 \, \Omega\text{-}cm$ (hence, $\tau_m = 30$ ms). The electrotonic length of the basilar dendrites is 0.8λ, and for the apical dendrites 1.0λ. Each dendritic compartment represents 0.1λ of membrane and is treated as a lumped circuit. It is assumed that the ends of the dendrites are sealed. We wanted the input resistance of the cell to be about 30 MΩ, and we knew anatomically that the radius of the apical shaft was relatively large (Lorente de Nó, 1934). We therefore specified $R_{input} = 90$ MΩ for the basilar dendrites and 60 MΩ for the apical dendrites. Using the formula $R_{input} = (\lambda R_i/\pi r^2)\coth(L)$ (Problem 2 in this chapter), we can then determine the radii of the respective dendritic cylinders, as well as the length. By specifying the input resistance of one of the apical branches, we can similarly determine its radius; then, by the $\frac{3}{2}$-power rule we can determine the radius of the other branch. If we assume impedance matching of the dendritic branches at the soma (i.e., if we assume that the $\frac{3}{2}$-power

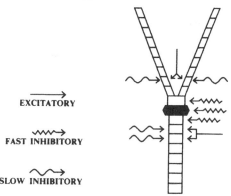

EXCITATORY

FAST INHIBITORY

SLOW INHIBITORY

Figure 4.2. Structure of the pyramidal-cell model. The soma compartment is black (it is compartment 9). The basilar dendrites are represented as an equivalent cylinder divided into eight compartments (below). The apical shaft, 0.1λ in extent, is compartment 10, just above the soma. There are two equivalent cylinders for the apical branches: one consists of compartments 11–18, the other compartments 19–28. The locations of synaptic inputs in network simulations are also shown. The soma contains conductances sufficient for burst generation. In some simulations, these conductances are also located in selected dendritic compartments. All other compartments are passive (i.e., the only membrane elements are capacitance and leakage conductance).

rule applies to the soma radius and to the radii of the dendrites), we can also determine the soma radius. These numbers in turn allow calculation of the areas of all of the compartments and hence the lumped leakage conductance (g_L) and capacitance for each compartment. To calculate the conductances that couple the compartments, we note that the internal resistance of a cylinder of length X and radius r is $XR_i/\pi r^2$. The input resistance of the final structure turns out to be 32.6 MΩ.

In a simulation, we replace the cable equation, a partial differential equation, by a coupled set of ordinary differential equations of the form

$$C_k \frac{dV_k}{dt} = \gamma_{k-1,k}(V_{k-1} - V_k) + \gamma_{k+1,k}(V_{k+1} - V_k) + I_{\text{ionic},k}$$

for each compartment k, where C_k is the capacitance of compartment k, $\gamma_{k-1,k}$ is the conductance (i.e., reciprocal resistance) between compartments $k - 1$ and k, and V_k is the potential across the membrane of compartment k (expressed relative to resting potential). (It is important to use a consistent system of units for time, voltage, current, conductance, and capacitance, e.g., ms, mV, nA, μS, nF.) We shall also assume that the extracellular space is isopotential,[6] allowing us to ignore extracellular currents. Much of the labor in this effort involves a reasonable specification of the $I_{\text{ionic},k}$, as discussed later. The γ values are determined by the electrotonic architecture of the model cell and by R_i.

For compartments capable of burst generation, we shall also need equations that govern the value of internal $[Ca^{2+}]$, designated χ, and that govern the coupling of χ and potential V to membrane processes. Internal diffusion, uptake, and release of Ca^{2+} are not considered in our formulation. Assume that Ca^{2+} in the cell is confined to a thin submembrane sheet of thickness d. For a membrane of area A (in appropriate units), we write

$$\frac{d\chi}{dt} = -\frac{c}{Ad}I_{Ca} - \beta_\chi \chi$$

Here, c is a constant for converting coulombs to millimoles, and β_χ is a constant. This assumes that the decay of χ, internal calcium, occurs via first-order kinetics, with no consideration of active pumping. We use a value of $\beta_\chi = 0.1$ ms^{-1}. With this 10-ms time constant, the decay of χ is fast relative to the removal of inactivation of the Ca current and is fast also with respect to the kinetics of the slow K current, as discussed later.

Summary of equations[7] (passive dendrites)

I. Cable equation (discrete version)

$$C_i\frac{dV_i}{dt} = I_{longit,i} + I_{ionic,i}$$

$$I_{longit,i} = \gamma_{i,i-1}(V_{i-1} - V_i) + \gamma_{i,i+1}(V_{i+1} - V_i) \qquad (i = 2\text{--}9,\ 11\text{--}18,\ 21\text{--}27)$$

$$I_{longit,1} = \gamma_{1,2}(V_2 - V_1)$$

$$I_{longit,10} = \gamma_{9,10}(V_9 - V_{10}) + \gamma_{11,10}(V_{11} - V_{10}) + \gamma_{20,10}(V_{20} - V_{10})$$

$$I_{longit,19} = \gamma_{18,19}(V_{18} - V_{19})$$

$$I_{longit,20} = \gamma_{10,20}(V_{10} - V_{20}) + \gamma_{21,20}(V_{21} - V_{20})$$

$$I_{longit,28} = \gamma_{27,28}(V_{27} - V_{28})$$

$$I_{ionic,i} = g_{L,i}V_i, \ (i = 1\text{--}5,\ 11,\ 13\text{--}20,\ 22\text{--}28)$$

$$I_{ionic,i} = g_{L,i}V_i + I_{synaptic,i} \ (i = 6,\ 7,\ 8,\ 10,\ 12,\ 21)$$

$$I_{ionic,9} = g_{L,9}V_9 + I_{synaptic,9} + I_{injected} + I_{active}$$

$$I_{synaptic,i} = I_{excit,i} + I_{slow\ inh,i} \ (i = 6,\ 7,\ 12,\ 21)$$

$$I_{synaptic,i} = I_{fast\ inh,i} \ (i = 8,\ 9,\ 10)$$

$$I_{excit,i} = \frac{c_e C_i}{C_6 + C_7 + C_{12} + C_{21}}s_e(t)(V_i - V_{ex}) \qquad (i = 6,\ 7,\ 12,\ 21)$$

$$I_{slow\ inh,i} = \frac{c_s C_i}{C_6 + C_7 + C_{12} + C_{21}}s_{slow}(t)(V_i - V_{slow}) \qquad (i = 6,\ 7,\ 12,\ 21)$$

$$I_{\text{fast inh},i} = \frac{c_i C_i}{C_8 + C_9 + C_{10}} s_{\text{fast}}(t)(V_i - V_{\text{fast}}) \qquad (i = 8, 9, 10)$$

$$I_{\text{active}} = I_{\text{Na}} + I_{\text{K}} + I_{\text{Ca}} + I_{\text{K[Ca]}}$$

$$I_{\text{Na}} = \bar{g}_{\text{Na}} m^3 h (V_9 - V_{\text{Na}})$$

$$I_{\text{K}} = \bar{g}_{\text{K}} n^4 y (V_9 - V_{\text{K}})$$

$$I_{\text{Ca}} = \bar{g}_{\text{Ca}} s^5 r (V_9 - V_{\text{Ca}})$$

$$I_{\text{K[Ca]}} = \bar{g}_{\text{K[Ca]}} q (V_9 - V_{\text{K}})$$

II. Differential equations for active membrane state variables and calcium

$$\frac{dm}{dt} = \alpha_m(V_9)[1 - m(t)] - \beta_m(V_9)m(t)$$

$$\frac{dh}{dt} = \alpha_h(V_9)[1 - h(t)] - \beta_h(V_9)h(t)$$

$$\frac{dn}{dt} = \alpha_n(V_9)[1 - n(t)] - \beta_n(V_9)n(t)$$

$$\frac{dy}{dt} = \alpha_y(V_9)[1 - y(t)] - \beta_y(V_9)y(t)$$

$$\frac{ds}{dt} = \alpha_s(V_9)[1 - s(t)] - \beta_s(V_9)s(t)$$

$$\frac{dr}{dt} = \alpha_r[1 - r(t)] - \beta_r(\chi)r(t)$$

$$\frac{dq}{dt} = \alpha_q(V_9, \chi)[1 - q(t)] - \beta_q q(t)$$

$$\frac{d\chi}{dt} = -\frac{c}{Ad} I_{\text{Ca}} - \beta_\chi \chi$$

Rate functions (in ms^{-1})

Variable	$\alpha(V, \chi)$	$\beta(v, \chi)$
m	$\dfrac{0.32(13 - V)}{\exp\left(\dfrac{13 - V}{4}\right) - 1}$	$\dfrac{0.28(V - 40)}{\exp\left(\dfrac{V - 40}{5}\right) - 1}$

h	$0.128 \exp(\dfrac{17-V}{18})$	$\dfrac{4}{\exp(\dfrac{40-V}{5})+1}$
n	$\dfrac{0.032(15-V)}{\exp(\dfrac{15-V}{5})-1}$	$0.5 \exp(\dfrac{10-V}{40})$
y	$0.028 \exp(\dfrac{15-V}{15})+\dfrac{2}{\exp(\dfrac{85-V}{10})+1}$	$\dfrac{0.4}{\exp(\dfrac{40-V}{10})+1}$

(Sometimes, $y \equiv 1$.)

s	$\dfrac{0.04(60-V)}{\exp(\dfrac{60-V}{10})-1}$	$\dfrac{0.005(V-45)}{\exp(\dfrac{V-45}{10})-1}$
r	0.005	$\dfrac{0.025(200-\chi)}{\exp(\dfrac{200-\chi}{20})-1}$
q	$\dfrac{\exp(V/27) \times 0.005(200-\chi)}{\exp(\dfrac{200-\chi}{20})-1}$	0.0004 to 0.002

Units: V in millivolts and expressed relative to resting potential; χ, the sub-membrane Ca^{2+} concentration, in millimoles per liter; see Traub (1982)

III. Equations for synaptic input state variables $[s_e(t), s_{fast}(t), s_{slow}(t)]$

For an excitatory cell,

$$\frac{ds_e(t)}{dt} = S(t) - \frac{s_e(t)}{\tau_e}$$

Note: A presynaptic action potential causes $S(T)$ to be held at 1 for 3 ms, in the case in which the postsynaptic cell is excitatory. In the absence of presynaptic activity, $S(t) = 0$. The effects of multiple simultaneous presynaptic action potentials add linearly (i.e., S can assume any positive integer value up to the total number of presynaptic inputs).

For an inhibitory cell,

$$\frac{ds_e(t)}{dt} = S(t) - s_e(t)$$

Note: A presynaptic action potential causes $S(t)$ to be held at 1 for 1 ms, in the case in which the postsynaptic cell is inhibitory.

$$\frac{ds_i(t)}{dt} = S(t) - \frac{s_i(t)}{\tau_i}$$

Note: A presynaptic action potential causes $S(t)$ to be held at 1 for 1 ms, in the case of fast inhibition.

$$\frac{ds_{slow}(t)}{dt} = S(t) - \frac{s_{slow}(t)}{\tau_{slow}}$$

Note: A presynaptic action potential causes $S(t)$ to be held at 1 for 40 ms, in the case of slow inhibition.

Glossary of terms

t: time
V_i: transmembrane voltage of compartment i, relative to rest
C_i: capacitance of compartment i
$g_{L,i}$: leakage conductance of compartment i
$\gamma_{i,j}$ ($= \gamma_{j,i}$): longitudinal conductance between compartments i and j
V_{Na}: equilibrium potential for sodium conductance, 115 mV positive to resting potential
V_K: equilibrium potential for potassium conductance, -15 mV (usually)
V_{Ca}: equilibrium potential for calcium conductance, 140 mV positive
V_{ex}: equilibrium potential for EPSP, 60 mV positive to rest
V_{fast}: equilibrium potential for fast IPSP, -15 mV
V_{slow}: equilibrium potential for slow IPSP, -25 mV
$\bar{g}_{Na}, \bar{g}_K, \bar{g}_{Ca}, \bar{g}_{K[Ca]}$: maximum conductance for respective ions; values are 3.32, 6.64, 3.98, and 0.10 μS, respectively.
$\tau_e, \tau_i, \tau_{slow}$: time constants for decay of excitatory, fast inhibitory, and slow inhibitory synaptic conductances, respectively; values are 3, 7, and 100 ms, respectively.
χ: $[Ca]_i$
c, A, d: constants for converting I_{Ca}, expressed in nA or 10^{-9} coulomb/s, into calcium concentration in some volume of cytoplasm beneath the membrane, expressed in mmol/liter; we use $c = 5.2 \times 10^{-12}$ mmol/nanocoulomb, A = area of soma membrane = 3,320 μ^2, $d = 5 \times 10^{-4} \mu$
β_χ: time constant for removal of $[Ca]_i$; equal to 0.1 ms^{-1}
s_e, s_i, s_{slow}: synaptic activation state variables for excitatory, fast inhibi-

tory, and slow inhibitory synaptic inputs, respectively; these variables
are computed for each cell by the network program, depending on the
activities of all of the various cells.

c_e, c_i, c_s: synaptic conductance parameters for excitatory, fast inhibitory,
and slow inhibitory conductances, respectively; c_e is varied from 3 to
20 nS; c_i is varied from 0 to 10 nS; c_s is typically 4×10^{-5} nS; note,
however, that a presynaptic action potential from a slow-inhibition
cell exerts an effect for 40 ms.

Behavior of the model

An example of a current-induced burst in the model pyramidal cell is
shown in Figure 4.3. This figure illustrates the four types of ionic currents,
together with the calcium signal that gates $g_{K[Ca]}$. Calcium-mediated spike
depolarizations occur in simulations, as do slow spikes and the long AHP.
Burst frequency increases as the resting potential depolarizes (Traub,
1982). Multiple dendritic burst-initiating sites can easily be incorporated

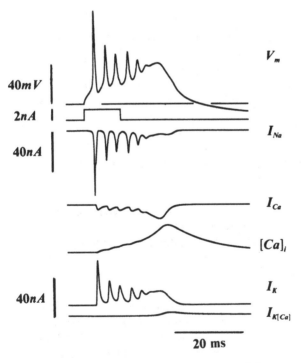

Figure 4.3. Membrane ionic currents and $[Ca^{2+}]_i$ during a current-induced
simulated burst. Note the relatively slow kinetics of I_{Ca} compared to I_{Na}.

in simulations. In network simulations, dendritic burst sites often are omitted to reduce computation time. The model thus reproduces most of the "essential" features of bursting listed earlier. Simulated burst morphology resembles the real situation closely.

A particularly interesting feature of intrinsic bursting in these cells is the ability to prevent a burst with a critically timed hyperpolarizing current (see Chapter 2). The protocol involves stimulating the cell with a brief current pulse that can reliably trigger an intrinsic burst of duration much longer than the duration of the triggering current itself. If this same trigger is followed by a small hyperpolarizing current, then the initial action potential is followed by a depolarizing afterpotential (DAP), rather than a complete burst (Figure 2.3) (Wong and Prince, 1981). The presumed physiological explanation for this is as follows: The inward currents (together, perhaps, with the longitudinal dendritic currents) that produce the DAP are relatively small compared with the regenerative currents underlying action potentials and calcium spikes. A small bias can therefore turn a net inward current into a net outward current. This same behavior is readily reproduced in our model (Figures 2.3 and 4.4). The hyperpolarizing current necessary to prevent a burst can be quite small if it is timed correctly. Once two or three action potentials have developed, a larger hyperpolarizing current is necessary to prevent the calcium spike (not shown).

We shall show that this exquisite control of pyramidal-cell bursting has important consequences for network behavior. Small differences in the timing or amplitude of inhibitory inputs can make the difference between bursting or not bursting in a particular pyramidal cell. With the powerful excitatory connections in the CA3 network, differences in output from one cell can be rapidly amplified and can radically alter subsequent network behavior. This important issue will be explored further in later chapters.

Interneurons. For simulation of interneurons, we sometimes use a variant of the pyramidal-cell model: calcium and calcium-dependent currents are removed, and g_K does not undergo voltage-dependent inactivation (in the foregoing notation, $y \equiv 1$). Such a model does not generate intrinsic bursts. It responds to injection of a steady current with a train of action potentials; see, for example, Figure 2 of Traub et al. (1987b).

Critique of the model

We should note certain deficiencies in both the behavior and structure of the pyramidal-cell model. Thus, with respect to behavior, the interspike intervals in simulations are short (3–4 ms, compared with 7–10 ms often seen experimentally). It does not respond to injection of large

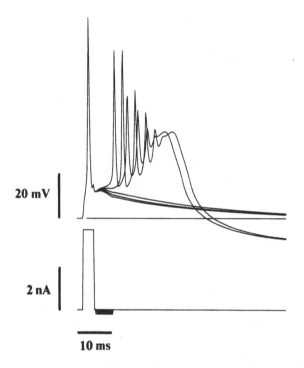

Figure 4.4. A prediction of the model: exquisite sensitivity of burst generation to a critically timed hyperpolarizing pulse; five superimposed traces (see
also Figure 2.3).

depolarizing currents by firing repetitive action potentials without evidence of calcium spikes (Wong and Prince, 1981). This may result from
inaccuracies in the voltage-dependent kinetics or spatial distribution of
g_{Ca}. The model cells do not produce a rebound burst after a transient
hyperpolarization (Kandel and Spencer, 1961b). This may be related to
inaccurate representation of inactivation of g_{Na}, to failure to include a
low-threshold Ca current (Jahnsen and Llinás, 1984a,b), or to other
factors. Finally, the model does not produce either multiple calcium
spikes during a single burst (Wong and Prince, 1978) or repetitive slow
spikes at 60–70-ms intervals as may occur during picrotoxin-induced
afterdischarges (see Chapter 6). This deficiency may result because we
do not generally use multiple dendritic regions with g_{Ca} [such as appear
to exist in Purkinje cells (Ross and Werman, 1987) and may exist also
in hippocampal pyramidal cells (Wong et al., 1979)]; another factor
may be inaccurate description of g_{Ca} inactivation and recovery from
inactivation.

With respect to structure, we are disturbed that the kinetics of the
simulated channels are not based directly on voltage-clamp data, but

rather are inferred indirectly from current-clamp data. Given this limitation, the model performs surprisingly well. Our g_K is a hybrid of several K currents: the delayed rectifier, the transient K current I_A, and perhaps a fast Ca^{2+}-dependent K current (Alger and Williamson, 1988; Storm, 1987; Zbicz and Weight, 1985). Some currents are not included at all, such as the M current[8] (Halliwell and Adams, 1982), a slow Na-dependent inward current (French and Gage, 1985), and a Ca-dependent Cl current (Owen, Segal, and Barker, 1984); slow inward currents can, however, be approximated by constant injected depolarizing currents. Many experimentally known effects are omitted, such as the voltage dependence of the decay of $g_{K[Ca]}$ (Segal and Barker, 1986). The time constant we use for removal of intracellular Ca, β_χ^{-1}, is 10 ms, whereas optical measurements of intracellular Ca removal suggest – at least under certain conditions – a much slower decay (Connor et al., 1988; Ross and Werman, 1987). However, optical measurements do not reveal the concentration of Ca^{2+} just beneath the membrane, and it is this quantity that enters into our model; furthermore, there has been a report of a calcium-removal time constant of under 100 ms in distal Purkinje-cell dendrites (Miyakawa, Lev-Ram, and Ross, 1988). Krnjevic, Morris, and Ropert (1986) estimated a time constant for decay of internal calcium transients of 7–14 s; those authors used an intracellular calcium-sensitive electrode. Again, the technique would not be expected to record calcium transients just beneath the membrane. Finally, as noted already, the model does not include an axon initial segment, a structure that appears to initiate Na spikes in motoneurons; see Dodge and Cooley (1973) and the references therein. The density of Na channels is higher in the initial segment than on the soma, at least for cultured cortical neurons (Angelides et al., 1988).

All of these deficiencies, and others besides, provide opportunities for further research. But to put the matter in perspective, the strictly phenomenological behavior of the model is quite good, and it suits most of our network modeling purposes well.

Comment on integration methods

We use the so-called Taylor series for integrating the differential equations for a single neuron (Daniel and Moore, 1978). This method is stable and allows us to use a reasonably sized integration step of 50 μs, compared with the 5-μs time step of our original publication (Traub, 1982), where a two-step Euler method was used (Traub and Llinás, 1977).

The idea of the integration method is as follows. Let the state variables of the neuron be $V_1, \ldots, V_K, V_{K+1}, \ldots, V_L$, where K is the number of compartments, the first K variables are true voltages, and the remaining ones are other state variables (m, n, h, etc.). The differential equations of the system can be written in the form $dV_i/dt = f_i(V_1, \ldots, V_L) + g_i(t)$. Here, the f_i incorporate terms for longitudinal currents, leakage currents, ionic currents, and so forth, for $i = 1, \ldots, K$, while the other f_i describe the time evolution of the other variables. For example, if V_i were to correspond to somatic state variable m, and V_9 to the somatic potential, then $f_i(V_1, \ldots, V_L) = \alpha_m(1 - V_9) - \beta_m V_9$. The $g_i(t)$ describe time-dependent inputs to the neuron, such as injected or synaptic currents. In what follows, we shall assume for the moment that all the g_i are zero. The equations are easy to modify for the case in which g_i is not zero.

If we formally apply a Taylor-series expansion to the function $V_i(t)$, retaining only terms up to order 2 in Δt, we obtain

$$V_i(t + \Delta t) = V_i(t) + \Delta t \frac{dV_i}{dt} + \frac{\Delta t^2}{2} \frac{d^2V_i}{dt^2} + \ldots$$

But, by assumption,

$$\frac{d^2V_i}{dt^2} = \frac{d}{dt}[f_i(V_1, \ldots, V_L)] = \sum_{j=1}^{L} \frac{\partial f_i}{\partial V_j} \frac{dV_j}{dt} = \sum_{j=1}^{L} \frac{\partial f_i}{\partial V_j} f_j$$

Hence,

$$V_i(t + \Delta t) = V_i(t) + \Delta t \frac{dV_i}{dt} + \frac{\Delta t^2}{2} \sum_{j=1}^{L} \frac{\partial f_i}{\partial V_j} f_j$$

Provided that we can compute the partial derivatives $\partial f_i/\partial V_j$, we therefore have an explicit formula for the values of all the V_i at the next time step, in terms of the present V_i, f(the present V_i), and partial derivatives of f(present V_i). It turns out that because the f_i do not depend explicitly on time, and the f_i all have a relatively simple form, the partial derivatives can be explicitly written down beforehand as functions $J_{ij} = \partial f_i/\partial V_j$. This is the basis, then, of our integration method. Its major disadvantage is that it makes it difficult to experiment with the rate functions, because new rate functions and their derivatives must be specified in the program. The method is most useful once suitable rate functions are specified in reasonably final form.

In order to make the integration most efficient, we want to avoid calculating the rate functions and their partial derivatives at each time step; such calculation is particularly disadvantageous because so many of the rate functions and partial derivatives involve time-consuming evaluations of exponential functions. To get around this, we construct tables of all these functions, at 0.25-mV voltage steps or 1-mmol Ca^{2+} concentration steps, before the actual simulation begins. These tables provide sufficient accuracy and speed up the calculation considerably.

Appendix: Hodgkin-Huxley theory

Our account of the single-cell model assumes the reader to be familiar with the principles of the Hodgkin-Huxley model of action-potential generation in the squid axon (Hodgkin and Huxley, 1952a–d). We therefore review this important subject.

The squid axon is a rare example of a system in which understanding of ionic membrane currents has allowed quantitative predictions of membrane potential as a function of time and space. Hodgkin and Huxley demonstrated that the action potential in the squid giant axon resulted from the interplay of two voltage-dependent currents (sodium and potassium) with the cable properties of the axon. Using a quantitative model, in the form of a set of differential equations, they reproduced the shape of the action potential and predicted the existence and properties of subthreshold responses, as well as the propagation velocity of an action potential along an axon. The experimental model involved several essential ingredients. First, wires were run through the interior of the axon so as to eliminate longitudinal currents and so that the inside of the axon could be maintained isopotential. This is called "space clamp"; it makes $\partial^2 V/\partial x^2$ identically zero in the cable equation. The cable equation can thus be written $C_m(\partial V/\partial t) + I_{ionic} = 0$. Next, they used electronic circuitry that would (except for brief transients) maintain the membrane potential at a constant level predetermined by the experimenter. Thus, except during a few brief intervals, $\partial V/\partial t = 0$, whereby $I_{ionic} = 0$. Because at a constant membrane potential the leak current will be constant, one can then measure directly the currents due to flow of voltage-dependent sodium and potassium currents. By using bathing media with different sodium concentrations, they could determine which part of this ionic current was due to sodium, and hence which part was due to potassium. (Nowadays, tetrodotoxin would also be used to block voltage-dependent sodium channels.)

Hodgkin and Huxley were able to show that a particular membrane current could be described by a generalized version of Ohm's law. For example, $I_{Na} = g_{Na} \times (V - V_{Na})$, where g_{Na} is a conductance (inverse resistance), V is the membrane potential relative to resting potential, and V_{Na} is the equilibrium potential for sodium relative to resting potential. V_{Na} is determined by the relative concentrations of Na^+ on the inside and outside of the membrane. At the equilibrium potential, the tendency of Na^+ to move inward by diffusion is balanced by the tendency to move outward caused by the electric field. Although this expression for membrane current seems obvious, it is by no means so. It suggests that the current is linear in V (on time scales too short for g_{Na} itself to change), that on a brief time scale g_{Na} is a well-defined constant, and that I_{Na} does not depend on other variables (e.g., K^+ currents) except insofar as these other variables effect g_{Na} and V. These are, in fact, important experimental issues. To show, for example, that g_{Na} is well defined, it is necessary to bring the membrane into a particular state (by clamping V), and then suddenly change V while measuring the instantaneous current. By performing this measurement for a number of different V values, the so-called instantaneous current–voltage relation can be obtained, and it must have a constant slope for this formulation to be meaningful. Likewise, the term $(V - V_{Na})$ is appropriate for squid axon, but the analogous term for potassium cannot adequately describe currents in other experimental systems (Frankenhaeuser, 1962).

The next problem is to determine how g_{Na} and g_K depend on the history of the membrane. Hodgkin and Huxley showed that these conductances could be modeled as functions of state variables that in turn depended only on membrane potential (rather than currents). How many state variables are required, and what is the nature of their dependence on membrane potential? Hodgkin and Huxley envisioned each state variable as corresponding to a fraction of particles located on the inside membrane border, versus the outside border of the membrane. (We might visualize the variables as corresponding to the fraction of membrane-protein pieces that lie with a particular orientation; these pieces might each possess a dipole moment and be connected to a molecular backbone via bonds with certain orientation preferences, so that the net energy of the orientation would depend on the electric field across the membrane. The concept of channel proteins as it now exists was not defined when the Hodgkin-Huxley model was formulated.) Because each state variable corresponds to a fraction of some sort of object in a particular state, each state variable will be a real number between 0 and 1. Each variable has a time dependence described by first-order kinetics, that is, a first-order differential equation with a "forward" term that increases the state variable, and a "backward" term that decreases it. Thus, for state variable n (on which g_K depends), we have $dn/dt = \alpha_n(V) \times (1 - n) - \beta_n(V) \times n$. Here, $\alpha_n(V)$ is the forward rate function, and $\beta_n(V)$ is the backward rate function. All of the rate functions are positive: $\alpha_n(V), \beta_n(V) > 0$. Thus, if $0 \le n \le 1$ at time 0, n will remain between 0 and 1, for if $n = 1$, then $dn/dt < 0$, and if $n = 0$, $dn/dt > 0$. Hodgkin and Huxley assumed that g_K was proportional to n^p, $g_K = \bar{g}_K n^p$, where $\bar{g}_K$ is the maximum K conductance, and p is a parameter to be determined. The form of $\alpha_n(V)$, $\beta_n(V)$, and p can be determined by voltage-clamp experiments using single voltage steps, or by using two steps, the first to force the membrane into a particular state and the second to measure the "tail current" that results when the voltage is forced to another level. Note that when V is clamped, α_n and β_n can be viewed as constants. In that case, $dn/dt = \alpha_n - (\alpha_n + \beta_n)n$, whence it is easy to show that n will tend to an equilibrium value $n_\infty = \alpha_n/(\alpha_n + \beta_n)$, with time constant $\tau_n = 1/(\alpha_n + \beta_n)$. Hodgkin and Huxley were able to fit their data with $p = 4$; α_n and β_n, and the other rate functions as well, were fit with functions of V involving elementary arithmetic operations (addition, subtraction, multiplication, division) and exponentiation.

It turned out that g_{Na} was more complex than g_K, because g_{Na} required two membrane state variables, m and h, to model it, rather than just one. Fortunately, m and h had different time courses and voltage dependences, so that they could be experimentally separated: m is the activation variable, which increases rapidly with depolarization (i.e., α_m is large at depolarized V); h is the inactivation variable, and it decreases at depolarized levels (β_h large), but more slowly than m increases [i.e., $1/(\alpha_h + \beta_h) < 1/(\alpha_m + \beta_m)$]. For I_{Na} to flow, however, both m and h must be large, because Hodgkin and Huxley found the most accurate formulation to be $g_{Na} = \bar{g}_{Na}m^3h$. At the resting potential, h is greater than 0.5, and m is small, and thus the effect of a sudden, adequate depolarization is to increase m rapidly. I_{Na} will flow inward, tending to further depolarize the membrane. This gives the upstroke of the action potential. Then h begins to decrease, diminishing I_{Na}. Finally, n begins to increase, turning on an outward K^+ current that repolarizes the membrane. The detailed kinetics of the rate functions influence the maximum rate of rise of the action potential, its height, its width, and the spike undershoot, as well as the possibility of repetitive firing in response to a sustained current stimulus, the dependence of firing rate on stimulus intensity, and so on.

A magnificent test of this formulation was the ability to predict the propagation velocity of an action potential, assuming uniform spatial distributions of $\bar{g}_{Na}$ and $\bar{g}_K$. Unfortunately, Hodgkin and Huxley were not able to integrate the cable equation in time and space. (Their calculations were done by hand!) They therefore looked for traveling-wave solutions: If the action potential everywhere has the same shape, then $V(x + y, t) = V(x, t - \phi y)$, where ϕ is a parameter that determines the conduction velocity. This allows one to express the cable equation as an ordinary second-order differential equation in t, rather than as a partial differential equation in x and t, for, using the basic definition of the partial derivative, one shows that $\partial^2 V/\partial x^2 = \phi^2(\partial^2 V/\partial t^2)$. Hodgkin and Huxley then solved the resulting cable equation for different values of ϕ until a nondivergent value of V was found.

5 Model of the CA3 network

This chapter concerns our methods. How do we translate the available data on the cellular physiology of the CA3 region into a useful model of the circuitry? By "model," we mean here a computer program. We must then consider how to organize and construct the computer program.

Specifically, we must decide the following: How many cells should we include, and of what types? How are the cells arranged in space? How can the communication between different cells be described? This last question is particularly complex, because it includes both functional and structural aspects. Functionally, we must model the transduction of soma membrane potential into axonal action potentials and axon conduction delays, and the transformation of arriving presynaptic impulses into postsynaptic conductance changes. Structurally, we must specify how the axonal outputs of each type of cell are distributed in space and how many synaptic inputs of each type (excitatory, $GABA_A$, $GABA_B$) each cell should have. We shall discuss these fundamentally physiological issues in turn and then analyze briefly how our simulation program actually works.

Cells

Types of cells. We use three basic types of cells: pyramidal cells (or e cells, for "excitatory cells"); inhibitory cells whose postsynaptic effect resembles that mediated by perisomatic $GABA_A$ receptors (i_1 cells); and inhibitory cells whose postsynaptic effect represents that mediated by dendritic $GABA_B$ receptors (i_2 cells). (See the discussion in Chapter 2 concerning the existence of two types of inhibitory cells.) The i_1 cells produce relatively fast IPSPs whose equilibrium potential is 15 mV hyperpolarized relative to rest. The unitary conductances produced by different i_1 cells usually (but not necessarily) are the same. Likewise, the intrinsic properties of the different i_1 cells are the same. This is quite a simplification, because cells mediating Cl^- IPSPs have a variety of firing patterns, and the resulting IPSPs have ranges of amplitude, latency, and

104

time course (see Chapter 3). Pyramidal cells and inhibitory cells are represented in network models in the ratio 10 : 1 (Dietz, Frotscher, and Abt, 1987), and we have arbitrarily set the number of i_1 cells equal to the number of i_2 cells.

How many cells? We aim for realism by using, to within a factor of 2 or 3, as many cells in our model network as are in the experimental preparation. The reason is that we would like to keep as many model parameters as possible within a physiological range. Such parameters include the number of synaptic inputs per cell, the strength of the unitary conductances, and the spatial distribution of synaptic connections. For these numbers to be self-consistent, we must then keep the total number of cells reasonable as well. Most of the simulations in this book are based on the longitudinal CA3 slice (Miles et al., 1988), which contains, we estimate, about 20,000 cells. Models of this system contain 9,000 pyramidal cells and 900 inhibitory cells. By using this large number, we can reproduce such phenomena as traveling waves of bursting that are synchronized locally, but have phase lags globally, as discussed later.

Another reason for using a large number of cells has come to light more recently. Suppose a population phenomenon, such as synchronized bursting, is triggered by a noise process whose probability distribution is known in individual cells. The "triggering cells" that initiate the population burst may be driven by the unlikely coincidence in them of closely timed random synaptic inputs. In order for this coincidence to occur at the correct intervals, it will be necessary to have sufficiently many cells. These considerations are relevant in the simulation of population bursts that occur in the presence of high $[K^+]$ (Chamberlin, Traub, and Dingledine, 1990; Traub and Dingledine, 1990).

Intrinsic properties of the cells. The intrinsic properties of model pyramidal cells were described in detail in the preceding chapter. We also mentioned a "generic" interneuron model, constructed from the pyramidal cell by omitting g_{Ca} and $g_{K[Ca]}$ and by not allowing voltage-dependent inactivation of g_K (i.e., $y \equiv 1$). We uniformly simulated i_2 cells as "generic interneurons" and simulated i_1 cells either as if they had the same intrinsic properties as pyramidal cells or as if they, too, were generic interneurons. (Usually, we used the former choice.) Excitatory synapses onto i_1 cells and i_2 cells behave differently than excitatory synapses onto e cells (see the equations for synaptic input state variables in Chapter 4 and later in this chapter).

Arrangement of cells in space. This is a feature that is important when the model includes axon conduction delays or spatial structure in the synaptic connectivity. We arrange the pyramidal cells into a rectangular array of size 40 × n, where n depends on the simulation ($n = 225$ for models of the longitudinal slice). The dimension 40 comes from the fact that slices are about 400 μ thick; CA3 cells have soma diameters of about 20 μ and are layered two or three deep in guinea pig stratum pyramidale; hence, one dimension of the array should be 40–60 cells. The inhibitory cells form a superimposed array of size 4 × n.

Intercellular communication

Transduction of soma potential into axonal output. Perhaps the most realistic way to do this would be to simulate explicitly at least a portion of the axon. That alternative, however, would introduce both new parameters and a significant increase in computation time (the small unit capacitance of axonal membrane and fast kinetics of axonal Na channels necessitating the use of a small integration time step). CA3 axons (or at least their Schaffer collaterals to CA1) have an absolute refractory period of about 3–4 ms (Grinvald et al., 1982); however, Andersen et al. (1978) found a refractory period down to about 2 ms. We therefore use the following rule: The cell sends an output if it is depolarized more than some threshold amount (20 mV depolarized relative to resting potential) and if no output has been sent for 3 ms.

Axon conduction delays. We must also consider the conduction velocity of pyramidal-cell axons (about 0.5 m/s along the longitudinal axis of the hippocampus) (Miles et al., 1988).[1] In a system such as the longitudinal slice, which is 5–10 mm long, a signal could be delayed as long as 10–20 ms through axon conduction alone, if individual axons run this far (Ishizuka, Krzemieniewska, and Amaral, 1986; Ishizuka et al., 1990). We allow for conduction delays of pyramidal-cell axons only, assuming that inhibitory axon collaterals are (for the most part) relatively localized (Finch et al., 1983; Seress and Ribak, 1985; Tamamaki et al., 1984). From a programming point of view, delays are a nuisance. They mean that the simulation must retain information about the past of the system; the longer the maximum possible delay, the more information must be retained. Furthermore, action potentials not only must be sent to all of the correct postsynaptic cells but also must arrive at the correct times. The arrival times will generally differ for the various postsynaptic target cells.

Synaptic actions. We consider four distinct types of synapses: (i) excitatory synapses on the dendrites of pyramidal cells; (ii) excitatory synapses on the somata of inhibitory cells (both i_1 and i_2); (iii) "fast" (Cl⁻, $GABA_A$ type) synapses on the somata and proximal dendrites of both e cells and i

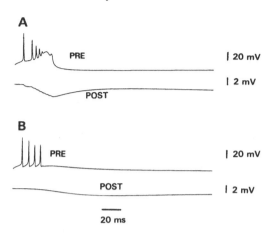

Figure 5.1. Firing properties of simulated i cells and their respective postsynaptic actions. A: The i_1 cell has the intrinsic properties of a pyramidal cell. Rapid, summating unitary IPSPs can be recognized. (Although some inhibitory cells in CA3 have this type of firing pattern, most do not; see Chapter 3.) B: The i_2 cell fires a nonadapting train of action potentials in response to injected current. The peak of the IPSP is delayed, and decay is slow. Unitary events are not recognizable. (In some simulations, all i cells have the firing properties shown in B.) (From Traub et al., 1987b, with permission.)

cells (Misgeld and Frotscher, 1986); these synapses are activated by the action potentials of i_1 cells; (iv) "slow" (K^+, $GABA_B$ type) synapses on the dendrites of both e cells and i cells; these synapses are activated by the outputs from i_2 cells. The equations describing unitary conductance for each type of synapse are given in the preceding chapter, and examples of IPSPs produced by i_1 cells and i_2 cells are shown in Figure 5.1. Here, we attempt to justify physiologically how we simulate the summation of multiple synaptic events impinging on a common postsynaptic cell.

We consider a synaptic action to consist of two processes: (i) an activation process, which represents the release of transmitter, its diffusion across the synaptic cleft, the interaction of transmitter with receptor, and the coupling between the receptor-transmitter complex and ionic channels (Land et al., 1984); we use the values of 3, 1, 1, and 40 ms for the four types of synapses that we consider, e → e, e → i, fast inhibition, and slow inhibition, respectively; (ii) a second process, with first-order kinetics, represents relaxation of the set of activated ionic channels. This relaxation process has the time constants 3, 1, 7, and 100 ms respectively for the same four synaptic species. When a signal arrives from a presynaptic neuron, it exerts a constant activating effect for 3, 1, or 40 ms, depending on the type of synapse. Synaptic conductance changes resulting from firing in different presynaptic cells, or from firing of the same presynaptic cell at different times, add linearly. This prescribes how different inputs are combined. We assume, in effect, that each synaptic input activates distinct receptors that are, in turn, coupled to distinct ionic channels, ruling out either occlusion or cooperativity between inputs. Once activated, the different ionic channels relax independently of each other and independently of whether or not they are being stimulated; hence the use of first-order kinetics.

To accomplish the "bookkeeping" required for this process, we proceed as follows. Each cell has associated with it three delay lines, one for each type of synaptic input. The program checks the synaptic inputs each 0.5 ms. Let us consider, for example, the delay line for cell L (an e cell) that saves excitatory inputs, called SYNINE (L, i), $i = 1, \ldots, 24$. SYNINE $(L, 1)$ represents the amount of excitatory input arriving now, SYNINE $(L, 2)$ the amount that will arrive 0.5 ms into the future, and so forth. We are saving, in effect, information about the last 12 ms of the system. Why use 12 ms? An excitatory input lasts 3 ms, or 6 steps in the delay line. Our longitudinal-slice model represents 4.5 mm of tissue, with maximum conduction delay 9 ms, or 18 steps in the delay, and 18 + 6 = 24. When an e cell presynaptic to cell L fires, we simply add six 1s into the delay line at a location determined by the axon conduction delay between the two cells. The delay line is shifted every 0.5 ms. In order to allow for different synapses having different "weights," that is, producing different postsynaptic membrane conductances, we can add into the delay line a string of numbers other than 1, depending on the pair of cells.

Arrangement of synaptic connections. The general structure of the network is shown in Figure 5.2. We construct the network as follows. First we specify the expected numbers of excitatory and inhibitory inputs each

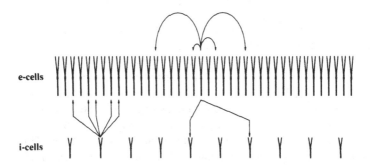

Figure 5.2. General structure of the network model. There are 10 times as many e cells as i cells. Connections are locally random, with i-cell outputs more spatially restricted than e-cell outputs. (Connections between i cells are also present, but are not shown in this diagram.)

kind of cell will have. Typically, all cell types receive an average of 20 excitatory and 20 inhibitory inputs in the 9,900-cell model. These numbers are based on estimates of connectivity from dual intracellular recordings and on comparisons of maximal synaptic inputs (e.g., during synchronized discharges) with unitary inputs (see Chapter 3). Then the program constructs the network by a sequence of independent random choices. There are two types of network topology that we use. In the first, the connection probability for any pair of cells of given types (say two e cells) is constant; this is a globally random network. In the second, a locally random network, the probability for a connection from cell M to cell L is

$$p(L)e^{-\frac{d(L, M)}{\lambda}}$$

where $p(L)$ is a scaling factor to ensure a constant expected number of inputs,[2] $d(L, M)$ is the distance between cells L and M (say, measured along the long axis of the array), and λ is a parameter that determines how localized the connections will be. We use different values of λ, depending on whether the presynaptic cell is excitatory (λ_e) or inhibitory (λ_i), and we keep (usually) $\lambda_e > \lambda_i$. Figure 5.3 gives a sense of the spatial distribution of the connections when $\lambda_e = 30$ and $\lambda_i = 6$. This connection scheme involves a minimum number of parameters to specify the structure of the network: We specify the statistical properties of the connections rather than a detailed wiring diagram. Nevertheless, the simulation program must have a particular wiring diagram (a particular sample network) in order to actually run.

Inhibition onto e cells compared with inhibition onto i cells. We do not have the same kind of quantitative information about IPSPs impinging onto i cells that we have for IPSPs onto e cells, although both fast and slow IPSPs are recorded in inhibitory cells (Misgeld and Frotscher, 1986). This means that arbitrary choices must be made for the strength of the maximum IPSP conductances onto i cells. These arbitrary choices may be important during a partial blockade of $GABA_A$-mediated IPSPs.

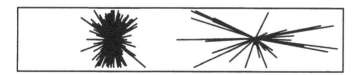

Figure 5.3. The outputs of an i cell (left) and an e cell (right) are shown. An i cell has, on average, 220 outputs: 200 to e cells and 20 to i cells. An e cell has an average of 22 outputs: 20 to e cells and 2 to i cells. The outputs of i cells are more localized than the outputs of e cells: $\lambda_i = 6$, while $\lambda_e = 30$. (From Traub et al., 1989, with permission; copyright AAAS.)

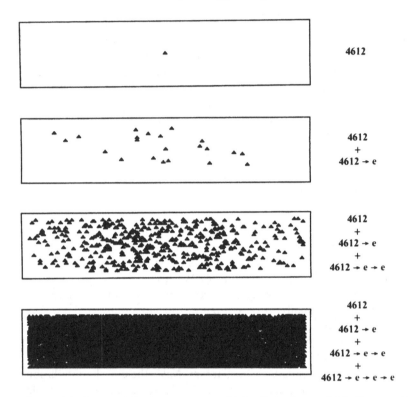

Figure 5.4. Connectivity between pyramidal cells in the model is illustrated by showing the e cells that can be reached from a selected e cell (4612) in chains of progressive length. Note that virtually all cells can be reached in three synapses.

Should IPSPs onto e cells and onto i cells be blocked in proportion? Our arbitrary choices are these: Slow IPSPs onto i cells (both i_1 cells and i_2 cells) have the same properties as slow IPSPs onto e cells; but the maximum conductance for fast IPSPs onto i cells (of both types) is kept at 0.4 of the corresponding conductance, c_i, for fast IPSPs onto e cells. This is done to limit the extent of disinhibition caused by i cells inhibiting each other.

Electrotonic synapses (gap junctions). In one early study (Traub and Wong, 1983b), motivated by the work on dye coupling and electrotonic coupling by MacVicar and Dudek (1980b, 1981), we included electrotonic synapses between pyramidal cells. These behaved basically as resistances between the somata of selected clusters of neighboring pyramidal cells. More recent anatomical ultrastructural data suggest that gap junctions exist between interneurons (Kosaka, 1983; Schlander and Frotscher,

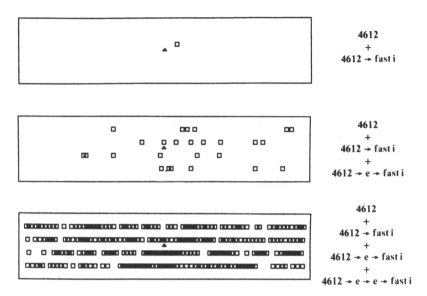

Figure 5.5. Inhibitory cells (squares) that can be reached from e cell 4612 through progressively longer excitatory chains. Because of the wide divergence of inhibitory-cell outputs, it is apparent that as more pyramidal cells become recruited into a synchronized event, all pyramidal cells will experience inhibition (see also Figure 5.6).

1986). Such junctions have not yet been incorporated into our model. Functional coupling between inhibitory cells may be important in some circumstances (Aram and Wong, 1989).

Illustrations of the model network: form and function. To visualize better the connectivity of this very large network, we illustrate how one cell (4612, in the middle of the array) can influence other cells, either directly or indirectly. Figure 5.4 shows the e cells monosynaptically excited by 4612, those disynaptically excited, and so on. Virtually all e cells are reached trisynaptically. Figure 5.5 illustrates the i_1 cells contacted directly by 4612 (top, i cells represented by squares), the i_1 cells contacted via another e cell, and so on. Finally, Figure 5.6 illustrates the e cells disynaptically inhibited by 4612 (top), those trisynaptically inhibited, and so on. Note that even with trisynaptic inhibition, there are "holes" in the system. Some cells are not inhibited, and so might receive polysynaptic excitation. The extent to which these holes actually exist is an important experimental question, because the holes determine the pattern for decay of activity after a local stimulus in the presence of normal inhibition.

In Figure 5.7 we compare experimental and model responses to a brief

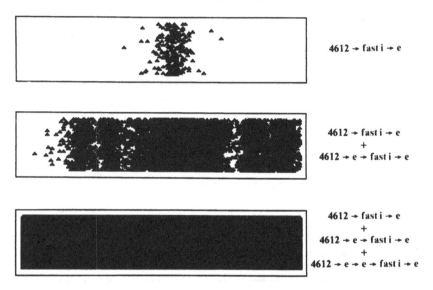

Figure 5.6. Pyramidal cells inhibited by e cell 4612, either disynaptically or through longer chains. Note the "holes" or noninhibited regions in the middle diagram. By the time all e cells disynaptic from cell 4612 are firing (third level in Figure 5.4), all e cells are being inhibited (bottom).

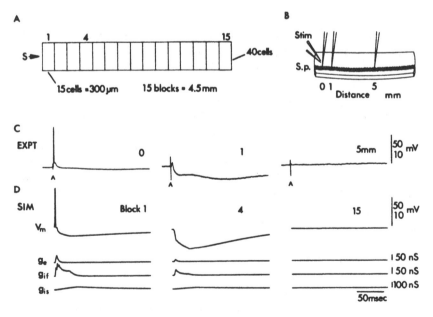

Figure 5.7. Responses of the model network and of the longitudinal CA3 slice to a stimulus at one end. A: Diagram of the model with subdivisions into 15

local shock. Functional behaviors are similar: (i) EPSPs in cells near the site of the shock generate a single action potential. Synaptic inhibition terminates the depolarization, and the action potential is followed by a long hyperpolarization (hundreds of milliseconds). (ii) About 1 mm away, the stimulus evokes a series of synaptic potentials: an EPSP, a fast IPSP, and a slow IPSP. These are all synaptically mediated, reflecting primary and secondary induced activity in excitatory and inhibitory cells. (iii) Sufficiently far from the stimulus, say 4–5 mm away, there is little or no apparent response. A local shock does not, in the presence of normal inhibitory circuitry, produce enough secondary effects to mediate synaptic responses at a distance. Blockade of inhibition will alter this situation (see Chapters 2 and 6) (Miles et al., 1988).

Technical computation aspects

We shall now attempt to convey a sense of how our simulation program works. Our code is written in FORTRAN. It is composed on an IBM 3090 with the interactive VM operating system. Simulations take so long to run that execution is done in batch mode on a different 3090 with the MVS operating system. This also makes it easier to store and catalog the extensive data that are generated by each simulation. The code is optimized to use the vector feature of the 3090, greatly increasing the efficiency of those sections of the program that integrate the differential equations. We have not succeeded in "vectorizing" those portions of the program that manage the communication between the cells, as discussed later. The overall structure of the simulation program is as follows.

Initialize cellular parameters. We start with the input resistance of the dendritic segments, the specific membrane resistivity and capacitance, the internal resistivity, and the electrotonic lengths of the dendrites. These define the radii and areas of the different compartments and, in turn, all the other passive parameters. We specify the maximum values

caption to Figure 5.7. (cont.) "blocks" (numbered on top of the diagram), each block containing 600 e cells and 60 i cells. The stimulus was a brief current pulse (3 nA, 2 ms) to all cells in block 1. B: Diagram of the longitudinal CA3 slice. The hatched region (S.p.) denotes stratum pyramidale. C: Near the experimental stimulus, cells fire a single action potential; 1 mm away there is an EPSP, a fast IPSP, and a delayed IPSP; 5 mm away from the stimulus there is no response. (Intracellular recordings.) D: The same sequence of responses is seen in the model. Below the voltage records are shown the synaptic inputs into the respective cells whose voltage responses are illustrated; g_e = excitatory conductance, g_{if} = GABA$_A$-type inhibitory conductance, g_{is} = GABA$_B$-type inhibitory conductance. The long duration of fast inhibition for cells in block 1 prevents them from bursting. (From Miles et al., 1988, with permission.)

of the active conductances, the equilibrium potentials of the active and synaptic currents, the axon conduction velocity, and so on.

Construct tables for the rate functions. This avoids having to calculate the rate functions at each time step. Note that computing exponentials is costly.

Construct the synaptic network. We specify the number of cells for each cell type, their geometric arrangement, the average number of excitatory and inhibitory inputs for each type of cell, and the parameters that determine how the connection probability depends on the intercellular distance, as discussed earlier. We then set the synaptic weights.

Simulation proper. The simulation proper has two main aspects: (i) managing the communication between the neurons; the program must compute, at each time step, all of the synaptic conductances for all of the cells; (ii) given all of the synaptic conductances and membrane state variables, the program must integrate the differential equations for some (relatively small) number of time steps, before repeating step (i). Steps (i) and (ii) are iterated in turn a number of times, saving selected data such as the somatic potentials of certain cells, the synaptic inputs to these cells, the firing times of all of the cells, and so on.

Comment on how the 3090 vector feature works. This feature of certain large computers is suited to algorithms in which the same sequence of operations is applied to multiple pieces of data (having all the same format) in turn. An example would be to compute $c_i = a_i + b_i$, $i = 1, \ldots, n$. In our simulation program, the relevant set of operations includes those required to perform one integration step for one neuron. But instead of computing first, say, V_9 and then V_{10} for a single cell, we organize the program to first compute $V_{9,l}$, $l = 1, \ldots, n$, and then $V_{10,l}$, $l = 1, \ldots, n$, and so forth (where n is the total number of cells). This method of program organization requires considerable extra storage in order to hold the values of intermediate variables for all of the cells; but on the other hand, it is extremely fast. The vector feature does not help much with other features of the computation, particularly the problem of routing cellular outputs to the correct synaptically connected cells with appropriate delays – these operations require branching decisions that are difficult to "vectorize," as discussed later.

Another approach to efficient simulation of neuronal networks would be to use a highly parallel computer with a large number of modules, each module dedicated to a (relatively) small number of neurons. Again, one must deal with the significant problem of how the neurons communicate with one another.

Comment on the management of intercellular communication. This issue is extremely intricate, because the conduction delays between pairs of cells are not the same for all cell pairs. Our solution involves the use of a delay line attached to each cell; that line will record inputs that will arrive at the cell up to 12 ms in the future; the maximum conduction delay is 9 ms. (Actually, there is, for each cell, a delay line for excitatory inputs, another for fast inhibitory inputs, and another for slow inhibitory inputs.) The length of the delay line is longer than the maximum conduction delay, because synaptic inputs produce effects lasting longer than one time step (effects that last from 1 to 40 ms, depending on the type of synapse). It is necessary that a synaptic input, when it does arrive at its destination, produce a postsynaptic conductance of the correct magnitude and time course. How ought the program to keep track of the past firings of all of the cells, making sure that the correct stimuli are delivered to all of the appropriate cells at the correct time? How much of the past history of the system must be saved? We shall illustrate our solution to these problems by presenting the "core" of our simulation program. We shall illustrate the case for excitatory synapses only. Fast and slow inhibitory synapses are treated separately.

Core of network integration code[3]

(Every 10 integration steps (0.5 ms), shift and update synaptic delay lines.)

```
DO L = 1 to N;
   DO K = 1 to 23;
      SYNINE(L, K) = SYNINE(L, K + 1);
   END;
   SYNINE(L, 24) = 0.;
(Do similar shift for fast and slow inhibitory delay lines.)
   END;
(Shifting completed.)
```

(Every 10 integration steps, process most recent outputs of excitatory cells.)
```
DO L = 1 to N;
   DO I = 1 to PNUME(L);
      K = PPE(I, L);
      IF ((TIME-OUTPUT(K)) ≤ 0.5) THEN DO;
         DELAY = 2. * STEPJ * ABS(JTAB(L) - JTAB(K));
```

(Delay = axon conduction delay between cell L and cell K, in units of 0.5 ms.)

```
        J1 = DELAY;
        IF (L ≤ NE) THEN DO J = 1 + J1 to 6 + J1;
            SYNINE(L, J) = SYNINE(L, J) + PWE(I, L);
        END;
        ELSE DO J = 1 + J1 to 2 + J1;
            SYNINE(L, J) = SYNINE(L, J) + PWE(I, L);
        END;
```

(If cell L is an e cell, the excitatory input is on for 3 ms. Otherwise, it is on for 1 ms.)

```
        END; (refers back to "TIME-OUTPUT(K)")
    END; (DO I)
```

(Do analogous processing of outputs of inhibitory cells; this code omitted.)

```
    END; (DO L)
```

(Processing of cell outputs completed.)

(Every integration step, update the synaptic state variables.)

```
        DO L = 1 to NE;
            SE(L) = SE(L) + DT * (SYNINE(L, 1) − SE(L) * ALFACT);
        END;
        DO L = NE + 1 to N;
            SE(L) = SE(L) + DT * (SYNINE(L, 1) − SE(L));
        END;
```

(Note that the excitatory input to e cells approximates an alpha function with time constant 1/ALFACT, or 3 ms, while the excitatory input to i cells is a pulse that decays with time constant 1 ms.)

(Now do similar processing of inhibitory synaptic state variables.)

(Every integration step, call the integration subroutine.)

```
        CALL EINT (membrane state variables, synaptic inputs, rate-
        function tables, other constants);
```

(Now update LASTOU and OUTPUT, every integration step.)

```
        DO L = 1 to N;
            IF ((VSTOR(L, 9) > 20.) & (LASTOU(L) > 3.)) THEN DO;
                OUTPUT(L) = TIME;
                LASTOU(L) = 0.;
            END;
```

ELSE LASTOU(L) = LASTOU(L) + DT;
END; (DO L . . .)

(Now repeat the whole process.)

Variables used in integration code

I, J, J1, K, L: indexing or "dummy" variables

N: total number of cells, typically 9,900

NE: total number of e cells, typically 9,000; cells 1 to NE are e cells, and cells NE + 1, . . . , N are i cells

DT: integration time step, 0.05 ms

SYNINE(N, 24): a set of delay lines, one for each cell, to record the number of excitatory presynaptic action potentials due to arrive in the future; SYNINE(L, I) = present value for the number of excitatory presynaptic action potentials due at cell L in I/2 ms in the future

PNUME(L): number of excitatory cells presynaptic to cell L; the maximum value this is allowed to be is called PNUMAX

PPE(PNUMAX, N) = a table of excitatory connectivity; PPE(I, L) = the Ith e cell presynaptic to cell L

TIME: time in milliseconds

OUTPUT(K): the most recent time that the soma of cell K was sending an action potential toward its connected followers

STEPJ: the time, in milliseconds, it takes an e-cell axon to conduct one cell diameter along the long axis of the cell array

ABS: absolute value function (negative conduction delays are meaningless)

JTAB(K): the position along the long axis of the array of cell K; JTAB(L) − JTAB(K) is the separation along the long axis of cells L and K

PWE(PNUMAX, N): a table of relative synaptic weights; PWE(I, L) is the relative weight of the Ith excitatory synaptic input to cell L; the usual value is 1

SE(L): the relative amount of excitatory conductance for cell L that is currently "on"; the actual conductance used in the integration program is $c_e \times$ SE(L); in response to a single action potential presynaptic to cell L, SE(L) will approximate an alpha function $te^{-\alpha t}$, with $\alpha =$ ALFACT in case cell L is an e cell, and $\alpha = 1$ in case cell L is an i cell

ALFACT: see above; ALFACT = 1/3 ms^{-1}

EINT: the name of the subroutine that integrates one time step for all of the cells

VSTOR:(N, 36): table of membrane state variables; VSTOR(L, 9) is the soma membrane potential of cell L

LASTOU(L): the time since the axon of cell L was last firing; this variable is reset to zero if the soma of cell L is depolarized more than 20 mV from rest and the axon has not fired for at least 3 ms (the assumed axon refractory time); that is, LASTOU(L) > 3

Our use of delay lines to store a partial history of the system – that part of the history necessary to reconstruct future synaptic inputs – has the significant advantage that it allows us to specify weights for all of the synaptic connections independently, without any additional computational work. On the other hand, our method does not record the time-dependent activity of individual synapses and thus does not lend itself to studies of how synaptic connections change with time as a result of ongoing neuronal activity. There are methods to handle this, at some extra cost in storage and computation.

6 Collective behaviors of the CA3 network: experiment and model

In this chapter and the next we shall analyze the interactions that take place between CA3 neurons in a large population (thousands of cells). The cardinal issues are these: Under what conditions does population firing become synchronized? What factors regulate the extent of synchronization? At one extreme, all cells might fire nearly simultaneously (complete synchrony), or alternatively small subsets of neurons might discharge at the same time (partial synchrony). How can one cell, or a small group of cells, influence the rest of the population? If synchronization is partial, rather than complete, what factors determine which selected cells participate?

It is well to consider why we so emphasize synchronization. After all, in principle, the firing pattern in any particular cell might resemble a Poisson process, and the correlation between firing patterns in different cells either might be weak or might assume some particularly complicated form. In that case, we would focus not on synchronization but on factors that, say, regulate the mean firing throughout the population. However, neuronal firing in the hippocampus in vivo (theta rhythm and sharp waves, described in Chapter 1) and in vitro (epileptiform population bursts and synchronized synaptic potentials, described in Chapter 3 and later in this chapter) tends to aggregate into (more or less) discrete "events" or waves. Thus, synchronization of population activity may represent a basic signaling mechanism. Furthermore, because unitary Schaffer-collateral EPSPs are small, synchronized firing within CA3 must occur for CA3 cells to influence firing of CA1 cells or to induce long-term potentiation of Schaffer-collateral synapses. We may note that synchronized rhythmical neuronal activity, at least during certain behavioral states, is characteristic of many parts of the brain (cortex, thalamus, inferior olive, and so on), so that the mechanisms that regulate synchrony are likely to be of general neurobiological significance. Of course, the relevant mechanisms need not be identical in every brain region.

Some general comments on synchronization

There are two reasons that a population of neurons might fire together: in response to an afferent input that is itself already synchronized; as a result of forces that couple the behaviors of the neurons together. For a synchronized burst in an isolated population of neurons, especially a burst in which the triggering stimulus excites only a small number of neurons, synchrony throughout the population can arise only because of cellular interactions.

Let us consider further how the interactions between cells might work. Suppose the "force" between any pair of neurons were weak, but that both neurons were oscillating spontaneously with periods not too different from each other. Then, it is conceivable that the neurons could eventually entrain one another so that the population would end up bursting in synchrony. Something like that appears to occur in the sinoatrial node of the heart, where the cardiac cells are coupled to neighboring cells via gap junctions (Delmar, Jalife, and Michaels, 1986; Jalife, 1984). But weak coupling between spontaneous oscillators seems unable to explain how a localized stimulus (such as stimulating one cell with a microelectrode, as described earlier, or locally injecting hypertonic KCl, as did Wong and Traub, 1983) could end up exciting the entire population. Another difficulty with the weak-coupling notion is this: Population bursts are not strictly periodic, and yet synchrony is "tight"; for example, cells may fire 50 ms out of every 10 s, or 0.5% of the time. This suggests that "strong" forces are required for synchronization (in the presence of picrotoxin).

In this chapter we shall restrict ourselves to interactions on a time scale of a few hundred milliseconds. This is done for reasons of conceptual simplicity. In the next chapter we shall consider time scales of many seconds. Again, for the moment and for the sake of simplicity, we assume that the population of cells begins at rest, whereas in the next chapter the population will be subject to a variety of influences that will permit more complex ongoing behaviors to occur.

Our main tool for this chapter will be computer simulations, but the problems themselves all derive from experimental observations. Our theoretical results have, in many cases, been checked experimentally.

Two-cell and three-cell circuits

Certain structural features of our 9,900-cell network model were described in Chapter 5. Before proceeding to population behavior in this large system, however, we need to consider some aspects of the behavior of small circuits: two or three cells, without loops or cycles. These small circuits provide the building blocks for understanding the behavior of large networks.

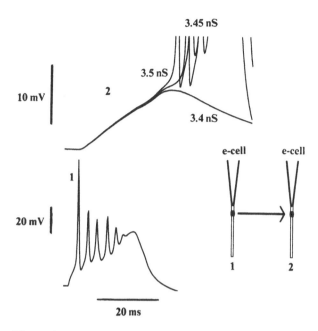

Figure 6.1. Burst transmission fails in all-or-none fashion as c_e (excitatory conductance parameter) is decreased. Two connected pyramidal cells were simulated (lower right) while the strength of the connection between them was varied. (Without the rest of the network, there is no opportunity for disynaptic inhibition or other polysynaptic interactions.) Cell 1 was induced to burst with a brief current. As c_e was varied over a narrow range, cell 2 responded with either a broad EPSP or a burst.

Burst transmission depends on the strength of the excitatory connections.
In Figure 6.1 we illustrate how the influence of one e cell (cell 1) on another (resting) e cell (cell 2) is critically dependent on c_e, the excitatory-conductance parameter. When c_e is above about 3.45 nS, a burst in cell 1 elicits a burst in cell 2. Experimentally (see Chapter 3), when two CA3 pyramidal cells are monosynaptically connected, a burst in the first cell elicits a burst in the second cell about half the time. The experimental situation, however, is more complicated than this simulation, for several reasons. In an experiment, the second cell will be subject to ongoing background synaptic inputs. If the second cell has just fired, it will be refractory and unlikely to fire again. In addition, real synaptic transmission is quantal, with significant variations in unitary EPSPs, whereas in the model synaptic transmission is not quantal. Finally, single presynaptic action potentials may on rare occasions elicit postsynaptic action potentials in experiments. This does not happen in the model when the postsynaptic cell is at rest.

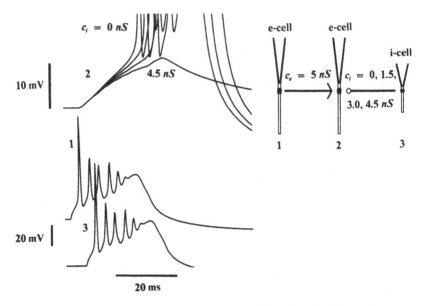

Figure 6.2. An IPSP can prevent propagation of bursting, but it must be strong enough. A three-cell network (upper right) was simulated, with cell 2 receiving an input from an e cell (cell 1, c_e = 5 nS) and an i_1 cell (cell 3, c_i taking on different values). Cell 3, the i cell, begins firing a bit later than cell 1 (bottom). With c_i = 4.5 nS, cell 2 does not burst. With progressively smaller values of c_i, cell 2 responds to cell 1 with a burst of progressively shorter latency.

Burst transmission depends on the strength of inhibition. In Figure 6.2 we illustrate how changes in the efficacy of inhibition affect propagation of bursting. The "target" cell (cell 2) is excited by a burst in a pyramidal cell (cell 1) and is inhibited by an i_1 cell (cell 3) that begins firing after cell 1 (lower left). Repeated simulations were done with different unitary inhibitory synaptic conductance (c_i, upper left). Note that cell 2 generates a burst when $c_i \leq 3$ nS; c_i also affects the latency of burst transmission. In our simulations of "normal" population behaviors, we use c_i of 5–12 nS (i.e., large enough to prevent burst propagation under these conditions). In experiments, unitary IPSP conductances range from about 1 to 10 nS (see Chapter 3).

Burst transmission depends on the timing of inhibition. Figure 6.3 shows that the timing of inhibition relative to a series of EPSPs can also be crucial for determining whether or not bursting propagates. In each simulation in this figure, c_i = 10 nS; what is varied is the onset of bursting in the i_1 cell (lower left). If the IPSP develops in cell 2 too late, cell 2 will already be "committed" to bursting.

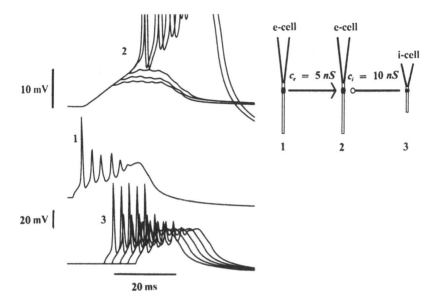

Figure 6.3. The relative timing of excitatory and inhibitory inputs also helps determine whether or not burst propagation will occur. We simulated the same three-cell network as in Figure 6.2, but with c_i = 10 nS. Cell 3, the i cell, was made to fire at various times after cell 1 (lower left). If inhibition begins too late after excitation, cell 2 generates a burst. (Note that the duration of the IPSP produced by cell 3 is rather long; see Figure 5.1, part A.)

Inhibition may not block burst propagation completely when excitatory synapses are powerful. Finally, Figure 6.4 shows that burst propagation can occur in the presence of inhibition if the effectiveness of the recurrent excitatory synapses is sufficiently high. In this case, c_i is held constant, as is the relative time of e-cell firing versus i-cell firing; rather, what is varied is c_e (upper left).

With these basic ideas from small circuits in mind, we are now ready to consider examples of behaviors that involve the entire neuronal population.

Synchronized population bursts (epileptiform bursts) with Cl⁻ IPSPs blocked: a chain reaction. A number of treatments can induce fully synchronous bursting in hippocampal slices (Table 6.1). All cells discharge simultaneously in response to stimuli or spontaneously in rhythmic fashion. In addition, animals may be injected with toxins or may be kindled (McNamara et al., 1984) to produce an epileptic syndrome, and slices from such animals can then be studied in vitro (Table 6.1). One such treatment is the blockade of $GABA_A$ synapses with penicillin,

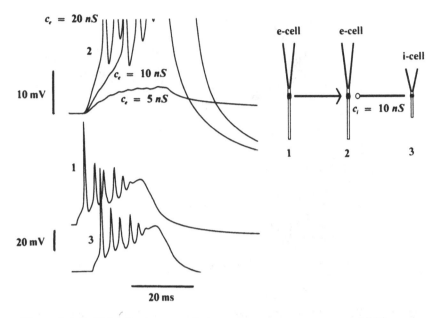

Figure 6.4. Sufficiently strong excitatory synapses can overcome inhibition. Same three-cell network as before, with $c_i = 10$ nS, and c_e varied.

bicuculline, or picrotoxin.[1] This reduces a system with three major classes of synaptic interactions (EPSPs, Cl⁻ IPSPs, and K⁺ IPSPs) to a system with only two classes of synaptic interactions.[2] We shall begin our analysis with penicillin and picrotoxin bursts; some of the other epilepsy paradigms will be considered later.

During a synchronous population burst, all of the pyramidal cells (and all of the interneurons as well) fire (Figures 3.11, 3.12, 3.13, and 6.5). Single events typically last 50–100 ms. Afterdischarges may also occur (see later in this chapter), to give a more complex event lasting a few hundred milliseconds. Events occur spontaneously with periods of 2–12 s. Synchrony of neuronal discharge can be demonstrated by the appearance of a large extracellular field potential. All intracellularly recorded cells fire in phase with the field.

Conceptually, we have two problems. First, how is a spontaneous population burst initiated? This is a difficult problem, because there is reason to think that the triggering event involves a small number of cells, and these cells might be difficult to locate within a large population. The particular cells involved may also have some distinctive properties, such as a tendency to burst spontaneously, or an especially large number of synaptic output connections. The second problem is to identify the mechanisms that come into play to synchronize the population.

Table 6.1. *Some methods of inducing synchronized epileptiform bursts in vitro*

Method	Mechanism	Acute/ chronic[a]	References (selected)
Penicillin	GABA$_A$ blockade	A	Schwartzkroin and Prince (1978)
Bicuculline	GABA$_A$ blockade	A	Wong and Traub (1983)
Picrotoxin	GABA$_A$ blockade	A	Miles and Wong (1983)
High $[K^+]_o$	Multiple	A	Rutecki, Lebeda, and Johnston (1985); Korn et al. (1987)
Low $[Mg^{2+}]_o$	Increased excitability, unblocking NMDA receptors	A	Mody, Lambert, and Heinemann (1987); Neuman, Cherubini, and Ben-Ari (1989)
4-AP	Multiple	A	Rutecki, Lebeda, and Johnston (1987); Ives and Jefferys (1990); Chesnut and Swann (1988)
Kainic acid	Decreased synaptic potentials, cell loss, & possibly rewiring	A, C	Westbrook and Lothman (1983); Fisher and Alger (1984); Franck and Schwartzkroin (1985)
Tetanization	Enhanced excitability (?), decreased inhibition	A	Miles and Wong (1987b)
Tetanus toxin	Decreased inhibition	C	Jefferys and Williams (1987); Calabresi et al. (1989)
Cholera toxin	Unknown	C	Jefferys and Williams (1989)
Kindling[b]	Unknown	C	McIntyre and Wong (1986)

[a]"Chronic" means here that a treatment is given to live animals, and slices are examined for epileptiform activity weeks later.
[b]Experiments done on pyriform cortex, not hippocampus.

Fortunately, population bursts can be elicited artificially, as, for example, with a localized extracellular current pulse, or even (sometimes) by stimulating a single cell (see Chapter 3) (Miles and Wong, 1983; Smith et al., 1988). We shall concentrate first, then, on stimulated population bursts.

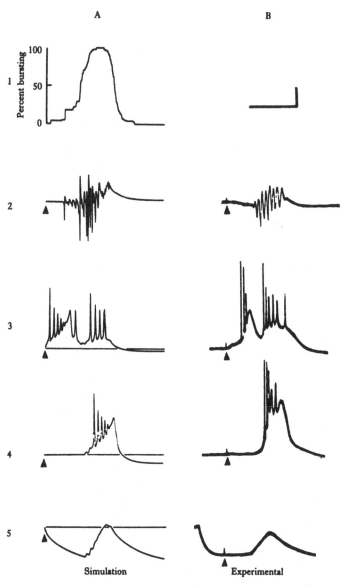

Figure 6.5. Synchronization via excitatory synapses. Simulation was of a 100-cell network, each cell connected to an average of 5 other cells, with synapses powerful enough to allow burst transmission. Four model neurons were excited to burst at the onset of the simulation. Experimental records were from the CA2 region of a transverse hippocampal slice, with a shock given to the fimbria (time marked by triangle), in order to evoke a synchronized event. A1: Rapid buildup of firing in the model as activity spreads across excitatory synapses. Cell firing ceases because of intrinsic AHPs. Row 2: Simulated and

What forces might be involved in synchronizing hippocampal neurons? There are at least four possibilities. First, and most important, we have synaptic interactions (MacVicar and Dudek, 1980a; Miles and Wong, 1986). These recurrent synapses are known to be powerful, in the sense that a burst in one pyramidal cell can, with probability about $\frac{1}{2}$, evoke a burst in a monosynaptically connected pyramidal cell (see Chapter 3). However, a number of other mechanisms may assist the synaptically mediated neuronal synchronization. Under pathological conditions wherein chemical synapses are blocked, these other mechanisms may lead to synchronization by themselves. Thus, high $[K^+]_o$ could excite all the cells; increases in $[K^+]_o$ are almost certainly involved in the triggering of, and perhaps in the spread of, so-called field bursts that occur in media that block synaptic transmission (Konnerth et al., 1984) (see Chapter 8); but it is difficult to explain how a mass effect of this sort would couple particular neurons to particular other neurons. Next, dual intracellular recordings show that there is electrotonic coupling between neurons (MacVicar and Dudek, 1981). However, dye-coupling experiments (MacVicar and Dudek, 1980b; Andrew et al., 1982) suggest that any one cell could be coupled to at most a few other cells. Thus, it should not be possible with electrotonic junctions alone to synchronize thousands of cells by exciting only one or a few cells. Finally, there are field effects, that is, coupling between neuronal activities mediated by extracellular currents (Jefferys and Haas, 1982; Taylor and Dudek, 1982) (see Chapter 8). Again, because the extracellular potentials produced by the firing of a single cell are known to be less than 1 mV, the effect any one cell can have on any other cell is small. We would expect, then, that field effects will have an entraining action when neurons are already firing and/or are excitable (i.e., are like the "weak" coupling forces mentioned earlier), and both experimental data and simulations are consistent with this view, as reviewed by Dudek, Snow, and Taylor (1986) and Dudek and Traub (1989) (see Chapter 8). It turns out that field effects do play a role in picrotoxin bursts, but they are not the "prime movers," as discussed later.

We suggest that chemically operated excitatory synapses between

caption to Figure 6.5. (cont.) recorded field potentials. (Field interactions do not take place in this model, so the field estimate is much noisier than the experiment; see Chapter 8.) Row 3: Cells that begin firing early may burst a second time, because of excitatory synaptic input during the peak of activity. Row 4: Most cells begin firing after a long latency, corresponding to the initial stages of spread of activity. Row 5: The responses of the cells of row 4 when they are held hyperpolarized. Large EPSPs are revealed; see Wong and Traub (1983) and Johnston and Brown (1981). Calibrations: 50 ms (simulation), 60 ms (experiment); 4 mV (A2 and B2), 25 mV (A3, A4, A5), 20 mV (B3, B4, B5). (From Traub and Wong, 1982, with permission; copyright AAAS.)

CA3 neurons are essential for synchronized bursts in picrotoxin. First, if synaptic transmission is blocked under conditions that still allow individual cells to burst, then synchronized activity disappears. This can be done by altering the ionic composition of the medium (Wong and Traub, 1983) or by using γ-glutamylglycine, a nonspecific blocker of excitatory amino acid transmission (Miles et al., 1984). Second, there is evidence of a powerful excitatory synaptic input during a synchronized burst. This evidence can be seen using a voltage clamp, which suggests an underlying conductance of as much as 180 nS (Johnston and Brown, 1981, 1984), or simply by means of extreme hyperpolarization of a cell so as to prevent engagement of regenerative currents (i.e., I_{Na} and I_{Ca}) (Figure 6.5).

A puzzle. Even if we assume that synaptic interactions are critical for picrotoxin synchronization, what is the origin of the 50–100-ms interval that may elapse between a localized stimulus and the resulting population burst? It was this question, posed by Robert K. S. Wong, that first led us to formulate the model shown in Figure 6.5 (Traub and Wong, 1982). We assumed that each of 100 pyramidal cells contacted, on average, 5 others chosen randomly (because it was known that the density of recurrent connections was low). The network was "statistically isotropic"; that is, the connectivity looked, on average, from any point the same as at any other point. This was done because experimentally a stimulus to any part of CA3 was capable of eliciting a synchronized burst. The connectivity was also "globally random," as seems likely for a relatively small local population of neurons (say fewer than 500–1,000), but not for much larger populations. However, including locality of connections does not alter the fundamental ideas, as discussed later. There were no inhibitory neurons. It seemed unnecessary to include i cells whose postsynaptic actions were mediated by $GABA_A$ receptors, because such actions were blocked pharmacologically. Those i cells whose postsynaptic actions were mediated by $GABA_B$ were omitted for the sake of simplicity, but were included in a later, more complicated model without affecting the basic principles, as discussed later. Finally, we assumed that excitatory synapses were powerful enough for a burst in one cell to cause bursting in synaptic follower cells. This was not known to be the case at the time, but this property of recurrent excitatory synapses has been carefully documented since.

As seen in Figure 6.5, this model accounts for the experimental data quite well. In both experiment and simulation, a synchronized event was triggered by a local stimulus (triangles, stimulus to four cells in the case of the model). The latent period between stimulus and population burst is evident in lines 1, 2, and 4. It corresponds to the initial stages of buildup of activity, during which most cells either receive no input or receive an input that is subthreshold. This is what would be expected in a chain reaction that has several stages of growth. The large excitatory synaptic input that occurs during a synchronized event is revealed by hyperpolarizing a selected cell (line 5: the same cell was hyperpolarized as shown in line 4). A cell that happens to burst during the earliest portions of a synchronized event may be reexcited to develop a second burst (line 3); in simulations, however, we have never observed three or more bursts in sequence under these conditions, even with a large neuronal population (9,000 pyramidal cells). That is, the simulated population does not oscillate unless new effects are introduced (Traub et al., 1984), either in the intrinsic properties of the cells or in the synaptic interactions.

To analyze the buildup process more carefully, we observe that if discharge begins with firing in one cell, then naively one would expect the buildup to occur in discrete steps: first the cells directly (monosynaptically) excited by the initiating cell, then the cells disynaptically excited, and so on. One can estimate the sizes of the monosynaptic, disynaptic, and subsequent populations as follows. Suppose we have N randomly connected neurons with connection probability p, and $q = 1 - p$. Define $s(k)$ to be the expected number of cells whose shortest path length from a fixed initiating cell is k. Define $r(k) = \Sigma_{i=1}^{k} s(k)$; $r(k)$ is the expected number of cells that have a path from the initiating cell of length $\leq k$. It is easy to see that $s(k + 1) = [N - r(k)] \times [1 - q^{s(k)}]$. To consider a particular example, suppose $N = 1,000$ and $p = .01$. Then we can calculate the following table:

k	$s(k)$	$r(k)$
0	1	1
1	10	11
2	95	106
3	550	656
4	343	999
5	1	1,000

The reasons that the buildup is not quite this simple are these: (i) Consider two cells each of which is connected to the initiating cell by at least one path of length 3, but each having no shorter paths. The first cell may have two such 3-paths, and the second cell may have only one. The first cell will then tend to fire earlier because of stronger excitatory drive, so that rigid relative timing will not be maintained. (ii) Because a burst lasts a relatively long time, the existence of long paths can modify the appearance of a burst once it is initiated by activity propagating along the shortest path(s). Thus, in the foregoing example, the first cell may have four paths of length 4, and the second cell may have six paths of length 4. (iii) Slow inhibition, as discussed later, may build up with different time courses in different cells.

The epileptiform field potential. Note in Figure 6.5 that the experimental field potential has an underlying slow positivity on which are superimposed relatively smooth notches. The simulated field potential is a crude approximation formed by taking a weighted sum of transmembrane currents; in this formulation, field effects between neurons do not take place. As a result, the simulated field potential is not smoothly notched the way the experimental field potential is (see Chapter 8).

Some network implications of epileptiform bursting. Because every pyramidal cell participates in a synchronized discharge, it follows that every pyramidal cell receives a number of recurrent excitatory inputs. It may be true anatomically that every CA3 cell has outputs that excite other CA3 cells in the slice (Ishizuka et al., 1990). We estimate physiologically that at least one CA3 cell out of three must have recurrent excitatory connections, because stimulation of this fraction of CA3 cells can evoke a population discharge (Miles and Wong, 1983). The remaining cells may have had axonal branches cut during the slicing procedure, or their recurrent connections may be weaker, or even absent. This remains an important open question; a relevant experiment would be to stimulate single cells in vivo, where all the connections should be viable. In a random network of 9,000 cells where each cell has an average of 20 outputs (such as we generally use), stimulation of any cell should excite the whole population, provided inhibition is sufficiently reduced. Thus, in particular, every cell lies on a cycle or loop in the network, indeed, on a large number of cycles. We do not know if this is true in the slice or in vivo. There are other statistical quantities that we would find interesting: (i) How many synaptic steps, on average, does it take to get from one CA3 pyramidal cell to another? (ii) What are the variances of the number of connections made by each cell, of the number of inputs per cell, and of unitary EPSP size? If we could approximate the connectivity of the CA3 region with a random graph, we might be able to apply some of the mathematical theory of such objects (Erdös and Rényi, 1960). This theory provides an estimate of the probability, as a function of the number of edges, that a graph with some large number of nodes will have certain properties (e.g., that the graph will contain a cycle of length k). (The theory of Erdös and Rényi, however, deals with nondirected graphs, whereas the connections between neurons are directed.)

Another interesting detail concerns the time required for firing to spread from cell to cell. At the beginning of a synchronized event, any cell that is being excited probably will be receiving input from a single cell. Presynaptic-to-postsynaptic transmission should then require 10–20 ms. Cells that begin to be excited later are more likely to have several synaptic precursors firing, and the latency from EPSP onset to the onset of firing will be correspondingly short. This explains why the onset of bursting appears so abrupt in Figure 6.5. The closer a cell is synaptically to the initiating cell(s), the more likely it is to receive a barrage of EPSPs preceding its burst. (These EPSPs will also be influenced by the presence of small degrees of synaptic inhibition and by cellular excitability, as discussed later.)

If this model is correct, one ought to be able to predict the minimum size for a cellular network in which stimulating a single cell will lead to bursting in the entire population. Experimentally, using CA3 wedges of different sizes bathed in picrotoxin, we have estimated that a minimum of about 1,000 cells is required (Miles et al., 1984). In order to make a proper comparison with experiment, it is essential to know something about the spatial distribution of the synaptic connections, so as to imitate properly the operation of cutting pieces of tissue. Modeling CA3 as a purely random network does not permit analysis of this question. We shall return to this issue after our discussion of propagating epileptic events, because it is those experiments that help to define the spatial structure of the excitatory synaptic connections.[3]

In summary, we can characterize CA3 as a "sparsely connected" network of rather "strong" excitatory connections. "Sparsely connected" means that the probability of a monosynaptic connection between a randomly chosen pair of cells is small (a few percent, see Chapter 3). But with "strong" connections that allow bursting to spread when inhibition is blocked, the "functional" connectivity is very high, because, in general, there are polysynaptic paths from any cell to any other cell. It is these paths that allow synchronized population bursts to occur when inhibition is blocked.

The principles underlying synchronization do not change when the model is scaled up in size or when slow IPSPs are included. Figure 6.6 illustrates the response of our 9,900-cell model when Cl^--dependent inhibition is blocked ($c_i = 0$) and a single cell is stimulated to burst ($c_e = 5$ nS). The same type of explosive buildup of activity occurs as illustrated in Figure 6.5. Single pyramidal cells receive a very large synaptic input, as occurs experimentally (Johnston and Brown, 1981). The important physiological idea here is this: Assuming that i_2 cells (the ones mediating slow IPSPs) are indeed recruited by recurrent excitatory synapses, the buildup of excitatory activity is capable of "outrunning" the development of slow IPSPs that might otherwise prevent or limit synchronization (bottom trace in Figure 6.6). In neuronal networks, timing can be

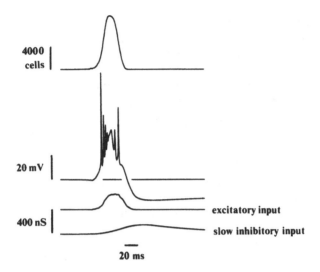

4000 cells

20 mV

400 nS

excitatory input

slow inhibitory input

20 ms

Figure 6.6. The basic principles of synchronization are not altered by using a larger model or by adding delayed inhibition (i_2 cells). This simulation was done in the full 9,900-cell model, with $GABA_A$ synapses blocked ($c_i = 0$). The stimulus was to one cell. The upper trace is the number of cells firing. Note that delayed inhibition develops after synchronization is fully developed. With the latency of burst propagation slowed by residual inhibition, or by weak excitatory synapses, delayed IPSPs might conceivably play a role in limiting synchronization (see Figure 6.7).

everything, and equilibrium conductances do not provide all the answers. However, it seems probable that delays in the spread of bursting between pyramidal cells might allow slow IPSPs to limit or even prevent the development of a synchronized burst (Figure 6.7).

The growth of synchrony depends critically on the strength of excitatory synapses. We ran a number of simulations in the 9,900-cell model, stimulating a single cell each time, with $c_i = 0$, and using a different value of c_e for each simulation (Figure 6.7). It is hardly surprising that a critical value of c_e was needed for population synchronization to occur, because with c_e below the threshold for burst propagation, stimulation of a single cell will have no effect on the population (Figure 6.1). We would expect, on the basis of Figure 6.1, that the population could become fully synchronized with $c_e \geq 3.45$ nS; yet Figure 6.7 shows that c_e must be about 4 nS for full synchronization to occur. Why the discrepancy? Figure 6.1 shows that the latency of burst propagation varies with c_e when c_e is near threshold for propagation. If burst propagation occurs too slowly (inset in Figure 6.7), slow inhibition builds up and limits the extent of synchronization. This idea was confirmed by blocking slow IPSPs as well as fast

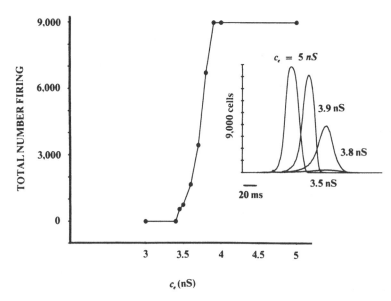

Figure 6.7. The extent of synchronization in the disinhibited model network is regulated by the strength of the excitatory synapses. The inflection is sharp and reflects two factors: (i) the ability of bursting to propagate from cell to cell at all (we know from Figure 6.1 that c_e must be above about 3.45 nS for burst propagation to occur); (ii) bursting must propagate fast enough to "outrun" delayed inhibition. This latter effect explains why the inflection in this curve does not begin until 3.5 nS and why it does not have a perfectly sharp corner. Note that increasing c_e shortens the population latency, as expected (inset). The stimulus was to one cell. What is plotted is the total number of e cells that fire at all, not the total number that fire at any one time.

IPSPs in the model. In that case, with c_e = 3.45 nS, stimulation of a single cell did initiate a synchronous population burst.[4]

Propagating synchronous firing and the local structure of synaptic connectivity

We shall now consider the propagation of synchronized firing in a distributed network. The reader will recall from Chapter 5 that we use a locally random connectivity in the 9,900-cell model. We were driven to choose a local connectivity by studies on the mechanisms of propagation of synchrony in large longitudinal slices of the CA3 region (10 mm in length). Under different conditions of inhibitory blockade, stimuli were applied, and responses at different distances were examined (Miles et al., 1988). We showed that synaptic responses to a fixed extracellular stimulus have two separable components, R_1 and R_2, each with its own special properties. For example, R_1 propagates at about 0.5 m/s, and its amplitude is reduced with distance from the stimulus, until no response can be detected at 2.5–4.5 mm from the stimulus (see Figure 3.7). The amplitude of R_1 is not affected by cellular excitability. It appears that R_1 is a monosynaptic population EPSP; it declines with distance from the stimulus because axons of passage do not all run the entire length of the slice. The progressive decline in R_1 with distance can be explained if the axonal terminations of any particular cell fall off (in a statistical sense) with distance from the soma. The "space constant" of this falloff is about 1 mm. Other explanations are logically consistent with the physiological data. For example, the termini from any particular cell might all be at a constant distance from that cell, but with a probability distribution on that distance, so that the connections from a group of cells would still fall off with increasing displacement. Such an explanation is inconsistent, however, with HRP injections of CA3 cell axons, which indicate that axons run for long distances (Tamamaki et al., 1984).

In contrast to R_1, R_2 propagates slowly (about 0.1–0.15 m/s). The expression of R_2 is dependent on the efficacy ·of both inhibitory and excitatory synapses. Thus, if Cl⁻ IPSPs are blocked in otherwise normal media, R_2 propagates along the entire slice without attenuation (Figure 6.8). In this case, R_2 behaves as the neuronal population analogue of a propagating action potential in an axon. There is a threshold stimulus required to elicit it, but once generated, it propagates at constant velocity and without decrement. If inhibition is only partially suppressed, then R_2 attenuates with distance and may disappear, and its propagation velocity also drops. Similar effects occur when inhibition is fully suppressed, and the efficacy of polysynaptic excitatory pathways is reduced by elevating divalent-cation concentrations to increase the neuronal firing threshold. R_2 evidently represents a polysynaptic population phenomenon, and indeed on a local scale it is the same phenomenon illustrated in Figure 6.5. (Note in Figure 6.8A that when two cells are recorded near to one another, they exhibit bursts that are synchronized with each other as well as with the population field potential.) On a larger spatial scale, activity is not precisely synchronized from place to place, because activity must traverse synapses along the way, given that connections are local.[5] Some time is needed for EPSPs to depolarize cells to firing threshold. This results in a slower velocity for the population wave (R_2) than for the axons themselves (R_1).

We constructed the locally random network model (described in Chapter 5) in order to demonstrate that the foregoing ideas were logically consistent. Thus, we incorporated an axon conduction velocity of 0.5 m/s and made the characteristic length for excitatory synaptic connections 0.6 mm. As Figure 6.9 demonstrates, synchronization in this model occurs locally, but the population wave propagates at 0.16 m/2. As expected, if the characteristic length of excitatory connections changes

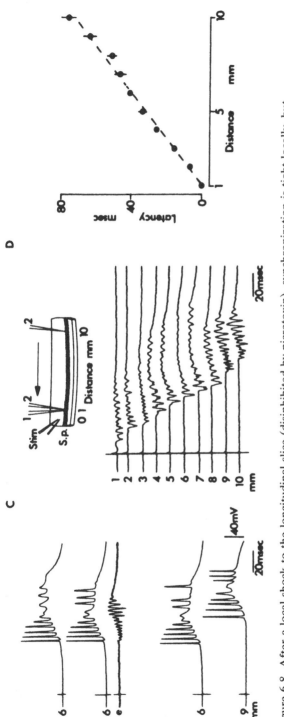

Figure 6.8. After a local shock to the longitudinal slice (disinhibited by picrotoxin), synchronization is tight locally, but there are phase lags on a spatial scale of millimeters. A shock was delivered to one end of the preparation. A: Dual intracellular recordings that are nearby (both 6 mm from the stimulus) show nearly simultaneous onset of firing, both in step with the local field potential (e). B: When the recorded cells are separated by 3 mm, the distal cell fires later than the proximal cell. C: Field potentials at different distances from the stimulus. D: From data such as in part C (repeated 12 times), one can estimate the conduction velocity of the wave of synchronized activity, 0.12 m/s in the present case. Recall that the conduction velocity of axons in this system is estimated to be about 0.5 m/s (Figure 3.7). (From Miles et al., 1988, with permission.)

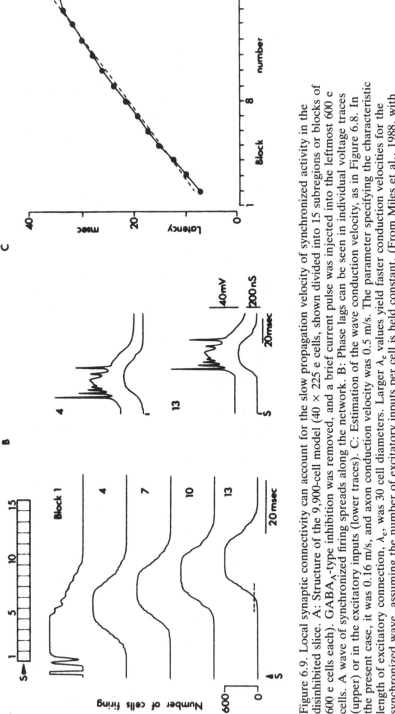

Figure 6.9. Local synaptic connectivity can account for the slow propagation velocity of synchronized activity in the disinhibited slice. A: Structure of the 9,900-cell model (40×225 e cells, shown divided into 15 subregions or blocks of 600 e cells each). GABA$_A$-type inhibition was removed, and a brief current pulse was injected into the leftmost 600 e cells. A wave of synchronized firing spreads along the network. B: Phase lags can be seen in individual voltage traces (upper) or in the excitatory inputs (lower traces). C: Estimation of the wave conduction velocity, as in Figure 6.8. In the present case, it was 0.16 m/s, and axon conduction velocity was 0.5 m/s. The parameter specifying the characteristic length of excitatory connection, λ_e, was 30 cell diameters. Larger λ_e values yield faster conduction velocities for the synchronized wave, assuming the number of excitatory inputs per cell is held constant. (From Miles et al., 1988, with permission.)

(something difficult to manipulate experimentally, but easy in the computer), so changes the velocity of R_2. When the connections are global, and enough cells are stimulated, the R_2 velocity becomes equal to the R_1 velocity; that is, synchrony spreads with the axonal conduction velocity (Miles et al., 1988).

In order to check the model, we made three types of manipulations. First, we examined the effects of focal block of inhibition in the center of the slice. That caused a localized synchrony, with complex, predominantly inhibitory synaptic potentials around the "focus" – the so-called inhibitory surround (discussed later in this chapter). Second, we showed that partial blockade of inhibition in the model produced attenuating population waves with propagation velocities slower than usual, consistent with experiment. Finally, we simulated the effects of a focal increase in firing threshold while inhibition was fully suppressed. Experimentally, GABA was applied locally in the presence of picrotoxin. Synchrony spread through the less excitable region, but after a pause longer than would be expected if the wave propagated through the block at constant velocity (Miles et al., 1988). We suggest that the pause results because only some of the connections cross the entire distance of the GABA-hyperpolarized region. Thus, the upstroke of the EPSP in the distal cells is slower than for cells proximal to the blocked region.

Thus, in summary, we believe that our 9,900-cell model is a reasonable representation of the longitudinal slice. We do not know, however, if excitatory synaptic connectivity is localized in the same fashion in vivo as it is in vitro. It is conceivable that the localization of connectivity is an artifact of the slicing procedure.[6]

The structure of the synaptic connections that we have postulated allows us now to examine synchronization in blocks of cells of varying sizes. To do this, we first constructed our usual 40×225 array. We then "cut away" the array except for a central block of cells, preserving the same connectivity within this block. With fast inhibition removed ($c_i = 0$), we stimulated a single cell and counted the total number of pyramidal cells that fired as a result (Figure 6.10). Note that there was little synchronization in blocks with fewer than 500 cells, whereas synchronization was virtually complete in a region with 1,400 cells. This result is in general agreement with experiment (Miles et al., 1984), and it also makes sense, at least qualitatively. Suppose that each pyramidal cell sent all of its 20 outputs to its immediate neighbors. Then, no matter how small the piece of tissue, stimulating one cell should recruit all the others. Consider now the opposite extreme, in which each pyramidal cell would excite no neurons that were less than 3 mm distant from it. Then, with a block 2.9 mm in length, all connections would be cut, and no cell could influence population activity. The real situation is somewhere between these two extreme "wiring" patterns. That is, most of the

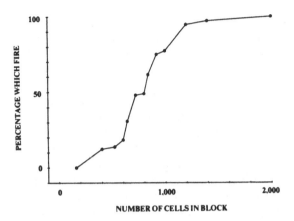

Figure 6.10. In a network with locally random connectivity, a critical size is necessary in order for synchronization to occur. Network parameters were as in Chapter 5 (specifically, λ_e = 30 cell diameters). A central block of cells, 40 × n in size (n varied), was retained, while all connections extending across the boundaries of the block were cut. GABA$_A$-type synapses were blocked (corresponding to picrotoxin application), and a single cell was stimulated to burst. We counted the total fraction of the e-cell population that fired as a result (ordinate). Somewhere between 1,000 and 2,000 cells are necessary for synchronization to occur with this connectivity. An experimental estimate from the transverse slice was 1,000 cells as the minimum necessary to support synchronization (Miles et al., 1984).

excitatory connections have a relatively short range, with an average displacement of perhaps 1 mm. It follows that there should be some critical size (which we expect would be less than 1 mm along the stratum pyramidale) below which at least most of the connections will have been cut. In such a piece, synchronization either will be impossible or will proceed so slowly that delayed IPSPs can terminate it.

Reducing cellular excitability may allow synchronization to occur only after stimulation of a threshold number of cells, generally more than one cell. One such case is illustrated in Figure 6.11. Here, we altered the intrinsic properties of the pyramidal cells so that they did not exhibit intrinsic bursting. We also used a value of excitatory synaptic strength c_e that, in combination with these modified intrinsic properties, did not permit transmission of burst firing at a monosynaptic connection. Instead, an average of about 2.5 presynaptic cells was needed to fire a train so as to elicit a train of action potentials in the postsynaptic cell. In this case, a threshold number of cells (about 80–100) must be stimulated before the population as a whole behaves in a regenerative fashion.

We can roughly estimate what the threshold number of cells ought to be as follows. Suppose that S cells are stimulated and that two inputs

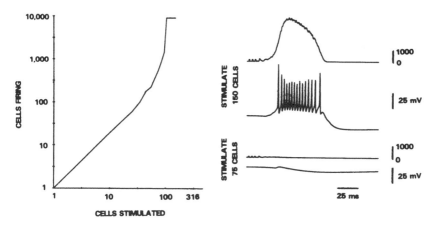

Figure 6.11. Synchronization in a population of 9,000 e cells that are not intrinsically bursting, wherein c_e is too small for firing to propagate from one cell to one other cell; a threshold number of cells ($\gg 1$) must be excited for synchronization to occur. Cells were made "repetitively firing" by reducing $\bar{g}_{Ca}$ fourfold and preventing inactivation of g_K. GABA$_A$-type synapses were blocked. A 2-nA, 10-ms depolarizing current was injected into various numbers of e cells (abscissa), and the number of e cells firing as a result was counted (ordinate, note log-log plot). This stimulus would cause, in one cell, a train of three action potentials; with the value of c_e used here (5 nS), such a train would evoke in a single connected neuron only an EPSP, not firing. In this case, 100 or more cells must be stimulated for regenerative activity to occur in the population. Right: The upper trace in each case is the number of cells firing, and the lower trace is the membrane potential of a particular neuron. Note subthreshold synaptic potentials only with stimulus to 75 cells (below), whereas there is a sustained burst after 150 cells are stimulated (above). This concept may be relevant to epileptiform activity in the cortex, which is difficult to evoke by stimulating a single cell, even with inhibition blocked.

must fire to drive a given cell to discharge. Let p be the connection probability for excitatory connections ($p = 20/9{,}000$), and let $q = 1 - p$. Define n to be the total number of e cells ($n = 9{,}000$), and ignore the locality of the connections. Finally, suppose T to be number of cells with two or more inputs among the S stimulated cells. The condition for growth of the response to stimulating S cells is $T > S$. But T is about ($n - S)(1 - q^S - Sq^{S-1}p)$. The smallest value of S for which $T > S$ with these parameters is 51. Similarly, if a cell requires three synaptic precursors to fire, then T is about $(n - S)[1 - q^S - Sq^{S-1}p - \binom{S}{2}q^{S-2}p^2]$. For T to be larger in this case requires that S be about 330 cells. We therefore expect the threshold number of cells to be between 51 and 330, as is the case.

This general situation may correspond, at least roughly, to the neocortical slice. Recurrent excitatory connections exist between pyramidal cells in neocortex (Mason et al., 1989), although not necessarily in the same pattern as in the hippocampus. The difference between resting potential and discharge threshold is significantly greater for neocortical than for CA3 pyramidal cells. Furthermore, stimulation of a single neocortical cell does not lead to a population discharge when inhibition is blocked (B. W. Connors, personal communication), although stimulation of a small group of cells and/or afferent fibers with an extracellular electrode can cause a population discharge (Connors, 1984; Gutnick, Connors, and Prince, 1982).

High $[K^+]_o$ alters the intrinsic properties of CA3 pyramidal cells so that single neurons do not fire in bursts, and it also induces synchronous firing (Chamberlin et al., 1990). This medium may increase cellular excitability, synaptic transmission, and the occurrence of spontaneous EPSPs in such a way as to compensate for the altered intrinsic properties (Traub and Dingledine, 1990). We shall return to this form of epileptiform activity in the next chapter.

Synchrony in CA1. Initial experiments, using penicillin, suggested that the isolated CA1 region could not generate synchronized bursts, but that the isolated CA3 region could (Schwartzkroin and Prince, 1978). The ability of the isolated CA3 region to produce synchronized activity has been repeatedly confirmed (Miles et al., 1984). Hablitz (1984), however, has observed synchronized bursts and even afterdischarges in the isolated CA1 region. The lesser tendency of CA1 to produce synchronized activity vis-à-vis CA3 could involve differences in cellular properties or synaptic organization or both. In general, CA1 cells, particularly CA1b cells, are less likely than CA3 cells to fire a burst after somatic stimulation (Masukawa et al., 1982). Instead, they tend to respond with one or two action potentials. Nevertheless, there are bursting neurons in CA1a and CA1c, and there are excitatory connections between CA1 pyramidal cells, although they seem to be less common than in CA3, or less effective, or both (Christian and Dudek, 1988b; Knowles and Schwartzkroin, 1981a). It seems likely, therefore, that both intrinsic and network properties contribute to the lesser ability of CA1 to generate a synchronized burst.[7] However, CA1 can readily respond to a synchronized discharge in CA3 with a synchronized discharge of its own (Wong and Traub, 1983), provided that inhibition is blocked in CA1 as well as in CA3 (Mesher and Schwartzkroin, 1980). Apparently, feedforward (possibly in combination with CA1 recurrent IPSPs) can prevent propagation of synchrony from one region to another (Dingledine, Roth, and King, 1987; Wong et al., 1979).

Partial synchronization in the presence of inhibition

Inhibition need not be completely suppressed for some degree of synchrony to occur. Synchronized bursting with inhibition blocked represents an extreme form of collective behavior, analogous to a chain reaction. Our view is that much of the normal activity of the CA3 region can be interpreted as a series of partially synchronized events. This view is suggested by the occurrence of theta rhythm and physiological sharp waves in vivo (Chapter 2) and synchronized synaptic potentials in vitro (Chapter 7). These behaviors seem to correspond to simultaneous firing in limited subsets of the cells in a larger neuronal population. Partially synchronized events will be modulated by the properties and history of the inhibitory neurons and synapses, as well as by the intrinsic refractoriness of the pyramidal cells. We shall explore how inhibition sculpts a partially synchronized event and, in the next chapter, how refractoriness from one event influences the cells that participate in the next event.

Two additional factors must be considered when $GABA_A$-mediated inhibition is functional. Without inhibition, one needs to visualize a large network with (for the most part) only one type of intercellular interaction. With inhibition, one needs to visualize what are really three interconnected networks (Figures 5.4, 5.5, and 5.6). Furthermore, the timing of signals in different pathways is important, and these times are influenced by neural integration properties at each step.

Motivation for studying synchrony when inhibition is not (completely) blocked. Several experimental results have motivated our studies on synchrony in the presence of synaptic inhibition. First, there have been several experimental epilepsy models in which inhibition has not been completely blocked, including models that feature the use of 4-AP and high $[K^+]_o$ (Table 6.1). In the presence of 4-AP, unitary IPSPs may even be augmented rather than reduced (Buckle and Haas, 1982; Rutecki et al., 1987). It is clearly necessary to develop theoretical tools in order to help understand such experiments. Second, it must be of functional importance that inhibition regulates the influence one cell may have on an entire population. Again, we need theoretical tools. Third, we know that inhibition in the hippocampus is labile and may be modulated by numerous factors. $GABA_A$-mediated inhibition is relatively suppressed by the following treatments: repetitive stimulation (Ben-Ari, Krnjevic, and Reinhardt, 1980; McCarren and Alger, 1985; Miles and Wong, 1987b; Thompson and Gähwiler, 1989a–c; Wong and Watkins, 1982), perhaps mediated in part by GABA-induced suppression of GABA release (Deisz and Prince, 1989); increases in extracellular K^+ concentration (Korn et al., 1987; Thompson and Gähwiler, 1989b); excitatory amino acids (Stelzer, Slater, and ten Bruggencate, 1987; Stelzer and Wong, 1989); intracellular metabolic factors activated by an elevation of intracellular calcium (Chen et al., 1990; Stelzer et al., 1988); peptide transmitters, such as neuropeptide Y (Colmers et al., 1987) and enkephalin (Masukawa and Prince, 1982). Some of these mechanisms, of course, may overlap.[8] We must therefore ask how hippocampal circuitry behaves as the "effectiveness" of synaptic inhibition is varied. From a clinical point of view also, synchrony in the presence of inhibition must be important. Inhibition may never be totally suppressed under physiological conditions, and the number of GABAergic terminals may even increase in hippocampal sclerosis lesions (Babb et al., 1989); yet interictal spikes and seizures, too, occur in patients.

An experimental example of inhibition controlling the effect one cell can exert on another. Figure 6.12 illustrates the effects on pyramidal cell 2 of stimulating pyramidal cell 1 at various times after adding picrotoxin. At first, there is no discernible effect. Then a slow, presumably polysynaptic EPSP occurs. Next (with probability less than 1), a second broad EPSP occurs at longer latency than the first. The second EPSP grows in size. Finally, there is an abrupt "switch," and stimulation of the first cell causes a population burst, which is reflected as a second burst in cell 1, a burst in cell 2, and an extracellular field potential. We suggest that as inhibition progressively fails, more polysynaptic paths become functional, until they all or almost all "open up."

Figure 6.13 illustrates a series of simulations in the 9,900-cell model that correspond to the experiment of Figure 6.12. Cell 4407 received disynaptic excitation from the initiating cell. The sequence of effects in cell 4407 as inhibition was blocked was remarkably similar to the experimental sequence, with the exception that the initiating cell could exert some influence on cell 4407 at any level of inhibition. (This may be an artifact of the situation in which the model always starts under perfectly resting conditions.) Furthermore, the model also showed a discontinuity in behavior between $c_i = 2.5$ nS and $c_i = 0$ (Cl^- conductance blocked totally). The relation between inhibitory synaptic strength and population activity is highly nonlinear. We can use the computer to reconstruct all of the functional paths between the initiating cell and cell 4407. This reconstruction shows that the first EPSP is caused by bursting in a particular intercalated cell (excited by the initiating cell and presynaptic to 4407). The second EPSP is caused by bursts in two cells presynaptic to 4407; in neither case is the path from the initiating cell to 4407 disynaptic, however. At intermediate levels of inhibition, the paths followed by activity as it spreads between cells begin to vary. This variability reflects details of the particular pathways between the initiating cell and the observed cell. Thus, with a relatively small total number of cells firing, and with such cells firing at different times, each cell will "see" a different temporal pattern of inputs. (Of course, if too few cells are firing, most cells will receive no excitatory input at all; and if all of the cells are firing together, then any cell will receive a large excitatory input. It is the intermediate regimes that are most complicated.) Details

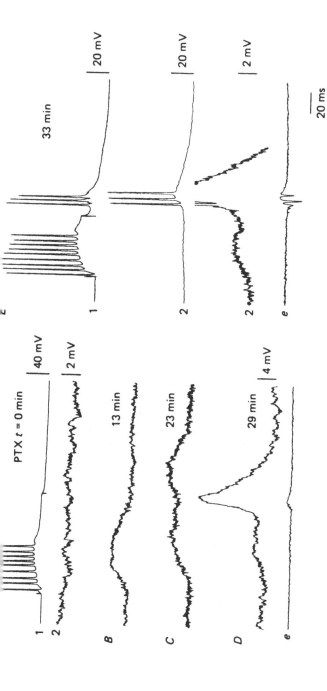

Figure 6.12. How inhibition can regulate the influence one particular pyramidal cell (cell 1) exerts on another particular pyramidal cell (cell 2). Experimental recordings were obtained from an isolated CA3 segment as picrotoxin (PTX) was washed in, progressively blocking GABA$_A$-type inhibition. Under resting conditions (A), a burst in cell 1 does nothing to cell 2. With progressive blockade of inhibition, cell 1 produces the following effects in cell 2: a broad EPSP of brief latency (B); intermittently, a pair of EPSPs, one separated from the other can be seen (C); the second EPSP becomes large, concurrent with some degree of population synchronization evident from the field potential (e) (D); the second EPSP is replaced by a burst of action potentials, concurrent with population synchrony (E). The latter is indicated by a second burst in cell 1 (cf. Figure 6.5), as well as a larger field potential. (From Miles and Wong, 1987a, with permission.)

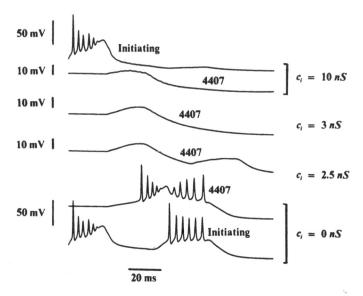

Figure 6.13. A similar sequence of effects of inhibition on polysynaptic circuits is seen in the model (cf. Figure 6.12). An "initiating cell" (112) is stimulated to burst, at different levels of c_i, the $GABA_A$ unitary conductance. We
illustrate the response in e cell 4407, which is disynaptically removed from
cell 112. Because the model begins "at rest" (i.e., no cells are hyperpolarized
from previous firing or IPSPs), disynaptic transmission is faithful in the
model, and an EPSP is seen even with c_i = 10 nS (unlike part A of experimental Figure 6.12). This disynaptic EPSP becomes a bit larger at c_i = 3 nS,
during which a total of 823 of the 9,000 cells fire. The EPSP is caused by a
burst in a single one of the e cells presynaptic to cell 4407 and postsynaptic to
cell 112. When c_i = 2.5 nS, a second EPSP appears. The first EPSP is caused
by a burst in one precursor to cell 4407, and the second EPSP is caused by
almost simultaneous bursts in two precursors. A total of 1,277 e cells fire
when c_i = 2.5 nS. Finally, with $GABA_A$ inhibition completely blocked (c_i =
0), all e cells burst; note the second burst in the initiating cell. (A second
discrete EPSP at intermediate levels of inhibition is not seen in all neurons in
the model. Sometimes there are complex excitatory–inhibitory mixtures at
intermediate levels of inhibition. Even experimentally, the late EPSP is seen
less than one-third of the time.)

such as these would be most interesting (although difficult) to observe
experimentally. Experimentally, responses of an individual cell do vary
at different levels of inhibition, but this variability could represent
quantal fluctuations in synaptic transmission, as well as variability in the
membrane potentials of intercalated neurons.

The current delivered to the initiating cell in Figure 6.13 can be
viewed as a special sort of afferent input that evokes a direct or primary
response, in this case a burst in one cell. The primary response, in turn,
elicits, through recurrent connections, a complex indirect, or secondary,

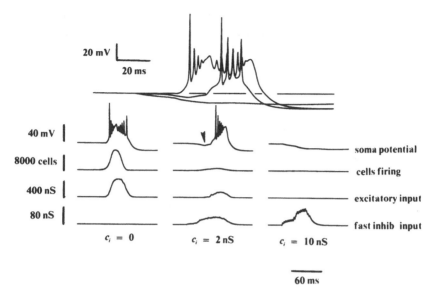

Figure 6.14. Population response after bursting in a single neuron at three levels of $GABA_A$ synaptic strength ($c_i = 0, 2, 10$ nS). The three voltage records are shown superimposed at the top. The response with inhibition blocked (left) is as previously described. With partial blockade of inhibition (center), a graded population response is seen. Note the leading hyperpolarization in the illustrated cell (arrowhead), a phenomenon seen in the "intermediate region" of the inhibitory surround (Dichter and Spencer, 1969a,b) (cf. Figures 6.18 and 6.19), as well as the delayed latency (top). Only about 25% of the e cells fire under these conditions. With "full-strength" inhibition, an IPSP is seen. The delayed component of this IPSP is, to some extent, an artifact of the resting state of the network (no cells hyperpolarized by previous firing or IPSPs); in this case, there is more firing than would occur under physiological conditions, and a number of i cells are recruited.

response. Figures 6.13 and 6.14 illustrate how changing inhibition can affect the secondary response. The next chapter will show how the secondary response also depends on the state of the network.

On the concept of inhibitory "holes" in the network. With the present connection parameters, an interesting form of propagation occurs in the presence of strong inhibition. Activity will spread sometimes to certain immediate descendants of an active cell at any level of inhibition. This odd behavior results because each pyramidal cell excites (in the model) only a few inhibitory cells. Suppose that cell 1 excites a single inhibitory cell, called I. The outputs of I, in general, will not include all of the outputs of cell 1. So a pyramidal cell monosynaptically excites some cells in which it does not evoke disynaptic inhibition. Sometimes this is also observed experimentally. Activity must then spread from cell 1 to these cells no matter how powerful the inhibitory synapses. We describe this by saying that "holes" exist in the model inhibitory system (see also Figure 5.6), and we wonder if such holes also exist experimentally. Recordings from monosynaptically connected pyramidal cells (as in Figure 3.8) suggest that such holes may in fact exist.

Another aspect of the system that makes straightforward analysis difficult is that inhibition does not control the spread of excitation in an all-or-none way. For example, an inhibitory input to cell 1 might block propagation caused by bursting in one of the cells presynaptic to cell 1, but cell 1 might nevertheless burst if more than one of its precursors burst simultaneously. This effect is important in the initiation of population bursts in cells that are only weakly excitable, even in the absence of inhibition (Figure 6.11).

Because timing is so crucial in neuronal network dynamics, the analysis must extend beyond the geometric factors considered in many, but not all (Schulman and Seiden, 1982), so-called percolation problems (see Chapter 9). Simulations remain essential, therefore, because a simulation so readily incorporates time. In simulations we can also reconstruct the entire history of a partially synchronized event. This is something we long to be able to do experimentally.

Another sequence of effects of one simulated cell on another cell as inhibition drops. Figure 6.14 shows another sequence of changes in the actions of one pyramidal cell on another as inhibition was suppressed. At first (c_i = 10 nS), stimulation of the "initiating cell" evoked disynaptic and polysynaptic IPSPs in the "target" cell. When c_i was reduced to 2 nS, a large summed polysynaptic event was apparent in cell 2, although its amplitude was smaller and latency longer than when Cl $^-$ IPSPs were completely blocked. The response was first an IPSP, then a burst, and then a second hyperpolarization. Both overlapping inhibitory and excitatory inputs (with the inhibition leading in time) and intrinsic conductances of the postsynaptic cell contribute to this complex response. The response resembles very closely events recorded in cells near to an epileptic focus, in particular the intermediate zone of the inhibitory surround of Dichter and Spencer (1969a,b), as discussed later in this chapter. Rutecki et al. (1985) illustrate a cell in high $[K^+]_o$ that exhibits a similar sequence of potentials. In high $[K^+]_o$, inhibition is reduced, but not blocked completely, although other effects may also become important (see Chapter 7).

Prepotentials before synchronized bursts. In general, when the spread of activity between excitatory cells is slowed, by residual synaptic inhibition for instance, prolonged barrages of excitatory synaptic events precede a synchronous burst in many cells. An example of this is shown in

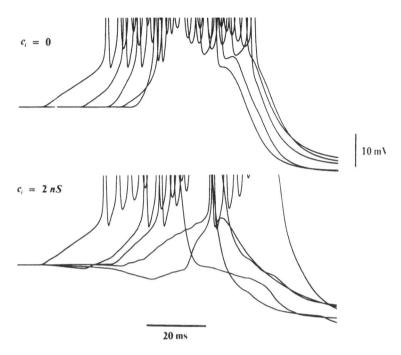

$c_i = 0$

$c_i = 2\,nS$

10 m\

20 ms

Figure 6.15. Different cellular prepotentials (simulations) during synchronized bursts with inhibition blocked completely (above) or partially (below). Note generally longer ramps below, with an occasional hyperpolarizing prepotential. This behavior may be relevant to the inhibitory surround, as well as to epilepsy models where some degree of inhibition is present [e.g., cholera toxin (Jefferys, 1990)].

Figure 6.15. Should this phenomenon prove to be of general validity, it may be useful in dissecting mechanisms of synchronization in other models of epilepsy besides GABA$_A$ blockade.

Critical behavior of the network as inhibition is blocked. Figure 6.12 suggests that a striking discontinuity in cell–cell interactions occurs as inhibition is weakened. Figure 6.16 shows a similar sharp transition in the number of cells that fire in response to activity in a single neuron. This figure was constructed by repeatedly stimulating a single cell using different values of c_i. The resulting graph may be divided into four regimes: (i) when c_i is large enough (say about 5 nS), a small baseline degree of synchrony occurs that is independent of c_i. This effect results from the existence of inhibitory holes in the network, so that baseline synchrony reflects a peculiarity of the topological structure of the network. Between 2 and 4–5 nS, small changes in c_i can produce significant effects on the number of cells firing. The response likely will not be called epileptiform,

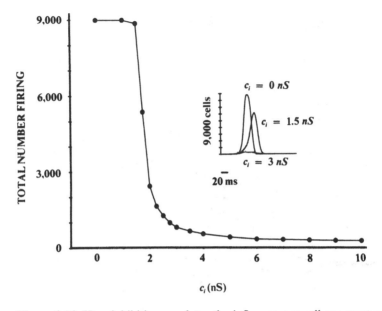

Figure 6.16. How inhibition regulates the influence one cell can exert on a large neuronal population. One pyramidal cell was excited using different values of the unitary $GABA_A$ conductance (c_i), and the total number of e cells firing was counted (ordinate). When $GABA_A$ synapses are sufficiently effective, varying c_i has little effect. Between 4 and 2 nS, small changes in c_i produce major changes in the population response. Below about 2 nS, there is an abrupt transition, so that stimulation of a single cell is able to excite the entire population. Inset shows sample simulations (number of cells firing as a function of time). Note that c_i affects the latency as well as the amplitude of the response. An interesting question arises: Is the brain itself able to regulate the effectiveness of recurrent inhibition within a local population? How is it accomplished?

however, because it is prolonged and involves only a fraction of the population (see, e.g., the 3-nS curve in the inset). Between 2 and 1.5 nS, there is a sudden switch to an epileptiform response of the population. Finally, below 1.5 nS, there is little change in the number of cells firing, although the peak and latency do change further (see the inset).

Interestingly, the three-cell network model of Figure 6.2 predicts that an inflection should occur at a c_i value of about 3 nS, when firing is just transmitted from cell 1 to cell 2. The graph of population firing, however, shows that the actual influence occurs at about 2 nS. Once again, this reflects the combination of slow propagation of bursting at $c_i = 3$ nS (inset) and the action of delayed IPSPs that suppress the spread of excitation.[9] Such a functional role for delayed K^+-mediated IPSPs in limiting the development synchrony when Cl^--mediated IPSPs are partially blocked remains to be demonstrated experimentally.

Although Figure 6.16 is useful in providing physical intuition, how are we to relate it to the physiology? In order to simplify the situation, we started the population in a perfectly resting state. We also arbitrarily chose a particular cell to stimulate. In real life, some cells will be refractory because of recent activity. The normal "drive" to the CA3 region in vivo presumably never consists of a stimulus to precisely one CA3 pyramidal cell, but rather of more or less coherent activities of granule cells, combined with perforant-path inputs, feedforward stimuli onto inhibitory cells (Frotscher, 1985, 1989), and so on. Because of the importance of Figure 6.16, we repeated this set of simulations under conditions of spontaneous activity (see Chapter 7).

Can strengthening excitation cause synchrony in the presence of inhibition? Figure 6.4 suggests that population synchrony might occur in the presence of inhibition, given sufficiently powerful excitatory synapses. We see in Figure 6.17 that this is partly true, but the size of the population response to stimulation of a single cell is graded. That is, up to $c_e =$

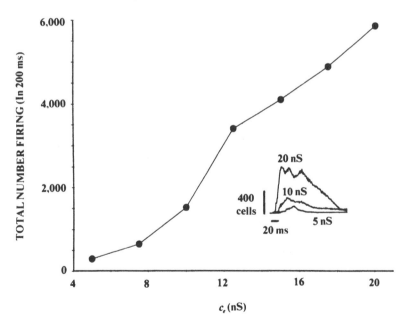

Figure 6.17. Sufficiently strong excitatory synapses (i.e., large c_e) allow a single cell to excite most of the neuronal population, even in the presence of inhibition ($c_i = 10$ nS). A single cell was excited, and the total number of e cells firing as a result was counted (ordinate). The effect of increasing c_e on the population response was relatively smooth (unlike the effect of decreasing c_i, see Figure 6.16). Inset shows sample simulations (number of cells firing versus time).

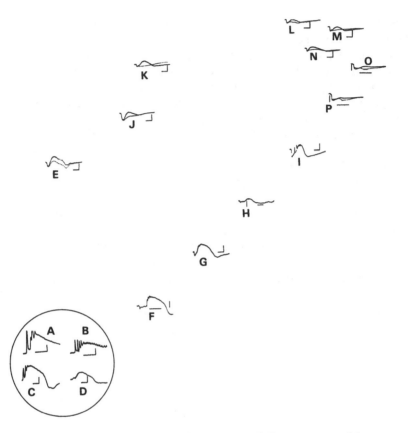

Figure 6.18. In vivo epileptic inhibitory surround. Data rearranged from Dichter and Spencer (1969a), with permission. Penicillin was applied locally to the exposed cat hippocampus. The center of the focus is indicated by the circle, and records are located in the figure according to the locations of the respective recordings. The dashed lines, where present, represent transmembrane potential (intracellular minus extracellular potential). Note large depolarizations within the focus (usually with superimposed firing), inhibitory-excitatory-inhibitory sequences around the focus (e.g., G and H), and predominantly inhibitory potentials at a distance from the focus (e.g., O). Calibrations are 50 ms and 10 mV.

20 nS, we still have not recruited the entire population. Of additional interest is that this curve is relatively smooth; that is, it lacks the sharp inflection evident in Figure 6.16. What is involved is not an all-or-none ability of bursting to propagate, but rather a competition between opposing forces in different cells. One would expect a similar type of behavior if, instead of increasing c_e, one were to enhance the excitability of the cells; we have not checked this in detail, however. This type of mechanism could be relevant in physiological sharp waves or in interictal

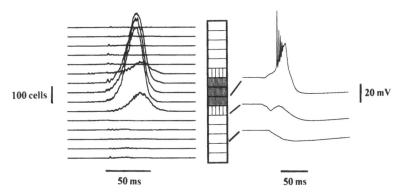

Figure 6.19. Simulation of the inhibitory surround in the longitudinal-slice model. At the center is a schematic of 9,900-cell model. Unitary IPSP strengths were distributed as follows: $c_i = 0$ in the central, darkly hatched region; $c_i = 12$ nS in the open region; c_i is linearly interpolated between 0 and 12 nS in the lightly hatched regions. On the left are shown the numbers of cells firing versus time in each of the 15 "blocks" or subregions of the model. On the right are selected membrane potentials: bursting in the "focus," an inhibitory-excitatory-inhibitory sequence in the near surround, and a prolonged hyperpolarization in the farther surround (cf. Figure 6.18). Similar potentials are seen when picrotoxin is applied locally to the center of a longitudinal slice (not shown).

spikes in epileptic patients. In both of these cases, synchronization is partial (Buzsáki, 1986; Wyler et al., 1982) (see Chapter 1).

The inhibitory surround. When in vivo inhibition is blocked in a region that is restricted but still large enough to support synchrony, rather complicated effects are seen in cells around the disinhibited area (Dichter and Spencer, 1969a,b; Prince and Wilder, 1967) (Figure 6.18). Near to the focus, cells tend to exhibit a hyperpolarization-depolarization-hyperpolarization sequence, possibly with firing during the depolarization (similar to what can occur with partially reduced inhibition, Figure 6.14). Cells farther from the focus usually show a prolonged hyperpolarization. Similar effects are seen when picrotoxin is applied locally to the center of a longitudinal CA3 slice. We originally explained the inhibitory surround by postulating a larger radius for inhibitory axonal arborizations than for excitatory axonal arborizations (Traub, 1983); this no longer seems tenable, however. At first sight, an inhibitory surround might seem likely if inhibitory axons had a larger average spread than excitatory axons. However, the available morphological data suggest, and our simulations use, a larger radius for excitatory axons than for inhibitory axons. The "trick" seems to be that excitatory axons also excite inhibitory cells and that this disynaptic e → i → e pathway is both stronger and faster than the disynaptic e → e → e pathway. The simulation in the 9,900-cell model of Figure 6.19 illustrates that this idea is plausible. Recall that in our model, long-range connections from firing pyramidal cells travel to inhibitory cells as well as to other pyramidal cells and exert a potent and rapid effect on such i cells, which in turn will each produce IPSPs in an average of 200 pyramidal cells near them. In addition, at least in the model, there is some very low level of e-cell firing in all regions (left of Figure 6.19), and this firing will recruit further inhibitory cells. Why, in the intermediate zone, is there a leading IPSP? The answer is that most of the depolarizing component represents a polysynaptic EPSP. Because of the relatively long delay in pyramidal-cell → pyramidal-cell recruitment, compared with pyramidal-cell → inhibitory-cell recruitment (Chapter 3), the IPSP tends, on average, to come first.

Afterdischarges in the presence of picrotoxin

In most of this chapter, we have discussed single synchronized bursts. That is, most cells fire a discrete burst at about the same time; only an occasional cell discharges in a double burst (Figure 6.5). Here, we summarize briefly some results on a more complex type of activity often seen in the presence of picrotoxin or other $GABA_A$-blocking agents. We call this activity "afterdischarges," although that term has been used in the epilepsy discipline to mean many different things. Important questions about the mechanism of picrotoxin afterdischarges remain unanswered.

Basic phenomenology of afterdischarges. In an individual cell, an afterdischarge appears as a prolonged (up to 200 ms or more) primary burst, followed by a depolarizing tail with briefer superimposed secondary bursts, generally fewer than about 10 (Figure 6.20, part A) (Hablitz, 1984; Miles et al., 1984). Secondary bursts occur with interburst intervals of about 60 ms. During the primary burst, the soma may be so depolarized that action-potential generation will appear to be blocked, although we presume the axon to be firing repetitively and at high frequency. Slow action potentials, presumably Ca^{2+}-mediated, usually underlie each secondary burst. The depolarizing tail during the period of secondary bursts may reflect an NMDA-activated current; such currents can last hundreds of milliseconds (Forsythe and Westbrook, 1988). The last secondary burst is followed by a prolonged AHP.

Synchrony of afterdischarges. Simultaneous records from cell pairs show that both the primary and secondary bursts are synchronized throughout the population, and the secondary bursts can generate a local field potential.

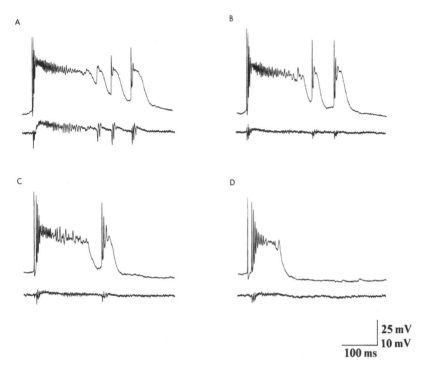

Figure 6.20. Afterdischarges in picrotoxin. Synchronized activity in the presence of picrotoxin (e.g., 0.1 mM) often consists of a series of bursts: a prolonged initial or primary burst, and a series of briefer secondary bursts. Both primary and secondary bursts are synchronized. As excitatory synapses are progressively blocked with γ-D-glutamylglycine (A → D), secondary bursts drop out one by one, and the primary burst shortens. This prolonged synchronized activity may depend on activation of NMDA receptors, but the mechanisms that cause the oscillating secondary bursts and determine the frequency are not known (see text). Upper traces are intracellular field potentials, and lower traces local field potentials (R. Miles and R. K. S. Wong, unpublished data).

Population size required. Afterdischarges can be generated in small wedges of CA3 tissue containing as few as 1,000–2,000 cells (Miles et al., 1984). This seems to exclude long reverberating synaptic loops as an essential requirement for their generation, as discussed later.

Elicitation by a small stimulus. As for single synchronized bursts, afterdischarges can also be elicited by stimulating a single cell in the disinhibited slice (see Figure 3.11).

Underlying synaptic input. We have repeatedly mentioned the large excitatory synaptic input that occurs during a synchronized burst. In analogous fashion, a large excitatory input occurs during the primary burst and during each secondary burst of an afterdischarge (Miles et al., 1984). Excitatory synapses appear to be necessary for the expression of afterdischarges, because nonspecific blockade of excitatory amino acid neurotransmission (with γ-D-glutamylglycine) leads to dropout of the secondary bursts, one by one (Figure 6.20). A medium high in $[Mg^{2+}]$ and low in $[Ca^{2+}]$ will have the same effect. Interestingly, afterdischarges in penicillin-treated slices from immature animals can last as long as 30 s (Swann and Brady, 1984), perhaps because there seem to be more recurrent excitatory connections in immature animals than in mature ones (Smith et al., 1988). On the other hand, extracellular K^+ accumulation has also been suggested to play a role in these prolonged events (Swann, Smith, and Brady, 1986b).

Spontaneous afterdischarges. Spontaneous afterdischarges occur in addition to evoked events. The spontaneous ones have interburst periods of several seconds. In the presence of picrotoxin, the primary burst and each secondary burst originate in or near CA2, and they each propagate toward the hilus at about the same velocity (average 0.13 m/s); the secondary bursts may die out before reaching the hilar end of CA3, whereas the primary burst usually propagates across all of CA3 (Knowles et al., 1987). In contrast, afterdischarges from rat hippocampal slices (the rats having been previously injected with tetanus toxin) originate toward the hilus (Jefferys, 1989).[10]

Considerations of the mechanism of afterdischarges. Our network model reproduces well single synchronized population bursts, but it does not generate, in the form described here, synchronized afterdischarges. This is true over a wide variation of the basic parameters. Why not? The model may be deficient in one or more of the following ways: (i) intrinsic cell properties; (ii) synaptic connectivity; (iii) the properties of intercellular communication (axons, presynaptic terminals, etc.); (iv) omission entirely of physiological effects that may be important. We shall discuss these in turn.

With respect to intrinsic properties, it is interesting that individual Purkinje cells (which are not interconnected by recurrent excitatory collaterals) can, in vitro, generate potentials that look rather like CA3 afterdischarges (Llinás and Sugimori, 1980a). In a Purkinje cell, a brief burst may be followed by a depolarizing plateau potential of duration 100 ms or more, followed in turn by a series of bursts. Each of the later bursts consists of a train of sodium spikes on a depolarizing wave, succeeded by an apparent calcium spike. This entire complex event probably is generated intrinsically by the Purkinje cell, without any apparent synaptic contribution. When potassium currents are suppressed, individual CA3 cells can also generate repetitive calcium spikes (Hablitz and Thalmann,

1987), as can CA1 neurons (Schwartzkroin and Prince, 1980a,b). Perhaps it is our single-cell model that is deficient in not being able to express such properties. A preliminary revised single-cell model that incorporates voltage-clamp kinetic data is able to generate repetitive dendritic calcium spikes (Traub et al., 1990). Another relevant experiment in cultured hippocampal neurons is this: If a cell is held depolarized, especially with potassium currents suppressed, 200-ms calcium spikes can occur; such an event could contribute to the primary burst (Segal and Barker, 1986); see also Figure 3 of Hablitz and Johnston (1981). On the other hand, Hablitz (1984) did not observe altered responsiveness of CA3 neurons to injected currents in the presence of picrotoxin. In particular, he did not see individual cells generate potentials that resembled afterdischarges unless the whole population was participating. Single cells do not discharge multiple calcium spikes in response to somatic intracellular stimuli, but only during synchronous events. However, potassium currents do not seem to be suppressed in the presence of picrotoxin (Hablitz, 1984).

With respect to connectivity, a series of cellular oscillations in a population suggests a reentrant loop. Such a loop could arise, for example, if most recurrent connections between CA3 cells were spatially restricted, but cells at one end of the slice selectively excited cells at the other end. We do not find this concept tenable, because it suggests the following result: Stimulation at the site of origin of the "bundle" should lead to the rapid appearance of synchronized bursting at the other end of the slice, However, experimentally, no difference seems to exist in the propagation velocities of bursts evoked from either end of a longitudinal slice. In transverse slices, synchronized bursts elicited at the CA4 end of the tissue do propagate somewhat faster than do bursts elicited at the CA2 end, but there is still no evidence of a jump from one region to another (Knowles et al., 1987). Timing is another problem with the reentrant-loop idea. As mentioned, synchronized afterdischarges can occur in small wedges of CA3 tissue that are only 1–2 mm along the stratum pyramidale. At 0.1 m/s, a synchronized burst should travel from one side of this wedge to the other in at most 20 ms; yet the period of the secondary bursts is more like 60 ms. A final problem with the reentrant idea is this: If there were a loop of activity, one ought to be able to find pairs of cells that would develop afterdischarges significantly out of phase with each other. We have not been able to find cell pairs with this property; dual intracellular recordings consistently reveal that the onsets of firing occur within 10 ms or so of each other.

With respect to intercellular communication, it is possible that excitatory synaptic interactions are phasically interrupted and that this leads to a population oscillation. Such interruption could result, for example, from desensitization of the glutamate receptor or inactivation of a channel coupled to it (Tang et al., 1989), or from block of conduction in the axons. Block of axonal conduction might result from an effect of increased $[K^+]_o$ (Poolos, Mauk, and Kocsis, 1987), or possibly from an extracellular field effect at points at which recurrent axons bend. This form of block has been demonstrated for climbing-fiber responses in turtle cerebellar Purkinje cells with an extracellular potential gradient artificially imposed (Chan, Hounsgaard, and Midtgaardt, 1989; Tranchina and Nicholson, 1986). We proposed a model (Traub et al., 1984) in which pyramidal-cell axons became refractory after a rapid train of action potentials. The recovery from that refractoriness was simulated with a time constant about half the period between secondary bursts. In spite of the fact that the axon blocking processes were all independent of one another, this model did generate synchronized afterdischarges. Furthermore, the afterdischarges were sensitive to the strength of excitatory synapses: In agreement with experiment, secondary bursts would drop out one by one as excitatory synapses were progressively blocked. Although extracellular K^+ provides a plausible mechanism for refractoriness in axons, it is not at all clear why this refractoriness should recover with a time constant in the tens of milliseconds. The model remains, therefore, tentative.

Our model does not include another effect that might phasically reduce population excitability. During the sustained primary burst, interneurons are maximally driven and are likely releasing GABA. Whereas $GABA_A$ effects presumably are blocked by picrotoxin, $GABA_B$ effects are not. In bullfrog spinal cord, presynaptic GABA receptors (of both A and B types) seem to exist and to be capable of mediating presynaptic inhibition (Peng and Frank, 1989a,b). This effect, were it to exist in the hippocampus, could also result in a phasic reduction of population excitability and possibly lead to population oscillations.

Afterdischarges thus pose a fascinating puzzle: Are new cellular or cooperative properties responsible, or both? Preliminary results favor the idea that cellular intrinsic properties, in combination with known excitatory synaptic circuits, are responsible (Traub et al., 1990). Afterdischarges are important to understand not just as an intellectual challenge. A brief series of secondary bursts represents a transitional behavior between an interictal spike (a single synchronized burst, which, in a patient, would not have behavioral concomitants) and a seizure. The cellular phenomenology of picrotoxin afterdischarges resembles that seen during certain experimental seizures in vivo, whether induced by penicillin (Matsumoto and Ajmone-Marsan, 1964b) or by electrical stimulation (Sawa, Nakamura, and Naito, 1968). We would guess that the mechanisms that generate afterdischarges in vitro might underlie certain human epileptic EEG phenomena, including polyspike and wave (an interictal EEG pattern seen in some generalized epilepsies), as well as paroxysmal fast EEG patterns that can be associated with brief tonic seizures (Brenner and Atkinson, 1982; Gastaut and Tassinari, 1975).

7 Collective behaviors of the CA3 network: spontaneous oscillations and synchronized synaptic potentials

Oscillatory synchronous neuronal population behaviors are generated in many parts of the mammalian brain. Such behaviors underlie rhythmical EEG waves in the cortex. Some other brain regions wherein repeating population events occur, with many of the cells firing synchronously, include the brain-stem respiratory pattern generator (Feldman and Ellenberger, 1988), various brain-stem nuclei during pontine-geniculo-occipital waves (PGO waves, an EEG correlate of REM sleep) (Steriade et al., 1989), the thalamus during spindle waves (Steriade and Llinás, 1988), and pools of motoneurons during swimming (Wallen et al., 1985) or during eye movements.

It is important to understand population oscillations, for several reasons. First, rhythmic population activities form the background "blackboard" on which afferent, associative, and motor activities must be written (Arieli and Grinvald, 1988; Eckhorn et al., 1988; Gray and Singer, 1989); see also the section on theta rhythm in Chapter 1. Understanding the initiation and synchronization of waves of activity in any one of these cases may shed light on underlying mechanisms in the others. Second, we would like to know the factors that determine the amplitude and period of the oscillation. Does each cell oscillate at the same frequency as the population? Can the frequency of the population behavior be inferred from the intrinsic properties of the cells (Llinás, 1988), or is population rhythmicity an emergent property that cannot be inferred from a single cell? What determines precisely which cells will fire during each population wave, and is there a recognizable structure in the sets of cells that fire during successive waves?

In this chapter we first consider repeating synchronized synaptic potentials, which are often observed in "resting" or slightly disinhibited slices. We must ask how these events emerge from a network organized as described in the preceding chapters. What is the relation between firing of cells in the population as a whole and synaptic potentials in individual cells? What factors determine the number of cells firing during a wave of activity, and what factors determine the intervals between waves? The issue of precisely which cells will fire during a particular wave of activity will turn out to be quite delicate. Because the waves of activity are repeating, is the population generating a behavior that is rhythmic (in a rigorous sense), or is the behavior actually chaotic? A second goal is to understand how spontaneous, fully synchronized population discharges are initiated. In Chapter 6 we studied synchronization itself, a stimulus playing the role of the initiator. Finally, we wish to determine if spontaneous oscillatory[1] activity in the slice might provide insight into the EEG *in vivo*.

Technical considerations

In Chapter 6 we confined ourselves to situations where the model network began in a resting state and was subjected to a localized stimulus. The resulting response, typically lasting a few hundred milliseconds at most, could be compared to corresponding experiments, although, of course, the experimental preparation is never truly at rest. We now consider the behavior of the network on longer time scales, seconds or tens of seconds, as it is spontaneously active. We need to have a way of producing spontaneous activity, and we hope that the collective behaviors that the network generates are not critically dependent on the details of how this spontaneous activity is generated. We shall consider two sources of underlying "drive" to the network: (i) The first source is steady depolarizing currents to the pyramidal cells, randomly distributed, so as to produce "spontaneous bursting" in some of the cells; these currents are intended to simulate slow inward currents that determine the specific resting potential of each cell. For low-amplitude population oscillations, we have the most experience with this form of stimulation of the network; (ii) The second source is excitatory synaptic noise, modeled as an independent Poisson process for each pyramidal cell. Sometimes the two methods are combined. We have also explored periodic inputs to random subsets of cells, but our experience is limited here.

Experimental background: synchronized synaptic potentials

It is remarkable that the CA3 region in vitro exhibits a strictly autonomous population behavior that is expressed in any pair of cells as repeating synchronized synaptic potentials (SSPs). SSPs can have excitatory or inhibitory components, or both. SSPs are larger than unitary synaptic potentials, indicating that they are induced by the (approximately) simultaneous firing of a group of cells. One cannot infer whether or not it is the same underlying group of cells that fires each time. We have not, however, found any individual cell that fires during each of a train of SSPs, suggesting that different groups of cells may elicit the individual SSPs. An example of SSPs was shown in Figure 3.13. In that case,

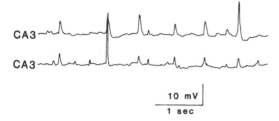

Figure 7.1. Synchronized synaptic potentials in a "resting" monkey hippocampal slice (dual intracellular recordings in CA3). The cells were held hyperpolarized. (From Schwartzkroin and Haglund, 1986, with permission.)

synchrony was not apparent until Cl^--dependent inhibition was partially blocked. As Cl-dependent IPSPs are blocked further and further, SSPs become larger (this effect is shown quantitatively in Figure 7.5), and the interval between them grows (Miles and Wong, 1987a; Schneiderman, Arnold, and Advani, 1989). We shall show that our model reproduces this phenomenon.

Repeating SSPs have been observed in several preparations and in other laboratories and probably represent a general phenomenon: (i) In biopsy samples of human lateral temporal neocortex, taken during neurosurgical procedures performed on epileptic patients, Schwartz-kroin and Knowles (1984) observed SSPs with periods typically about 0.5 s. (ii) Hippocampal slices taken from normal (i.e., not known to be epileptic) monkeys exhibited SSPs in the CA3 region, although not in the dentate gyrus (Schwartzkroin and Haglund, 1986). (iii) Schneider-man (1986) obtained indirect evidence suggesting the existence of SSPs. Using field-potential measurements in the apical dendritic layers of in vitro CA3, he recorded repeating small potential transients, with inter-vals again a few hundred milliseconds. These small fields were most likely to occur in the presence of penicillin concentrations too small to allow synchronization of the entire population; at larger concentrations wherein full population events did occur, the small fields might still be seen, particularly in the latter part of the interburst interval (an example of Schneiderman's recordings that illustrates these phenomena is shown in Figure 7.2). He interpreted the miniature field events to reflect synaptic currents elicited by the (more or less) synchronized firing of small groups of cells. In the resting slice, the field potential tended to be irregular, but it became regular with slight blockade of inhibition (Schneiderman et al., 1989); these authors then found the power spec-trum of the field potential to be broad, but not flat: There was a clear peak in the neighborhood of 2–3 Hz in the resting slice. There were also distinct peaks around 6 Hz in the presence of low-dose penicillin (0.085–0.17 mM). (iv) In *neocortical* slices that were partially disinhibited,

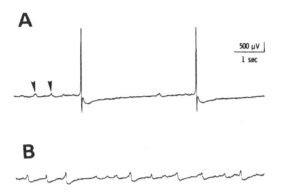

Figure 7.2. Field-potential records from the guinea pig CA3 region in the distal apical dendrites, obtained by Dr. J. H. Schneiderman. A: The slice was bathed in 1.7-mM penicillin. This caused synchronized bursts to occur, evident as field-potential transients >1.5 mV, with period about 2 s; in addition, small (<0.6-mV) field potentials occurred (arrowheads), with period about 0.5 s. B: The slice was bathed in 0.425-mM penicillin; only the "small" events occurred, with period about 0.5 s. These small events were believed to represent synchronized synaptic events in a subpopulation of the neurons. (From Traub et al., 1987c, with permission.)

Chagnac-Amitai and Connors (1989) observed what may be a limited version of this same phenomenon: A brief localized shock would sometimes elicit a 20–50-Hz train of up to seven SSPs.

It appears that in all preparations SSPs have the following features: (i) The morphology of the SSPs is complex and often consists of both depolarizing and hyperpolarizing components (Figures 5.12, 7.1, 7.3, and 7.4). This suggests that the subset of cells whose firing generates each SSP includes both pyramidal cells and inhibitory cells. (ii) pyramidal cells do not generally fire during any given SSP, so that pyramidal-cell firing tends to be at a much lower rate than the rate of the SSPs themselves (Figure 7.3); a few cells may fire in successive SSPs if the latter are not too closely spaced (upper trace in Figure 7.4A). (iii) Interneurons are much more likely than pyramidal cells to fire during an SSP (Schwartzkroin and Haglund, 1986) (see Figure 7.7), a phenomenon also noted during theta rhythm (Buzsáki et al., 1983). (iv) Schwartzkroin and Haglund (1986) found that synaptic potentials were tightly synchronized in nearby cells, but that in separated cell pairs a relatively constant time lag existed between the potentials. The interval between onset of the potentials tended to increase with intercellular separation. (v) The average amplitude ot SSPs becomes larger as inhibition is blocked, and so does the variance of the amplitude, at least until full-population synchronized bursts occur (Figure 7.5).[2]

The observation that firing in single pyramidal cells occurs at a slower

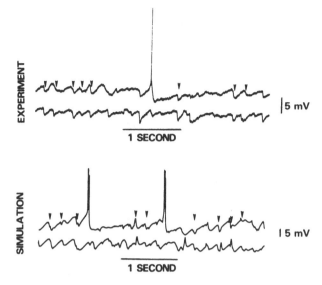

Figure 7.3. SSPs. Experiment: Dual intracellular recordings from two CA3 cells about 200 μ apart in a guinea pig hippocampal slice. Note the recurring SSPs, generally hyperpolarizing, and infrequent firing. Simulation: Soma potentials from two cells in the 9,900-cell model, with random distribution of bias currents (bias 0–1.2 nA, c_e = 5 nS, c_i = 10 nS). In our experience with slices, it is usually (but not always) necessary to reduce inhibition slightly (e.g., with low-dose picrotoxin or with tetanization) in order to "bring out" SSPs. (From Traub et al., 1989, with permission; copyright AAAS.)

frequency than the population rhythm is interesting because it is characteristic of theta waves in vivo (Alonso and Garcia-Austt, 1987b) (see Figure 1.5). Thus, during theta, a population rhythm continues at one frequency, while the individual cells fire at a lower frequency, and irregularly at that. Of course, during theta there is a periodic input into limbic structures from the septal nuclei that seems to impose the rhythm on the hippocampus, and irregular firing of pyramidal cells might simply reflect irregular inputs from other structures and have nothing to do with the rhythmic activity per se. But in the slice, there is no septal input. We therefore have an intriguing physical question: how to generate a population rhythm without rhythmicity in the principal neurons, where the population frequency is faster than the mean firing frequency that any of the cells exhibit. Note that the spontaneous bursting rate of individual CA3 neurons usually is at less than 1 Hz (Hablitz and Johnston, 1981). Although we have occasionally seen spontaneous bursting at about 3 Hz, population rhythmicity can occur as fast as about 4 Hz. Bursting at higher frequencies can be seen in individual cells when the slice is bathed in cholinergic drugs (Leung and Yim, 1988), but we do not routinely use

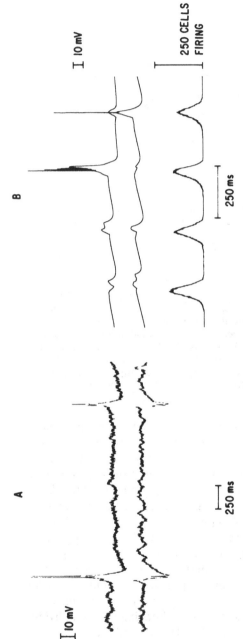

Figure 7.4. Rhythmic EPSPs and firing are more common after partial blockade of inhibition. A: Recurrent inhibitory pathways were partially suppressed by tetanic stimulation (50 Hz, 5 s × 2) (Miles and Wong, 1987b). Dual intracellular recordings in CA3. B: Simulation in the 9,900-cell model with same parameters as in Figure 7.3, but c_i reduced from 10 nS to 4 nS. Note the low-amplitude oscillations in the numbers of cells firing; it is this activity that directly and indirectly leads to the synaptic potentials. (From Traub et al., 1988, with permission; © 1988 IEEE.)

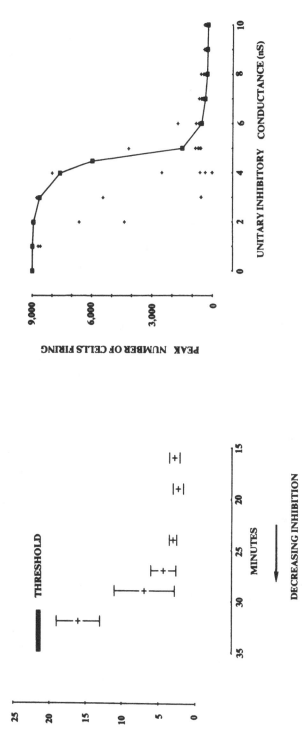

Figure 7.5. Inhibition regulates the amplitude of spontaneous as well as evoked synchronized events (cf. Figure 6.16). A: Amplitude of synchronized intracellular EPSPs as picrotoxin is washed into the slice (recordings from CA3). The bar marked "threshold" indicates the onset of synchronized population bursting. B: Simulations in the 9,900-cell model, 4 s of activity, with $c_e = 10$ nS and bias currents 0–0.3 nA. Note in each case that the variance of the amplitude is large at intermediate values of inhibition: With inhibition powerful, all events are small; with inhibition almost gone, all events are large; but in between there is indeterminacy. (Data in part A rearranged from Figure 10B of Miles and Wong, 1987a.)

such agents. Pacing by a single cell seems unlikely, because any one cell could contact only a very small fraction of the population and so could not induce widespread SSPs without first producing firing in other cells; rhythmic firing would then be apparent in those cells.

Approach to modeling population oscillations

These experimental data and our computer simulations suggest that the oscillatory activity is best visualized as a series of partially synchronized population bursts (Figure 7.6) (Traub et al., 1987c, 1989). There are several differences between these waves and the events described in Chapter 6. Each wave may be initiated by spontaneous bursts in a number of cells, not just one, and these initiating cells may be scattered throughout the array (or tissue).[3] The initiating cells need not discharge at precisely the same time, and bursts in single cells may occur at any time during a partially synchronized burst. Propagation, furthermore, will be limited not only by recurrent synaptic inhibition but also by long-duration AHPs in those pyramidal cells that have fired recently. Recall that the interevent period is hundreds of milliseconds, whereas the time constant for relaxation of $g_{K[Ca]}$ may be as long as 2 s (Numann et al., 1987). In some cases, also, a cell may be just about to fire spontaneously as its AHP decays, but then it receives an EPSP and fires during a partially synchronized burst. Then the AHP will be reset, and the next spontaneous burst will be deferred for hundreds of milliseconds or more. Because of the interplay of these factors, cells that in isolation might burst periodically will then not fire periodically because of the bombardment of EPSPs and IPSPs. Figure 7.6 shows that all individual cells discharge irregularly, despite the rhythmicity of population firing. We also took advantage of the model to isolate synaptically all of the cells in the simulation. The isolated cells fell into three categories: those that did not fire spontaneously at all, those that burst once only, and those that burst rhythmically. The shortest period for the rhythmically bursting cells was between 400 and 500 ms, and the average period of the population rhythm was only 210 ms (Traub et al., 1989).

These findings show that collective network behaviors need not be equivalent to behaviors exhibited by a so-called lumped system, wherein a small number of neuronal elements will each represent the average behavior of a larger ensemble of similar elements. We were able to demonstrate this directly by constructing a network that was equivalent to a lumped system. In this network, each of the three cell types (e cells, i_1 cells, and i_2 cells) had stereotyped properties, without any intercellular variability. In addition, the number of inputs for each cell (excitatory, fast inhibitory, and slow inhibitory) was kept precisely constant for each cell type. This network did not generate collective oscillations that re-

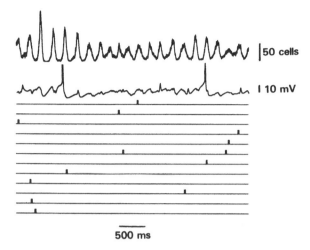

500 ms

Figure 7.6. In simulations with inhibition present, rhythmic behavior occurs in the population as a whole, but not in any one cell. Same simulations as in Figure 7.3. The upper trace shows oscillations in the number of e cells firing; note the small amplitude of the oscillations (there are 9,000 e cells in all). The middle trace is potential from a particular cell; it fires during a minority of the population waves (cf. Figure 1.5 for this kind of behavior in vivo). Below: "Unit activity" in 12 different neurons. Again note the apparent irregularity. (From Traub et al., 1989, with permission; copyright AAAS.)

sembled the data: All behavior was "all-or-none." By "breaking the symmetry," as, for example, by allowing dispersion of intrinsic cell properties and variability in the details of the connectivity (both of which are realistic assumptions), we constructed a class of networks that do exhibit behaviors similar to those seen experimentally. We shall now concentrate on the problem of how such model networks generate low-amplitude collective oscillations.

The occurrence of correlated synaptic events in randomly chosen pyramidal-cell pairs during partially synchronous population events results from the divergence of excitatory and inhibitory axons. Suppose, for example, that 2% of the 9,000 pyramidal cells (i.e., 180 cells) burst during an event. Each pyramidal cell excites, on average, 20 other pyramidal cells, so that about 3,600 cells receive EPSPs. The 180 cells also excite an average of 360 inhibitory cells (half generating "fast" and half "slow" IPSPs). Because of the wide divergence of inhibitory axons (one inhibitory cell contacting 200 pyramidal cells), all of the pyramidal cells will be more or less simultaneously inhibited. In conclusion, SSPs, at least those with an inhibitory component (and often those with an excitatory component as well), will appear throughout the population if subsets of a few hundred cells discharge at the appropriate intervals. The

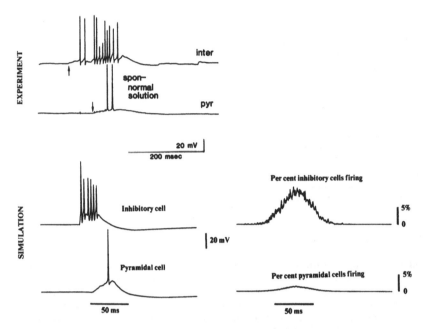

Figure 7.7. Simultaneous records from inhibitory and pyramidal cells during oscillatory activity. The experimental record is from a slice where cells were exhibiting spontaneous SSPs (data from Schwartzkroin and Haglund, 1986, with permission); the interneuron was identified by its firing pattern. The parameters in the simulation were $c_e = 5$ nS, $c_i = 8$ nS, and bias currents 0–0.3 nA. A larger fraction of inhibitory cells than pyramidal cells fire during any given event (right: data from simulation), and inhibitory-cell firing usually leads the pyramidal-cell firing. This gives the impression that inhibitory cells "drive" the rhythm, but, at least in the model, that is not so; the first few cells firing are always pyramidal cells. Such "ancestral" cells would be most difficult to locate experimentally.

subsets of discharging cells need to be the same for each event, and in the model they are not.

An intuitive explanation of the effects of inhibitory blockade is this: If "fast" IPSPs (i.e., Cl⁻-dependent IPSPs) are partly blocked, more pyramidal cells will burst during an event, increasing the number of cells receiving EPSPs; furthermore, each EPSP will on average be larger, because it will be generated by more bursting precursors. Although each pyramidal cell may also receive a larger number of unitary IPSPs, the individual IPSPs will be of reduced amplitude; hence, the synaptic events become more predominantly excitatory.

In Figure 7.7 we compare the behavior of an inhibitory cell with that of a pyramidal cell during these population oscillations; the experimental data are from Schwartzkroin and Haglund (1986). Usually, i-cell firing leads e-cell firing. Furthermore, i cells are more likely to fire than e cells, at least if we plot the data as fractions of the respective cell populations (lower right in Figure 7.7). This creates the impression that partially synchronized bursts results from activity in inhibitory cells and even are somehow initiated by the inhibitory cells (a phenomenon that appears to be possible, at least under special circumstances) (Aram and Wong, 1989). Nevertheless, at least in the model, every population wave is initiated by the pyramidal cells. The lower right part of Figure 7.7 is deceptive, because there are 10 times more pyramidal cells than inhibitory cells. Magnification of the lower trace shows the very first cell firing to be a pyramidal cell.

We can use the computer to study the initiation of a partially synchronized event in more detail. To identify the initiating cells in a simulation, we first define, by eyesight, the time of onset and termination of a partially synchronized event. This is easy unless the excitability of the pyramidal cells is very high. The computer keeps a record of all cells that fire and the times at which they fire. One then makes a raster plot of all the pyramidal cells that fire during an event (as in Figure 7.8). The computer also stores the synaptic connectivity. Superimposed on the raster plot, one can draw in "lines of causality," which join the dots representing firing in cell 1 to the dots representing firing in cell 2. A line is drawn if (i) cell 1 is monosynaptically connected to cell 2, (ii) cell 1 begins firing before cell 2, and possibly (iii) cell 2 begins firing within, say, 25 ms of the time cell 1 ceases firing. That is, a line is drawn if one reasonably believes that cell 1 contributed to the firing in cell 2. (These plots are quite complex and do not reproduce well.) Cells in the raster that fire, but have no lines of causality leading into them, are presumed to fire spontaneously, and thus to be initiating cells for the event. If there is any doubt, the whole simulation can be repeated, saving the membrane potential and the synaptic inputs of the presumed initiating cell(s). These lines of causality demonstrate that at the beginning of a synchronized event, propagation is "one-to-many" from the initiating cells, but at the end of the event, propagation is many-to-one, because of the buildup of inhibition. The longest synaptic path from initiating cell to firing cell, to another firing cell, and so on through the event, may be five synapses or more. Depending on the excitability of the pyramidal cells, that is, on the depolarizing bias currents, the number of initiating pyramidal cells for an event can range from only one to a hundred or more. There will be only one initiating cell if the excitability is just above threshold for population activity to occur at all.

The relatively few pyramidal cells that, in the model, initiate a synchronized event rapidly recruit inhibitory-cell firing: The latency for propagation of firing from pyramidal cells to inhibitory cells is much faster than the latency for propagation to other pyramidal cells; this is

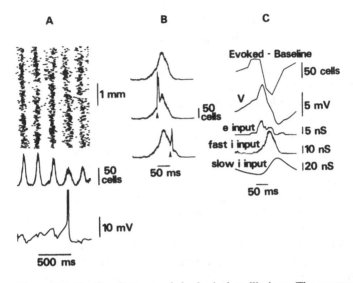

Figure 7.8. Further features of rhythmical oscillations. The parameters are c_e = 5 nS, c_i = 10 nS, and bias currents 0–1.2 nA. A: Raster plot of cells firing during spontaneous activity. This plot again indicates that different cells fire during each wave (as can be checked by identifying each cell in each wave); furthermore, the waves are coherent, in a statistical sense, along the entire length of the model (225 cells), as are sharp waves and theta waves in the hippocampus in vivo (see the data of G. Buzsáki in Chapter 1). The average behavior and a single-cell potential are plotted below the raster. B: The amplitude of an evoked response (stimulus was 2 nA for 10 ms to 600 cells) depends on the phase of the underlying oscillation. The top trace is a spontaneous wave. This simulation was repeated multiple times, with a stimulus given at different phases of the wave (arrowheads). C: The responses to the different stimuli are summarized in the upper plot ("Evoked − Baseline"). The reason for the phase variation in the response is apparent from the average behavior of 15 cells, shown below ("V" is average somatic membrane potential): The cells, on average, receive a wave of excitatory input, followed by and overlapping an inhibitory input.

true both in the model and experimentally (see Chapter 3). This mechanism also contributes to the apparent early predominance of inhibitory-cell firing.

The issue raised here is both important and delicate. Our understanding of the origin of spontaneous partially synchronized events depends on identifying the initiating cells and on studying the initial stages of propagation of firing from these cells. Although this is not difficult to do in a computer simulation, it seems most difficult to accomplish experimentally, and it will prove especially so if in the slice, as in the model, different cells initiate each partially synchronized event. For the moment, at least, we must rely on relatively indirect means of confirmation of our model.

Each synchronized event in Figure 7.8A can be divided conceptually into two portions. The firing of the initiating cells can be viewed as the primary response, and the subsequent evoked firing is the secondary response. Note that it is difficult to predict precisely which cells will participate in the secondary response, even with complete knowledge of the network connectivity, because propagation from the initiating cells is modulated both by synaptic inhibition and by the differing degrees of refractoriness in the various cells.

In a network in which many cells may be refractory, and in which inhibition is at least relatively intact, how can synchronized firing occur at all, even at a low level? Inhibition may fail to contain the growth of population firing in two ways. First, the inhibitory synaptic strength may be decreased to some extent (see Chapters 3 and 6). Second, even with strong inhibition, our estimates for network topology suggest that inhibitory holes will exist (see Chapter 5). The network that we most often use in simulations contains many inhibitory holes. Inhibitory holes may exist in the slice, because the probability of observing any disynaptic IPSPs between two randomly chosen e cells (within 400 μ) is only about 0.3 (see Chapter 3). However, inhibitory holes alone cannot explain partially synchronized bursts, because usually there is more than one initiating cell. One must consider, in addition, more complicated probabilities (i.e., of finding an e cell excited by at least one initiating cell, but not disynaptically inhibited by any of them). Although this makes it plausible that propagation could occur to at least some followers of the initiating cells, it is important to realize that propagation in the model takes place to only a small fraction of any one firing cell's followers, provided that inhibition is retained (i.e., c_i greater than about 2 nS). We therefore suggest that the occurrence of partially synchronized bursts should be diminished by reducing the number of inhibitory holes in the network. Doubling the average number of both excitatory and inhibitory inputs to all cells has this effect and does suppress spontaneous oscillations, although they are not eliminated entirely.

A raster plot of simulated oscillatory activity in the 9,900-cell model is shown in part A of Figure 7.8. It is remarkable that this activity is so spatially coherent, especially because the initiating cells (not shown in the raster) are scattered across the entire array. This, it seems, must be an emergent property of the system (How do the initiating cells "know" to discharge at about the same time?), yet it simply reflects that the level of pyramidal-cell firing that develops can recruit most or all of the i_2 cells, coherently across the array, and these in turn produce prolonged IPSPs in all of the pyramidal cells. Although the relatively localized connectivity of the pyramidal cells (see Chapters 3 and 6) makes the wide coherence intriguing, it is not so totally mysterious. The wide spatial coherence of activity shown in Figure 7.8 is robust to many parameter changes, but it can be altered under special conditions: (i) When pyramidal-cell excitability is low, synchronized events may be initiated by a single cell, and a propagating wave is produced (Traub et al., 1989); such an event might account for the phase lags in synaptic potentials in the separated cells that Schwartzkroin and Haglund (1986) observed. Slow propagation along polysynaptic pathways has been observed in longitudinal slices after partial blockade of inhibition and a localized stimulus (Miles et al., 1988). (ii) When the excitability is, in contrast, high (e.g., twice that of Figure 7.8), spatially coherent waves are difficult to define. (iii) When synchronized activity is suppressed by increasing the synaptic connectivity, coherence across long distances is again lost.

Figure 7.8 also shows that excitability itself oscillates during rhythmic events, as it does during in vivo theta rhythm (Buzsáki et al., 1981; Rudell, Fox, and Ranck, 1980). The upper trace in part B of this figure shows an individual wave from the same simulation as in part A (plotted as number of cells firing versus time). The simulation was repeated multiple times, but with a stereotypic stimulus given to 600 cells, at a different phase of the wave for each stimulus; examples of the evoked responses are shown in the lower two traces of part B. The evoked amplitudes are plotted in the upper trace of part C; to construct this trace, the amplitude of the baseline underlying wave at time t was subtracted from the amplitude of an evoked stimulus given at time t. How can the biphasic shape of the evoked-response curve be explained? The lower traces of part C, obtained by averaging data from 15 cells taken during the "baseline simulation," demonstrate that the answer is simple: The average SSP is itself biphasic, consisting of an initial EPSP, an overlapping Cl^- IPSP, and a further overlapping K^+ IPSP. By stimulating sufficiently many cells, one simply measures the average "synaptically induced state" of the population.

The coherence of activity along the entire array (Figure 7.8) indicates that the entire distributed circuitry contributes to each wave of activity. But is the entire circuitry required to express oscillatory activity? To address this question, we performed the simulation of Figure 7.9. At the time indicated by the arrowhead, the 40 × 225 array was separated into two: a 40 × 112 array and a 40 × 113 array. Inhibitory cells and connections were similarly separated. Note that the oscillatory activity in the two separated pieces continues at the same frequency. Because the pieces are disconnected, and because the synchronized events are not precisely periodic, their oscillations drift in and out of phase with each other. Waves that are out of phase are shown by the vertical lines. In summated activity for the whole system (upper trace) the out-of-phase waves appear as notches (small arrowheads). This indicates that subarrays can oscillate at the same frequency. The frequency must therefore arise from

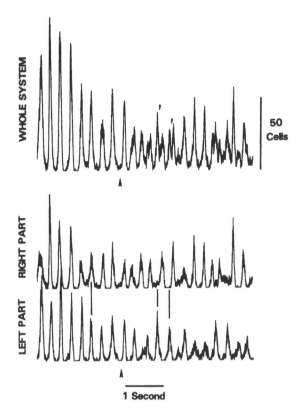

Figure 7.9. The frequency of the simulated oscillation depends on intrinsic cell properties and local (not global) connectivity. The parameters were c_e = 5 nS, c_i = 10 nS, and bias currents 0–0.6 nA. At the time marked by the arrow, all synaptic connections were cut between two halves of the model (one 40 × 112 cells, the other 40 × 113 cells). Each half continues to oscillate at the same mean frequency, but the two halves drift in and out of phase with each other (vertical lines); note notched waves in the curve for the whole system (small arrowheads).

intrinsic cell properties and (relatively) localized synaptic circuitry properties, rather than population size per se – provided the population size is above a threshold amount. When the array is subdivided sufficiently, the oscillatory activity becomes irregular and fragmented. This is not surprising, because we know that sufficiently small pieces of the CA3 region will not support synchronized activity even with inhibition blocked (Miles et al., 1984) (see Chapter 6).

Further insight into the mechanisms involved in collective oscillations, and SSPs, can be obtained by altering various of the basic model parameters. For example, a sudden reduction in the pyramidal-cell excitability (i.e., the bias currents) slows the rhythm (Traub et al., 1989). Increasing the excitability has the opposite effect. [Schneiderman (1988) increased the excitability in slices bathed in low-dose penicillin by dropping the Mg^{2+} concentration; that likewise increased the frequency of rhythmical field potentials.] Provided that c_e is large enough that excitability is above a threshold value, increasing the excitability further causes, in the model, a decrease in the amplitude of the waves (measured as the number of cells firing) (Traub et al., 1989).

Figure 7.10 illustrates the effects of changing various synaptic strengths. First, and not surprisingly, excitatory synapses between pyramidal cells are essential for the oscillatory activity. This result in consistent with experimental data suggesting that nonspecific blockade of excitatory amino-acid-mediated synaptic transmission, with kynurenic acid, will completely abolish spontaneous rhythmical field potentials in the in vitro CA3 region (J. S. Schneiderman, personal communication). Interpretation of the experimental result is complicated by the fact that excitatory amino acid blockers may also prevent the recruitment of inhibitory cells. For example, 6-cyano-7-nitroquinoxaline-2,3-dione (CNQX) (Blake, Brown, and Collingridge, 1988; Honoré et al., 1988) not only blocks the quisqualate type of glutamate receptor on pyramidal cells but also blocks EPSPs onto inhibitory cells (Miles, 1990). Second, total blockade of slow IPSPs disrupts the rhythm and leads generally to augmented cell firing. This notion could be checked with phaclofen (Dutar and Nicoll, 1988) in doses sufficient to block delayed IPSPs completely. Next, we illustrate the effects of a partial reduction in the unitary Cl^--IPSP conductance (third tracing from the top, Figure 7.10); as discussed previously, events become larger and less frequent. Finally, reducing the efficacy of recurrent inhibition by reducing the strength of excitatory synapses made onto inhibitory cells also increases the amplitude and reduces the frequency of the oscillations. Plasticity at these synapses may be induced by strong tetani (Miles and Wong, 1987b) and could be important in synaptic plasticity (Figure 7.19).

Why does reducing inhibition lead to slowing of the rhythm? The results reported in Chapter 6 show that reduced Cl^- IPSPs will lead to a larger individual synchronized event. Let us suppose, for the sake of concreteness, that the event grows from 100 cells to 200 cells. Two mechanisms then come into play. First, cells will be recruited into the larger synchronized event that might otherwise have initiated the next event. The long duration of AHPs implies that a cell recruited into one event is unlikely to initiate the next event. But this effect will be small (assuming a reasonable degree of cellular excitability), because the 100 additional pyramidal cells recruited will represent only 100/9,000 or about 1% of the population. Second, the 100 cells firing during the original event will recruit about 100 out of 450 i_2 cells that produce slow IPSPs. The 200-cell event will recruit about twice as many i_2 cells, and

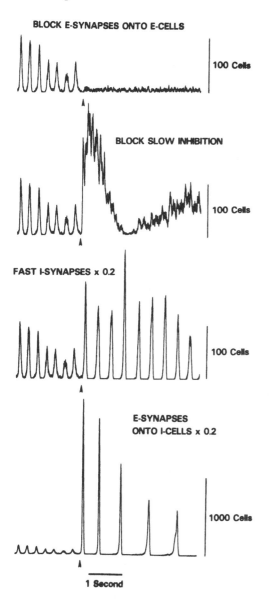

BLOCK E-SYNAPSES ONTO E-CELLS

100 Cells

BLOCK SLOW INHIBITION

100 Cells

FAST I-SYNAPSES x 0.2

100 Cells

E-SYNAPSES
ONTO I-CELLS x 0.2

1000 Cells

1 Second

Figure 7.10. Effect on simulated oscillations of parameter changes involving synapses. Basic parameters were $c_e = 5$ nS, $c_i = 10$ nS, and bias currents 0–0.6 nA. At the time marked by the arrowhead, a parameter was changed as indicated. Note that oscillatory activity is abolished when recurrent excitation is blocked. It changes form markedly by complete (but not necessarily partial) blockade of slow IPSPs. Partial block of $GABA_A$-type IPSPs (either by diminishing the unitary IPSP conductance or by diminishing excitation onto i cells) leads to an increase in amplitude, and decrease in frequency, of the waves.

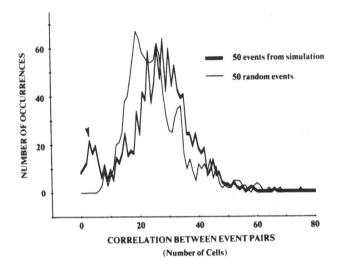

Figure 7.11. The cells that fire during any particular wave are similar to what would be expected by picking cells at random (even though the system is deterministic!). A simulation was run for 12 s to generate 50 waves ("events"); c_e = 5 nS, c_i = 5 nS, and bias currents 0–1.2 nA. The cells firing during each event were identified, so that to each event i is attached a binary vector $E_i(1, \ldots , 9,000)$, where $E_i(j) = 1$ if and only if cell j fires during E_i. The correlation between two events is the number of ones (i.e., cells) they have in common; the dark line in the figure is a histogram of the correlation between all event pairs, an indication of the statistical structure of the successive events. To construct random events, the computer generated 50 binary vectors R_i, where each R_i has the same number of ones as E_i, and each cell j is in as many R_i as it is in E_i; an iterative algorithm was used to do this. The histogram of correlations for the random events (thin lines) was similar to the histogram for oscillatory events, except at small correlations (arrowhead); this anticorrelation for the simulation reflects the fact that once a cell bursts, it is unlikely to do so again for a number of interevent periods simply because of intrinsic refractoriness. In particular, successive events are likely to have no cells at all in common.

these i_2 cells will fire longer than before. The larger resulting IPSPs will then slow the rhythm. When excitability is so low that spontaneous bursts will occur less frequently than a typical slow-IPSP duration, then the excitability will be the dominant effect in setting the frequency.

The discussion to this point has mainly concerned the amplitude and frequency of the population rhythm. We shall now consider the composition of the subsets of cells that fire during the different partially synchronized events. We call the subset of pyramidal cells that fire during such an event a *cluster*. From data of the sort displayed in the raster plot of Figure 7.8, we know that (in the model, in runs lasting as long as 12 s and displaying dozens of different events) clusters do not repeat. In fact, the cellular composition of clusters appears to be almost random. To demonstrate this, we analyze the data using an idea suggested by L. S. Schulman (Figure 7.11). If there are repeating subsets of neurons that tend to discharge together (neural groups, neural assemblies, or the like), they should be demonstrable by analyzing the correlations between different clusters. The correlation of two clusters is defined as the number of cells that form part of both clusters. A simulation was performed to generate 50 events, correlations were calculated for all 1,225 event pairs, and a histogram was constructed of the correlations (thick line in Figure 7.11). The problem is this: Does this histogram reveal meaningful structure, or not? To answer this, we constructed a set of 50 "random" events that satisfied two contraints. The number of cells in the ith random event was the same as the number of cells in the ith "real" event, and each cell in the population participated in the same number of random events as real events. The correlations between the random events are shown by the thin line in Figure 7.11. The statistical structures of the real events and the random events are quite similar, except in the region of zero correlation (arrowhead). The nonrandomness in the real events results because cells firing during one event are unlikely to fire during the next one; this anticorrelation produces the peak shown. This result implies that little knowledge of past events can be derived from identifying the cells that fire during a particular event, except that these cells probably did not fire during the last event. On the other hand, if recurrent CA3 connections have a low threshold for potentiation, an effect not included in our model, then this result need not necessarily be correct.

These considerations make it compelling to devise methods (perhaps optical) that will identify experimentally precisely which cells in a large population are the ones to fire during rhythmical activity. Such experiments would provide a test for this model.

If the clusters firing during rhythmical population oscillations are almost random, then the cellular composition of the repeating events carries considerable information, in the formal sense of information. This suggests that the cellular composition of the clusters, if not of the overall oscillation, might be sensitive to small perturbations of the system, a property of so-called chaotic dynamical systems.

Dynamical-systems aspects of hippocampal oscillations

In order to test the sensitivity of the model network behavior to small perturbations, we performed the simulations shown in Figure 7.12. A "basic" simulation was run, and the output (in particular, the number of cells firing at each time) was stored. The simulation was then repeated with identical initial conditions. The new simulation was superimposable upon the first one, until the time indicated by the arrowhead. At that

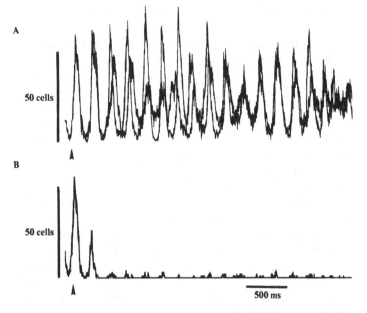

Figure 7.12. Exquisite sensitivity of the fine structure (but not the population frequency) of simulated oscillations to small perturbations. Two simulations were run with identical parameters (c_e = 5 nS, c_i = 10 nS, bias currents 0–1.2 nA), except that at the time indicated (arrowhead) a current was injected into one cell (2 nA, 25 ms), causing that cell to burst when it would not otherwise have done so. The upper curves are the superimposed traces of the number of cells firing in the two runs; note how they drift in and out of phase. This drift is not transient, but rather continues indefinitely. The bottom curve is the correlation between the two runs; that is, at each time, we count the numbers of individual cells firing in both runs. This correlation is lost within a few hundred milliseconds of the disturbance. What this means is that even though the average behaviors of the perturbed and unperturbed simulations often appear similar, the cellular compositions of the events are totally differ- ent in the two cases. This simulation suggests that information cannot be encoded solely in autonomous firing patterns in a CA3-type network on a time scale of seconds.

time, a 2-nA, 25-ms current was injected into one cell; let us call this the "perturbed" simulation. The population oscillations for the perturbed and unperturbed cases are displayed superimposed in the upper part of Figure 7.12. The mean frequencies and amplitudes of the waves are the same, but they drift in and out of phase with each other – not tran- siently, but persistently. (The simulations were continued for 9 s after the perturbation.) Because certain properties, but not the details, of the signal are preserved, this suggests that the "motion" that produces this output lies near to an attractor in some high-dimensional space. It seems reasonable to guess that the perturbation has just moved the orbit so that it winds around the attractor in a different way. Let us now consider the cellular compositions of the clusters in the perturbed and unperturbed cases. The lower tracing plots the correlation of the two simulations, that is, at each time, the number of cells firing in common during each run. Note that the correlation between the runs falls off rapidly (within hundreds of milliseconds) and stays minimal, even though only one cell was perturbed.[4] We emphasize that these simulations are deterministic; that is, noise was not included. At the level of cellular composition, then, our model hippocampal network, under the current conditions of a distribution of depolarizing bias currents to the pyramidal cells, does appear to be a chaotic system (Ott, 1981).

In view of the structural features of this network, it is perhaps not so surprising that there is such sensitivity to initial conditions. First, there are positive feedback and high gain. The recurrent excitatory connections are powerful enough to allow burst propagation, each cell participates in multiple cycles of the network, and the bursts themselves are a form of amplification. Second, a delicate balance of excitatory and inhibitory inputs into each pyramidal cell can determine whether or not it will burst (Figure 6.3). So each pyramidal cell may be sensitive to small perturbations. Together, these features ensure that a small perturbation will produce consequences that will propagate throughout the system. However, if inhibition is reasonably intact, the propagating disturbance does not consist of an unbounded increase in firing, but rather in different "decisions" as to which cells will fire.

We next examined the power spectrum of the simulated collective oscillations. Our guess was that with such complex underlying dynamics, the spectrum would not be sharp; but features of the system such as slow IPSPs might introduce one or more peaks. A 40-s run was performed with a somewhat reduced network (4,000 pyramidal cells and 400 i cells, with other network parameters as described in Chapter 5, and with a random distribution of bias currents into the pyramidal cells). This was done so as to obtain a large number of events. Examples of the raw data (above) and power spectrum (below) are shown in Figure 7.13. A reasonable degree of rhythmicity of the population is shown by the relatively broad peak between 3 and 4 Hz. There appears to be fine structure to this spectrum that we do not know how to interpret. In comparing this spectrum to the spectra of field-potential recordings, which possess considerable power below 3 Hz (Schneiderman et al., 1989), remember that this signal represents the number of cells firing, rather than extracellular potential. It is not practical to compute extracellular potentials (at least in a reasonably detailed way) in a 40-s run. We would expect that field-potential records would have a smoother and broader spectrum than would the signal corresponding to the number of cells firing. The reason is that the synaptic currents induced by a cell firing are slow compared

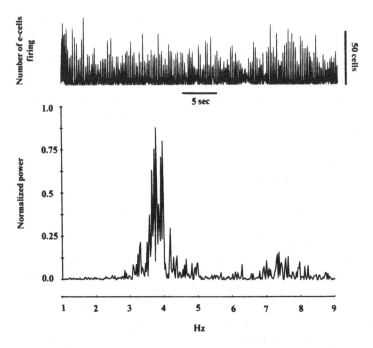

Figure 7.13. The power spectrum of the simulated oscillation has a peak, but not a sharp one. A 40-s simulation was run for a model with 4,000 e cells, 400 i cells, c_e = 5 nS, c_i = 10 nS, and β_q = 1/2,000. The number of cells depolarized more than 20 mV ("firing") was counted every 5 ms. Upper trace: Raw data. Lower trace: Power spectrum. The power spectrum of field-potential signals recorded from "resting" hippocampal slices is even broader than that from the simulation (Schneiderman et al., 1989).

with the firing per se and are dependent on the states of all the postsynaptic cells to which any given cell is connected. We do not yet have quantitative information on this, however. In any case, the spectra of experimental field-potential records are broader than the one illustrated in Figure 7.13.

The cellular composition of event clusters is complicated. However, consideration of the number of pyramidal cells firing as a function of time, $x(t)$, allows some simplification. In the model, $x(t)$ is calculated by explicit simulation of the activities of 9,900 interconnected model neurons, but the form of $x(t)$ might be equivalent to a function produced by a motion in a much smaller space, possibly even one with less than 20 dimensions. We attempted to compute the correlation dimension of $x(t)$ (Grassberger and Procaccia, 1983) to explore this idea. Correlation dimensions calculated from human EEG data include 2 for the EEG during an absence seizure (Babloyantz and Destexhe, 1986), and about 5 and 4.05–4.37 for sleep stages 2 and 4, respectively (Babloyantz, Salazar, and Nicolis, 1985). Here, also, the idea was to determine if the time series in question was equivalent to or indistinguishable from one generated by a motion in a relatively low-dimensional space.[5]

Following Babloyantz et al. (1985), let us denote the time series $x(t)$, where t is discrete time. Consider some displacement τ (in practice, several different τ must be examined) and positive integer n. From the original time series we construct a new one, $\vec{x}(t)$ by the identification $x(t) \rightarrow (x(t), x(t + \tau), \ldots, x(t + (n - 1)\tau)) = \vec{x}(t)$. We are interested in the correlations of $\vec{x}(t)$. To quantify these, first define $E(x(t), x(u))$ as the usual n-dimensional Euclidean distance between $\vec{x}(t)$ and $\vec{x}(u)$. Now construct the correlation function

$$C(r) = \frac{1}{N^2} \sum_{t \neq u} \theta\{r - E(x(t), x(u))\}$$

where the sum is taken over all nonidentical pairs of points in the time series, and θ is the Heaviside function [$\theta(x) = 0$ if $x \leq 0$, and $\theta(x) = 1$ if $x > 0$]. Basically, $C(r)$ counts the number of pairs of points of distance at most r apart. If there is an attractor, $C(r)$ may, for small r, behave like a power of r, $C(r) \sim r^d$, where d can be thought of as a dimension. This so-called embedding method is applied in practice by estimating d for a number of different n. If d converges to some constant value as n increases, this limiting value is viewed as the dimension of the attractor for the time series. The smallest n for which d reaches this asymptotic value can be viewed as the dimension of the "smallest" space in which the derived time series $\vec{x}(t)$ exhibits the appropriate attractor. A further issue is whether the attractor is a "strange" or "chaotic" attractor or is more like a toroidal (of perhaps dimension > 2) attractor for a periodic or quasi-periodic motion. A strange attractor is one for which, as orbits approach the attractor, in the sense that the distance between a point moving on the orbit and the attractor set approaches zero as time approaches infinity, the orbit does not approach any particular orbit lying within the attractor. The dimension of a strange attractor is, in general, not an integer. Strange attractors usually are fractal objects. To determine the nature of the attractor, one can calculate the largest Lyapunov exponent of the motion, or one can show that nearby orbits tend to diverge from each other (as in Figure 7.12), even though they both tend to the attractor. See Eckmann and Ruelle (1985) for a review of these matters.

A "noisy" time series $x(t)$ would be one generated by a motion in a space of large or of infinite dimension. For our model, it is not clear what to expect. The underlying dynamics might, in principle, be irreducibly complicated, or the whole system might be reducible to a much simpler one. On the one hand, $x(t)$ is very roughly periodic, but with a

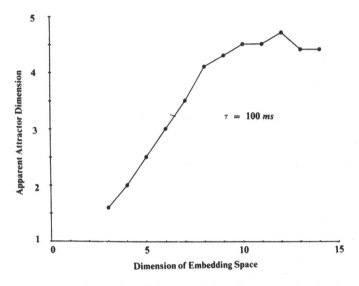

Figure 7.14. Estimation of the correlation dimension of a chaotic attractor for the signal illustrated in Figure 7.13 (number of cells firing over 40 s) using the embedding method. The asymptotic value for the dimension was about 4.2; τ was 20 data points (or 100 ms, because points were saved every 5 ms).

rather complex spectrum (Figure 7.13). On the other hand, $x(t)$ is produced by a deterministic system with many thousands of degrees of freedom (recall that there are 9,900 cells, each with a number of membrane potentials and membrane state variables). As we have suggested (Figure 7.12), the existence of a chaotic attractor is suggested because a small perturbation of the system (stimulating one extra cell briefly) leads to an $x(t)$ that is, in most regions, not superimposable on the $x(t)$ of the unperturbed system; yet, the two $x(t)$ have very similar spectra. In preliminary calculations, using the embedding method described earlier, we have estimated that the correlation dimension of a particular 40-s time series $x(t)$ is about 4.2 (Figure 7.14). This result suggests that our very complex model system is producing an average output equivalent to what could be produced by a much simpler system. The problem is to deduce the structure of this simpler system. Of course, the simple system would not be able to reproduce the detailed composition of the cellular clusters firing during each wave. It will be interesting to determine if the correlation dimension of $x(t)$ remains unchanged in the model when synaptic transmission is quantal, a more physiologically realistic representation, but one that is not deterministic.

These results raise the large question as to the function of the circuitry that generates, at the population level, rhythmic firing in nonoverlapping clusters of CA3 cells. We imagine that if CA3 is used to respond to a brief input, say from the granule cells, the response should be "read out" within a few hundred milliseconds at most. This follows because ongoing activity lasting more than a few hundred milliseconds is too sensitive to initial conditions to carry useful information (Figure 7.12), unless the useful output is not the particular cells that fire, but rather the amplitude and frequency of the entire population response. The fact that individual neurons, such as place cells, in the hippocampus seem to carry specific information about the outside world must make us cautious about this latter possibility, that it is the total number of cells firing that is important.

How robust is the phenomenon of population oscillations? We would also like to know that the basic phenomena we have been discussing are not accidents of a particular choice of parameters. We have shown previously (Traub et al., 1989) that population oscillations continue when the following parameters are varied over at least a 50% range: c_e, c_i, the strength of excitatory synapses onto i cells, $g_{K[Ca]}$, and the range over which bias currents are distributed. We can also make connectivity global rather than localized, decrease the size of the population, reduce slow IPSPs or alter their time constant (but not reduce them too much), or scatter the values of unitary IPSPs throughout the system. The time constant for relaxation of $g_{K[Ca]}$ can be set at the same value throughout the population, or scattered randomly over a fivefold range. We have even seen similar oscillations when there has been prominent synaptic noise, as in our high-$[K^+]_o$ model, as described later, under conditions such that c_e has been too small to permit full population discharges. We therefore believe that low-amplitude oscillations are properties of brain regions that possess recurrent excitation, (possibly) intrinsic bursting, recurrent inhibition of both fast and slow time courses, and a source of spontaneous firing or bursting. This is not to say that the population oscillations survive all manipulations of the parameters; particularly when the pyramidal cells do not have intrinsic bursting properties, and when c_e is small and inhibition intact, spontaneous population behavior can appear "disorganized."

Additional comparisons of in vitro oscillations with in vivo theta. Our simulated network oscillations share two further properties with theta rhythm. The first property is phase resetting. When a sufficiently large stimulus is given in the model, before a partially synchronized burst is due to occur, the phase of subsequent events is reset (Traub et al., 1988). The mechanism appears to be this: A sufficiently large stimulus will recruit (through pyramidal-cell firing) a set of i_2 cells that will fire synchronously. The resulting slow IPSPs delay the initiation of the next event, and so reset the cycle. Phase resetting has been observed in vivo

(Buzsáki et al., 1979, 1981), and there is also suggestive experimental evidence for it in slices (Schwartzkroin and Haglund, 1986). The mechanisms may be similar to the model, but that remains to be demonstrated. A stimulus pulse in vivo will also (antidromically and via afferent fibers) excite the septum, and phase resetting could be taking place there. The second property concerns the correlation between cellular firing and population waves. Figure 7.7 demonstrates that a much larger fraction of the i-cell population fires during a partially synchronized event than is the case for the e-cell population. Schwartzkroin and Haglund (1986) observed that interneurons were much more likely to fire during a partially synchronized event than were pyramidal cells. This relationship is also observed during theta in vivo (Buzsáki et al., 1983); it is conceivable, however, that the mechanism in vivo is totally different. For example, the septal inputs might periodically depolarize inhibitory cells in vivo during theta states (see Chapter 1).

Spontaneous synchronized population bursts

The mechanisms that underlie synchronization of cellular firing during $GABA_A$ blockade seem to be reasonably understood (see Chapter 6); yet the initiation of these events is not fully understood. The post-burst refractoriness factors must all be cataloged and preferably studied quantitatively (delayed IPSPs, $g_{K[Ca]}$, perhaps electrogenic Na-K pumps, etc.), and so must the sources of spontaneous firing or bursting that would initiate the synchronized event. Spontaneous firings could result (i) from a single spontaneous EPSP or train of EPSPs, (ii) from intrinsic pacemaker currents, or (iii) from random events in pyramidal-cell membranes. Spontaneous EPSPs, in turn, conceivably could be generated by ectopic action potentials originating in axons or presynaptic terminals, or by random quantal EPSPs; random EPSPs have been recorded in CA3 neurons in the presence of TTX (Brown et al., 1979).

In contrast to the case of synchronized bursts during $GABA_A$ blockade, we have a plausible, although not complete, model of the initiation of spontaneous synchronized bursts in high $[K^+]_o$ (Traub and Dingledine, 1990). High-$[K^+]_o$ bursts are instructive also as a kind of counterpoint to picrotoxin bursts; although many of the details of the experimental situations are different, the underlying principles, for synchronization at least, seem similar.

Basic phenomenology of high-$[K^+]_o$ synchronized bursts. These events have been studied by Rutecki et al. (1985), Korn et al. (1987), Chamberlin and Dingledine (1988, 1989), and Chamberlin et al. (1990). The following discussion applies to the CA3 region of rat hippocampal slices bathed in 8.5-mM $[K^+]_o$. In this medium, isolated spontaneous bursts are rarely observed in individual neurons. The resting potential of the cells is somewhat depolarized (about 55 mV) (Chamberlin et al., 1990), and this may contribute to the tendency of the cells not to burst. In this system, synchronized bursts occur, consisting in each cell of a large underlying depolarization and multiple action potentials. The bursts occur spontaneously at intervals of about 1 s.

During the interburst interval, EPSPs occur in an apparently random pattern, with mean interval in any given cell typically a few hundred milliseconds. On the other hand, just before the onset of a synchronized burst, the frequency of EPSPs rises more than twofold (Chamberlin et al., 1990).

Each cell develops an AHP following a burst that decays (at least in terms of the hyperpolarization, if not the membrane shunt) during the latter half of the interburst interval. The AHP duration is significantly correlated with the interburst interval in any particular slice. Reducing the AHP amplitude with phorbol-12,13-diacetate in the bath reduces, in turn, the interburst interval (Chamberlin and Dingledine, 1989).

Although Cl^- IPSPs are not blocked by high $[K^+]_o$, their reversal potential is shifted toward the resting potential (Korn et al., 1987). The unitary synaptic conductance may also be reduced somewhat (Thompson and Gähwiler, 1989b).

Alteration in Cl^- IPSPs cannot completely explain these synchronized events. If the extracellular $[Cl^-]$ is reduced so as to shift the Cl^- reversal potential in a manner comparable to that induced by 8.5-mM $[K^+]_o$, synchronized bursts will occur much less frequently than they do in the high-$[K^+]_o$ solution (Chamberlin and Dingledine, 1988). This suggests that K^+-induced changes in membrane potential and/or in synaptic transmission are also significant.

When CNQX is added to the bath, spontaneously occurring and evoked EPSPs are reduced in amplitude (and frequency). Concomitant with this, the population burst frequency is reduced, and bursts become less intense. Eventually, in most cases, detectable synchronized activity ceases (Chamberlin et al., 1990).

Residual Cl^- IPSPs partly regulate high-$[K^+]_o$ bursts, because bicuculline, a $GABA_A$ blocker, increases their "intensity" and decreases their frequency; burst intensity has been defined by Korn et al. (1987).

Model of high-$[K^+]_o$ synchronized bursts. We began with the 9,900-cell model described in Chapter 5, but made the following changes. Cell membrane properties were modified so that intrinsic bursting would not occur; $E_{IPSP(Cl)}$ was set at the resting potential, and E_K and $E_{IPSP(K)}$ were shifted in a depolarizing direction. Depolarizing bias currents of up to 0.45 nA were injected into each pyramidal cell, and, in addition, each pyramidal cell was subjected to randomly occurring spontaneous EPSPs.

These events followed Poisson statistics with a mean inter-EPSP interval usually of 250 ms. The amplitude of spontaneous EPSPs was assumed equal to the amplitude of recurrent action-potential-evoked EPSPs. The combination of spontaneous EPSPs and cellular depolarizations guaranteed that action potentials would begin to occur in various neurons once AHPs had decayed sufficiently. Details of the methods for this model are given by Chamberlin et al. (1990) and Traub and Dingledine (1990).

This model reproduces all of the basic experimental observations summarized earlier. Figure 7.15A illustrates synchronized activity that occurs when c_e = 7 nS and c_i = 5 nS. The potentials from two different cells are displayed. The arrowheads indicate population bursts. Note that EPSPs occur during the interburst interval, growing in size, on average, as the AHP decays, because of the progressive reduction in the shunting conductances associated with delayed IPSPs and $g_{K[Ca]}$. The mean interval between population events here is 1.3 ± 0.3 s. Figure 7.15B shows the relative frequency of excitatory synaptic stimulations. There is a constant background, with a suggestion of an increasing trend toward the burst, and then a sudden jump just before a population burst. The reason for this is indicated in Figure 7.16, which uses data from the same simulation, but displays the number of cells firing during bursts and between bursts (lower of the two top traces, at high gain). Note that firing of cells begins, at a rather low level, during the latter half of the interburst interval, and there is a sudden acceleration as the burst starts. This firing produces widespread EPSPs (because of axonal divergence, each pyramidal exciting, on average, 20 others in the network). The increase in EPSP frequency is evident in the voltage records of two cells (below, note arrowheads).

Detailed analysis of the initiation of a population burst showed that the burst began with spontaneous firing (induced by background EPSPs superimposed on the bias currents) in fewer than five cells. Synchronization then proceeded via excitatory recurrent collaterals just as described in Chapter 6. We found that propagation of firing from one neuron to another was state-dependent. When two of our model neurons (as used in the high-$[K^+]_o$ simulations) were connected together in the resting state, a train of action potentials in one would induce only a summated EPSP in the other. On the other, the depolarizing bias currents are such that eventually each cell will begin firing spontaneously with no synaptic input. It follows that at some point in its refractoriness cycle, and before a spontaneous action potential occurs, each cell can be discharged by excitatory synaptic inputs from presynaptic action potentials. It is at this point that random EPSPs can trigger action potentials in a few cells, and in turn these cells can "set off" the whole population. The decay of AHPs and intrinsic depolarizations reduce the firing threshold and

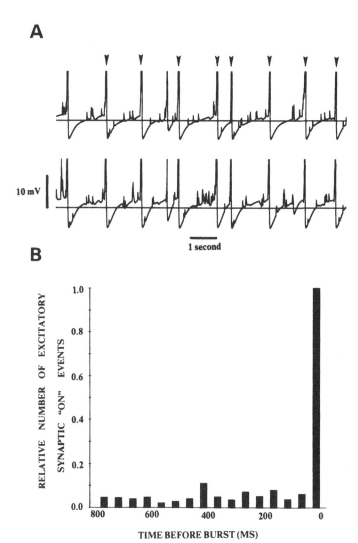

Figure 7.15. Simulation of high-$[K^+]_o$ synchronized bursts. A: Dual intracellular records. Arrowheads indicate population events where virtually all
of the 9,000 pyramidal cells fire (approximately) simultaneously. Note the
AHPs after each burst, and the EPSPs (and an occasional IPSP). The interval
between bursts was 1.3 ± 0.3 s for this 12-s simulation. EPSPs late in the
AHP generally are larger than those early in the AHP. Note the truncation of
action potentials. B: Excitatory synaptic events occur most frequently just
prior to a population burst. Averaged data for 16 cells and six bursts. The
computer counted the total number of time steps during which excitatory synapses were activated. The time bins are 50 ms. Data from the same run as for
part A. (From Chamberlin et al., 1990, with permission.)

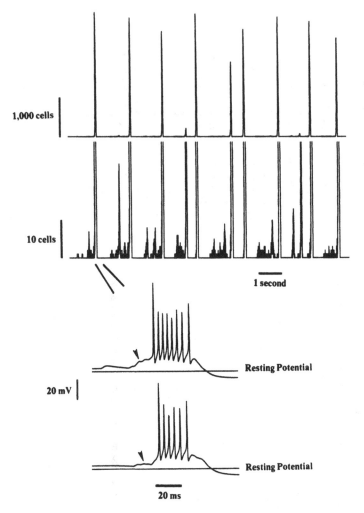

Figure 7.16. Model of high-$[K^+]_o$ synchronized bursts. The upper two traces show, as a function of time, the numbers of cells firing at two different gains. The high-gain tracing illustrates the low-amplitude buildup of firing prior to a population burst. The bottom two traces are simultaneous somatic membrane potentials during a burst. These records demonstrate the depolarizing envelope, repetitive firing, and succeeding AHP. Note the EPSPs prior to the bursts (arrowheads). (From Traub and Dingledine, 1990, with permission.)

thereby make the cells more easily triggerable by background spontaneous EPSPs or by firing of presynaptic neurons.

Support for this model comes from three parameter manipulations. First, partial blockade of $g_{K[Ca]}$ increased burst frequency (Traub and Dingledine, 1990; compare Chamberlin and Dingledine, 1989). Sec-

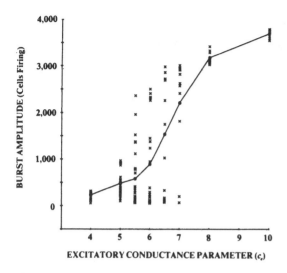

Figure 7.17. Model of high-$[K^+]_o$ synchronized bursts. Reducing the conductance of the excitatory synapses between pyramidal cells reduces burst amplitude (measured by peak number of cells firing at once). Both recurrent and spontaneous EPSPs are reduced in tandem by reducing c_e (as would be expected in CNQX). The crosses mark the amplitudes of all population events with peaks greater than 50 simultaneously firing cells, counted for 12-s runs; the first event, however, was excluded. The line is drawn through the mean. Note the large variance at intermediate values of c_e. (From Traub and Dingledine, 1990, with permission.)

ond, when $GABA_A$ inhibition was blocked, burst amplitude increased, and the interburst interval was prolonged, as occurs experimentally with bicuculline (Korn et al., 1987). Finally, when excitatory synapses were progressively blocked to imitate the CNQX experiments, burst amplitudes dropped progressively (Figure 7.17; compare Chamberlin et al., 1990). Note further in Figure 7.17 that the variance of burst amplitude increases as the bursts become attenuated, as also observed experimentally (Chamberlin et al. (1990). This is reminiscent of the increased variance of synaptic events in the "midrange" of synchronization induced by picrotoxin (Figure 7.5).

What is especially attractive about the high-$[K^+]_o$ system is that one can describe both interburst refractoriness and a source of interburst generation of action potentials, both in a reasonably plausible way. It will be interesting to see if the principles demonstrated generalize to other experimental systems wherein synchronized firing occurs.

An application of the model to synaptic plasticity: recurrent excitatory synapses. We have begun to employ our model to questions involving synaptic plasticity in the CA3 region. The first question concerns the

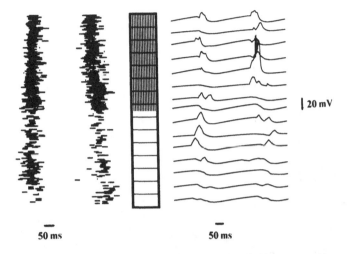

Figure 7.18. Increasing the conductance of recurrent excitatory synapses ($\times$ 2 in this case) increases the amplitude of population oscillations without affecting the frequency or phase. Center: Diagram of the model with 40 $\times$ 225 cells; c_e was 5 nS in the clear region and 10 nS in the hatched region. Left: Aligned raster plot of cell firings during two population waves. Note the clearly increased amount of firing in the upper region; the waves occur at the same frequency and are in phase. Each wave is initiated by cells in both regions of the array. Right: Somatic potentials in 15 cells at locations corresponding to the central diagram. Note the generally larger EPSPs extending into part of the lower half of the array; this extension is a consequence of the fact that excitatory connections have spatial extent (average = 30 cell diameters) and of the increased firing in the lower portion of the hatched region. Action potentials truncated.

recurrent excitatory synapses. Suppose that all of the recurrent excitatory synapses in a region of CA3 are "potentiated." How is ongoing autonomous oscillatory activity (as discussed in this chapter) affected? To be specific, we let c_e for synapses in one half of our network model be 10 nS, while c_e remained 5 nS in the other half. Partially synchronized events continued as before, with both model halves locked together (Figure 7.18), but firing was much more frequent in the "potentiated" half. The events were initiated by spontaneous bursts in both halves of the model. Although firing frequency was increased in the upper half of the model, even there the probability was low that a pyramidal cell would fire during any particular event. Producing potentiation within one region of CA3 will provide an interesting way to apply the network model to in vivo problems.

Synaptic changes in CA3 induced by repetitive stimulation. The model may also be useful in further studies on the synaptic changes induced in CA3 by repetitive stimulation, changes that may be more complex than just long-term potentiation of the excitatory synapses (Brown et al., 1988b; Gustafsson and Wigström, 1988). By way of background, we note that something analogous to kindling (McIntyre and Racine, 1986; McNamara et al., 1984) occurs in vitro, when stimuli lasting for seconds are delivered every 5 min. The responses to stimuli become altered, and eventually spontaneous epileptiform events are seen. Altered behavior persists for those hours during which slices can be maintained. The studies of Yamamoto and Chujo (1978) consisted of repetitive stimulation of the dentate gyrus while recording in CA3. The evoked population spike was transiently depressed and then potentiated. Intracellular excitatory-inhibitory synaptic sequences were altered so that the excitatory component grew and the inhibitory component shrank. Eventually, stimuli would evoke brief afterdischarges. An intracellular response seen at that time could consist of an oscillating potential, with period about 20 ms, that grew in amplitude. Such potentials are not observed, to our knowledge, in the presence of picrotoxin. Stasheff, Bragdon, and Wilson (1985) excited CA3 dendrites with 2-s, 60-Hz stimuli given every 5 min. They observed afterdischarges toward the end of later stimuli, abnormal bursting responses to single shocks delivered later, and spontaneous synchronized bursts (detectable with field potentials). Anderson, Swartzwelder, and Wilson (1987) demonstrated that 2-amino-5-phosphonovalerate (2-APV) blocked epileptogenesis induced by repetitive stimulation, but not synchronization itself once the slice had been "kindled"; see also Stasheff et al. (1989). A similar phenomenon has been described in pyriform cortex by Hoffman and Haberly (1989).

The cellular basis of changes induced in CA3 by repetitive stimulation was studied by Miles (1988) and Miles and Wong (1987b), using dual intracellular recordings. Strong tetani, to mossy fibers or to longitudinal fibers, sometimes led to the development of afterdischarges. Before such afterdischarges, oscillatory intracellular potentials could be seen in one cell that were evoked by intracellular stimulation of another cell (Miles and Wong, 1987b); an example of such a response is shown in Figure 7.19. At the unitary level, we have observed an increase in efficacy of monosynaptic EPSPs that may originate presynaptically. Disynaptic IPSPs, induced in one pyramidal cell by another pyramidal cell, show biphasic changes. The probability that disynaptic IPSPs are elicited increases sharply for several minutes after a tetanus and then declines, often to levels below control. This suggests that excitatory synapses terminating on inhibitory cells may exhibit short-term potentiation succeeded by long-term depression.

Simulation of tetanically induced plastic changes in CA3. We therefore wondered if a relatively small increase in unitary EPSP size, coupled

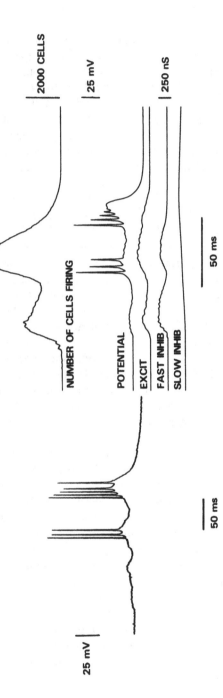

Figure 7.19. Left: Membrane-potential oscillations can occur in the CA3 region after tetanization of afferent pathways. The concomitant synaptic changes that occur are these: a decrease in the failure rate of recurrent EPSPs and an increase in the failure rate of disynaptic IPSPs (Miles, 1988; Miles and Wong, 1987b). Right: Similar membrane-potential oscillations occur in the model when the strength of excitatory synapses onto i cells is decreased sixfold. In that case, the i cell will not fire after a single presynaptic action potential; instead, two or more inputs are required. This delays the onset of recurrent inhibition and allows population (and cellular) oscillations to occur after stimulation of a single cell. Other parameters: $c_e = 8$ nS, $c_i = 10$ nS, $\beta_q = 1/500$.

with a significant decrease in the size of EPSPs onto i cells, could account for the cellular oscillations of the type shown in Figure 7.19. In the model, the e → i synapse is powerful enough for a single EPSP to cause an action potential (in a resting cell). If the unitary synaptic conductance at this synapse is reduced about fivefold, then two closely spaced excitatory synaptic inputs are required to cause firing; the consequence in the population is that the onset of inhibition is delayed. Figure 7.19 illustrates a simulation where the unitary e → i synaptic conductance was reduced sixfold, and a single cell was stimulated. Some of the cells (including the one illustrated) generated membrane-potential oscillations very similar to those observed experimentally. During the simulated oscillation, there are overlapping waves of excitatory and fast inhibitory synaptic input, and synchrony in the population increases with each wave. Experimentally, also, the last wave may be correlated with a small extracellular field potential. Once excitatory synapses onto i_1 cells are blocked sufficiently, the functional effect is indistinguishable from those of setting c_i equal to zero, and a fully synchronized population burst will occur. As we discussed in Chapter 6, the model in the form used here will not generate afterdischarges. If excitatory synapses onto i_2 cells are also completely blocked, cellular bursts that develop in synchrony will not repolarize.

In conclusion, we suggest that tetanic stimuli may induce changes in recurrent synaptic circuits as well as in afferent synapses. Both recurrent excitation and recurrent inhibition may change, possibly via opposing effects at excitatory synapses that terminate respectively on pyramidal cells and on inhibitory cells. In consequence, population synchrony is enhanced, as seems also to be possible if excitatory synapses alone are potentiated sufficiently (Figure 7.19). We would expect that reducing inhibition would lead to a greater enhancement of synchronization than would just an augmentation of excitatory synapses (compare Figure 6.17 with Figure 6.16).

Appendix: What does the EEG measure?

We have been concerned with the mechanisms underlying the EEG. This is so because the EEG (or, in general, extracellular-potential measurements) is one of the simplest methods of assessing rhythmic activity in a population of neurons. By "EEG" we mean a potential measured either within the extracellular space (but not inside a neuron or glial cell) or on the surface of the brain, the dura, or the scalp – but only potentials are considered that represent neural activity (something not always easy to prove conclusively). In clinical practice, most EEGs are taken at the scalp (possibly supplemented by nasopharyngeal or sphenoid electrodes), but in special situations electrodes may be placed on the surface of the brain or in brain parenchyma. In experimental animals and in brain slices, electrodes are placed directly into the tissue of interest.

To understand what extracellular electrodes are measuring, we must first define the time scale of interest. In this book, we do not consider slow or DC potential shifts (with time constants of seconds or more), which depend on slow changes in extracellular ion concentrations and their induced glial currents (Dietzel, Heinemann, and Lux, 1989; Somjen and Giacchino, 1985), as well as on membrane-pump-induced currents and other slow processes. Rather, we consider time scales of hundreds of milliseconds or less. Here, potentials in the extracellular space reflect (largely) currents flowing across neuronal membranes, through the extracellular space, and back through neurons. These currents are of two general types, not always possible to distinguish cleanly: those due to active membrane processes (e.g., action potentials, voltage-gated calcium currents), and those induced by synaptic currents; see Pedley and Traub (1990) for a review. Action potentials are recorded in the extracellular space as "unit activity." This activity is expected to induce smaller voltage disturbances in the extracellular space than is activity related to slower synaptic currents. The physical basis for this expectation is as follows.

The effective space constant λ_f of a dendritic cable (i.e., the distance for the potential induced by a point steady-state sinusoidal current of frequency f to fall to $1/e$ of its value at the current source) is related to the cable space constant λ by the formula

$$\frac{\lambda_f}{\lambda} = \sqrt{\frac{2}{1 + \sqrt{1 + \omega^2 \tau_m^2}}}$$

where $\omega = 2\pi f$, and λ, the DC space constant, is $(rR_m/2R_i)^{1/2}$, r is the cable radius, and τ is the membrane time constant (see Chapter 4). With $r = 3 \times 10^{-4}$ cm, $R_m = 10,000$ Ω-cm^2, and $R_i = 100$ Ω-cm, then $\lambda = 1.2$ mm. For a 3-ms action potential corresponding to $f = 170$ Hz, and $\tau = 30$ ms $= 0.03$ s, we obtain $\lambda_f = 295$ μ. For a slower synaptic potential, say one approximatable as a 30-Hz sinusoid, then $\lambda_f = 660$ μ. Roughly, λ_f falls off as $1/\sqrt{f}$. Now suppose we approximate the membrane current distribution along the cable as a dipole current source. The induced extracellular potential at some distance from the cell is proportional to the dipole separation (assuming the dipole current is kept constant) (Reitz and Milford, 1960, p. 38). This is the reason that faster membrane processes (at least those induced by localized membrane current flows) tend to produce smaller extracellular potentials. A more detailed analysis of this issue, with relevant experimental results, is given by Humphrey (1968).

In summary, the extracellular potential records a complex weighted sum of activities, weighted toward synaptic inputs rather than action potentials, and weighted also with distance and orientation of the active neurons with respect to the electrode (Creutzfeldt and Houchin, 1974; Creutzfeldt, Watanabe, and Lux, 1966; Humphrey, 1968; Plonsey, 1969). Quantitative understanding requires both a model of neuronal activity (which cells fire when, what synaptic currents flow, etc.) and a model of current flow in the extracellular space, that is, a means of solving some form of Poisson's equation given the membrane currents defined by the "neuronal activity model."[6] In turn, a major difficulty in understanding the neuronal-activity part of this picture is that synaptic inputs in some cells are themselves caused by action potentials in other cells (or perhaps the same cells!). This problem can be ignored if the synaptic currents in the population under study are all generated by neuronal firing in a separate and distant neuronal population. This is the approach most commonly taken for in vivo studies of theta rhythm, where the rhythm in hippocampus, for example, is assumed to be projected from rhythmic oscillations in the septal nuclei and the entorhinal cortex. Taking advantage of the lamination of synaptic inputs onto hippocampal pyramidal cells, and the well-defined layering of these cells, one can try to reconstruct the different synaptic inputs from measurements of extracellular potentials at different levels along the axis of the pyramidal cells (Buzsáki et al., 1986; Leung, 1982, 1984).

It is important to understand that in this book we have taken a different approach. We have emphasized EEG waves generated within an isolated, autonomous population of neurons. Neuronal population oscillations, producing a local EEG, have been demonstrated in hippocampal and temporal neocortical slices, as well as in the in vivo isolated nucleus reticularis thalami (Steriade et al., 1987). With the aid of a model, one can hope to sort out the intricate relations between the firings of certain neurons (generally a small fraction of the population during any EEG wave) and the synaptic currents thereby induced in neurons (generally a large fraction of the population). Note that in the model it is not necessary to compute the actual extracellular potential as a function of time. Although it is possible to do so (see Chapter 8), it is a computationally difficult exercise. Rather, we can follow population activity in other ways, such as determining the number of cells depolarized beyond some point, the intracellular potentials of particular cells, the synaptic inputs to particular cells, and so on.

As the population of neurons under study becomes larger and larger, one can, in principle, understand EEG waves, first in slices, and eventually perhaps in vivo.

8   Field effects[1]

Thus far, we have concentrated on collective neuronal behaviors in which the only interactions have been mediated by chemical synapses. Another type of neuronal interaction is clearly of importance during hyperexcitable states and may exert at least subtle influences even under normal conditions. Influences between neurons may be mediated by the flow of transmembrane current through the extracellular medium: field effects (Dudek and Traub, 1989). Field effects provide a means for the synchronization of action potentials in different neurons on a time scale of about 1 ms. Slow or DC extracellular fields can also bias a large population of neurons, rendering them all more excitable. The general subject of electrical field effects in the brain has been reviewed by Faber and Korn (1989). We shall restrict our attention here to the hippocampus.

There are several structural features and electrophysiological observations suggesting that field effects might be important in the hippocampus.[2] First, there is the large amplitude of extracellular population spikes that can be obtained after synchronized stimulation of an afferent pathway. Amplitudes of 5–10 mV or more are not unusual in the stratum pyramidale during epileptiform activity in vitro, and population spikes of 20 mV and more in vivo are not unusual (Somjen et al., 1985). These extracellular negative potentials would be expected to produce transmembrane positivities. It is important to remember that voltage-dependent membrane channels "see" the local electric field, which depends on the local gradient of potential across the membrane. Such transmembrane transient positivities might, especially when a cell is near threshold, make the difference between a cell's firing or not. Second, extracellular potential gradients can alter cellular excitability (Jefferys, 1981; Taylor and Dudek, 1984a). Extracellular potential gradients of 5–10 mV/mm are sufficient to alter the excitability of a population of granule cells, and larger gradients than that occur in the hippocampus during synchronized population spikes. Third, the extracellular resistivity of the hippocampus proper is high. Whereas the longitudinal resistivity (i.e., parallel to the axis of the dendrites and orthogonal to the stratum pyramidale) is about 125 Ω-cm in dendritic

194

layers (J. G. R. Jefferys, personal communication) – probably similar to intracellular resistivity – the extracellular resistivity within the stratum pyramidale itself is about three times higher (Jefferys, 1984). High extracellular resistivity within the stratum pyramidale favors the flowing of extracellular currents across membranes into neurons, as opposed to flowing out into the dendritic extracellular spaces and into the bathing medium. Fourth, at least in the rodent, hippocampal pyramidal cells are aligned with each other, so that extracellular currents induced by a somatic (or initial-segment) action potential in one cell will maximally influence the corresponding membrane regions of nearby cells. Finally, the shape of the epileptiform field potential (e.g., as in Figure 3.13), with its slow positivity and superimposed notches suggestive of a train of population spikes, indicates that the firing times of action potentials in nearby cells must be highly correlated. However, excitatory synapses have actions that seem too slow (several milliseconds and more) to provide synchrony on a time scale of only 1 ms or so. (Recall that in Figure 3.13, fast inhibitory synapses are blocked, and slow inhibitory synpases are much slower even than excitatory synapses.) Perhaps field effects provide a means to synchronize action potentials on this fast time scale.

Synchronization with chemical synapses blocked

Strong evidence that field effects generate at least one type of synchrony came from observations of large population spikes in the in vitro CA1 region bathed in media that both blocked synaptic transmission and, additionally, increased cellular excitability (Jefferys and Haas, 1982; Taylor and Dudek, 1982) (Figure 8.1). Those publications were themselves synchronized, appearing within a week of each other. Similar effects were subsequently demonstrated in other hippocampal regions (Snow and Dudek, 1984a, 1986). Further studies have shed light on the underlying mechanisms: Taylor and Dudek (1984a,b), Haas and Jefferys (1984), Konnerth et al. (1984, 1986a).

Figure 8.1 shows trains of action potentials in a single cell that are tightly phase-locked to large extracellular population spikes. Action potentials in many nearby cells are synchronized. These events occur spontaneously and can be evoked by a localized shock. Note that individual action potentials often are preceded by a brief negative notch (Figure 8.1B). In transmembrane recordings, this notch corresponds to a membrane depolarization (Taylor and Dudek, 1982, 1984a). This observation is crucial for understanding synchronization under these experimental conditions. The trains of synchronized action potentials represent true population events. An individual cell can be hyperpolarized so that it will not fire, but removing the hyperpolarization will allow the cell to

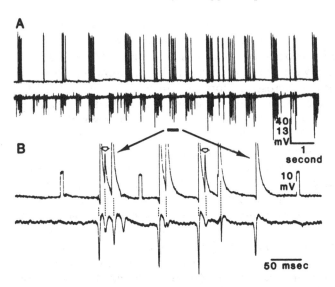

Figure 8.1. Synchronized action potentials in a medium that blocks synaptic transmission (0.5-mM $[Ca^{2+}]_o$, 2.3-mM $[Mn^{2+}]_o$). Recordings in CA1 region of hippocampal slice, on different time scales. Upper traces are intracellular referenced to ground; lower traces are local extracellular potential (transmembrane potential can be calculated from the difference). Note the very large field-potential transients (population spikes), sometimes more than 15 mV. Most action potentials are phase-locked to population spikes; most action potentials are preceded by a brief negativity in the intracellular record; subtraction of the extracellular record shows this brief potential to be a transmembrane positivity. (From Taylor and Dudek, 1982, with permission; copyright AAAS.)

participate once more in synchronized action potentials (Taylor and Dudek, 1984b). The spike train can last for seconds. Spontaneous trains of action potentials (called "field bursts" by Jefferys and Haas) usually begin near the subicular end of CA1. Events that begin locally gradually propagate along CA1 at low velocities (0.001–0.010 m/s), but individual population spikes propagate across the tissue considerably faster (0.04–0.15 m/s) (Haas and Jefferys, 1984). The latter velocity is similar to the propagation velocity for picrotoxin-induced synchronized bursts (see Chapter 6), but the mechanism seems to be different, because excitatory synapses are crucial in the picrotoxin-induced activity but are blocked during field bursts.

There are two major factors to be considered in understanding the physiological mechanisms of field bursts. First, how does the CA1 pyramidal-cell population become excitable so that at least some of the cells will fire spontaneously? Second, once some of the cells are firing spontaneously, what forces between cells can cause the firing to be synchronized? These two issues are not completely independent, because the synchronizing forces may lead to action potentials that would not occur otherwise, but we shall, for the moment, pretend that excitability and synchrony are separate (recall from Chapter 7 how we treated separately the sources of spontaneous bursting – slow inward currents and/or synaptic noise – and the sources of intercellular communication). Regarding the two issues as somewhat independent is also justified by the observation that field-burst-like events have been observed without simultaneous large population spikes (Konnerth et al., 1984).

Concerning the first issue, overall neuronal excitability depends on the ionic milieu. Lowered $[Ca^{2+}]_o$ will increase membrane excitability (Frankenhaeuser and Hodgkin, 1957). In addition, extracellular $[K^+]$ rises as cells fire synchronously, up to 9–10 mM (Haas and Jefferys, 1984). An advancing wave of increased $[K^+]_o$ probably underlies the slow propagation (about 1 mm/s) of certain field bursts (Konnerth et al., 1984). It appears that $[K^+]_o$ rises slowly preceding a field burst, which then causes a still further rise. In addition, the velocity of propagating field bursts can be increased by increasing $[K^+]_o$ (Yaari et al., 1986). Increased $[K^+]_o$ would be expected to depolarize neurons and to reduce the hyperpolarization caused by the opening of voltage-dependent K channels. Both effects would increase neuronal excitability. Extracellular $[K^+]$ probably also increases secondarily consequent to neural activity itself in nearby cells. The increase is maximal in the stratum pyramidale and would correlate with the slow extracellular negativity during a field burst that is also maximal in the stratum pyramidale (Haas and Jefferys, 1984; Konnerth et al., 1984). During a field burst, neurons are indeed observed to develop a simultaneous depolarization (Taylor and Dudek, 1984b) that may reach 10–12 mV (Haas and Jefferys, 1984).

It may be clinically relevant that events closely resembling field bursts also occur in CA1 in vitro bathed in media containing elevated $[K^+]_o$ with normal extracellular $[Ca^{2+}]$ (Jensen and Yaari, 1988; Traynelis and Dingledine, 1988). However, the intense presynaptic activity associated with synchronized bursts that occur simultaneously in the CA3 region might lower extracellular $[Ca^{2+}]$ somewhat (Heinemann et al., 1986). High-$[K^+]_o$ field bursts have been compared to tonic seizures, because of the associated slow extracellular negativity, the long duration, the intense neuronal firing, and the tendency for synchronized "clonic" bursts to follow the field burst (Jensen and Yaari, 1988; Traynelis and Dingledine, 1988). Once high-$[K^+]_o$ field bursts are occurring, excitatory synaptic transmission seems not to be required (Jensen and Yaari, 1988), in contrast to the case of synchronized bursts and afterdischarges induced by picrotoxin (Miles et al., 1984). Both low-$[Ca^{2+}]_o$ (Yaari et al., 1986) and high-$[K^+]_o$ field bursts are preceded and possibly initiated by small further rises in extracellular K^+ concentration (Traynelis and Dingledine, 1988). Repeated synaptic drive in CA1 from CA3 synchronized bursts may be the stimulus that induces the triggering increase in $[K^+]_o$.

Concerning the second issue, field effects seem to be critical in synchronizing action potentials. Experimentally, a transmembrane depolarization that is correlated in time with the extracellular field transient often occurs prior to action potentials. This transmembrane potential is not affected by the act of hyperpolarizing or depolarizing the cells. Extracellular current sinks occur in the stratum pyramidale during the large negative portion of the population spike, associated with dendritic sources, possibly due to current flow into cells bodies, along the interior of dendrites, and out dendritic membranes (Taylor and Dudek, 1984a,b). Furthermore, increasing the extracellular osmolarity in CA1 bathed in high $[K^+]_o$ decreases tissue resistivity, blocks field bursts, and reduces the amplitude of population spikes (Tasker and Dudek, 1989; Traynelis and Dingledine, 1989a). Field effects should be more potent as extracellular resistivity increases, so this result supports a role for field effects in synchronizing action potentials. In a way, field effects act as both cause and effect. Synchronized firing leads to large extracellular potentials, which further enhance synchronization.

The influence of field effects on synchrony was examined in detail using a model of a population of cells (each described using the principles outlined in Chapter 4) that also attempted to simulate the electrical properties of the extracellular space. Extracellular ionic gradients and shifts were not modeled explicitly. From a technical point of view, this model is tricky. Thus, in "classical" approaches to the EEG (see the Appendix to Chapter 7), the extracellular potential is regarded as passively reflecting the transmembrane currents of a population of neurons (and possibly glia). This vastly simplifies the analysis, because one can compute the extracellular potential at a single spatial location of interest, and because one need compute the extracellular potential no more frequently than it would be sampled experimentally (say at 1 or 2 kHz). But to understand how extracellular potentials themselves influence neuronal activity, extracellular potentials must be computed throughout the tissue of interest. The potentials must also be computed on a time scale at least as fast as field-induced interactions actually take place. In our experience, stable computations occur only when field potentials are updated every single time step, that is, every 50 μs. In combination, these two requirements present a daunting challenge.

Approach to simulation of the extracellular space. Our approach is schematically indicated in part A of Figure 8.2. The extracellular space is described as a three-dimensional lattice of "nodes." Internal nodes are connected by resistors to each of the six neighboring nodes. Two boundaries of the lattice are distinguished in that the nodes in these two faces

A   B

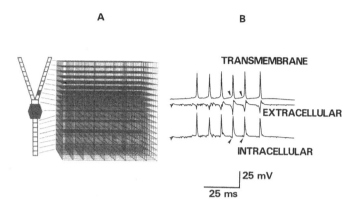

Figure 8.2. Simulation of action-potential synchronization via field-potential interactions. A: Structure of the calculation; 100 compartmental neurons were embedded in a three-dimensional resistive lattice representing the extracellular space; two faces of the lattice were grounded. Currents flowing through the extracellular space, caused by transmembrane currents, can perturb the membrane potentials of the cells. B: Synchronization of action potentials can occur provided the cells are excitable enough and provided the extracellular resistivity is sufficiently high. (From Traub et al., 1985b, with permission.)

are connected, through resistors, to ground (these faces are the ones in contact with the bathing medium). The other boundary faces are closed. The potential at node (i, j, k) represents the extracellular potential at "level" k for the neuron i, j (the neurons are arranged into a square or rectangular lattice). For neuron compartments 1 through 10, level k corresponds precisely to compartment k. For levels $k = 11-19$, we imagine compartment 11 as superimposed on compartment 20, 12 superimposed on 21, and so on. In effect, a node represents a *region* of extracellular space around some subsection of the neuronal membrane. By using a lattice as shown in Figure 8.2, and the definition of nodes given earlier, we are ignoring both the lateral spread of the dendrites and the packing of several neurons on top of each other in the stratum pyramidale. The next question is how to choose the resistances between lattice points. Here, we can attempt to use experimental measurements of tissue resistivity (all of which, to our knowledge, are along the axis orthogonal to the stratum pyramidale) and the fact that resistivity increases within the stratum pyramidale itself, as described earlier. Also, the model of a single cell is represented in electrotonic coordinates, with one compartment corresponding to 0.1λ of electrotonic length of dendrite; but electrotonic length is not so easy to define in the extracellular space, and it seems best to describe it in geometrical coordinates. In that case, because of dendrite branching, layers of the extracellular lattice get closer together as one moves away from the soma. In smaller dendrites, 0.1 λ corresponds to a smaller length of dendrite than for a larger dendrite (see Figure 4.1). [Although this approach is correct physically, our experience indicates that it is not essential for the qualitative demonstration of field interactions (Traub et al. (1985b).] In any case, the correspondence between our model and the actual slice was imprecise enough that we performed multiple simulations using a variety of extracellular resistivities and demonstrated that field effects become significant once the extracellular resistivity was larger than a threshold value.

Algorithm for simulations of field interactions. Chapter 4 presented the equations that describe the behavior of a single model neuron. Some of the variables in those equations were the membrane potentials $V_1, \ldots,$ V_{28}. Let us define new variables $V_1^{in}, \ldots, V_{28}^{in}$, which represent the potentials of the various compartments relative to a distant ground. We also have the local extracellular potentials, $V_1^{ex}, \ldots, V_{19}^{ex}$. The equations for one neuron are the same as before, except that where a transmembrane voltage appears (such as an argument for a rate function, or in an ionic-current term), we replace V_i with $V_i^{in} - V_i^{ex}$ ($i = 1$–19), or with $V_i^{in} - V_{i-9}^{ex}$ ($i = 20$–28). Likewise, in longitudinal current terms such as $\gamma_{i,i+1}(V_i - V_{i+1})$, we use instead $\gamma_{i,i+1}(V_i^{in} - V_{i+1}^{in})$.

The overall calculation proceeds as follows. First, we take an individual neuron. It has its membrane state variables, intracellular and extracellular potentials, injected currents, and synaptic inputs (if there are any) all defined. We can therefore integrate the differential equations that describe that neuron for one time step. All the transmembrane currents across all the membrane compartments of that neuron for that time step (both capacitative and ionic currents occur), as well as the new transmembrane potentials, can be calculated. We repeat this integration for all of the neurons. We now know all of the transmembrane currents everywhere. The next step is to calculate the new extracellular potentials. This involves applying Kirchhoff's law to all of the nodes in the extracellular lattice: We find a set of extracellular potentials so that at each node, the extracellular currents flowing into that node are exactly balanced by the transmembrane currents flowing into the node. Mathematically, this involves solving as many linear equations as there are extracellular nodes; a so-called iterative overrelaxation method has been used (Traub et al., 1985b; Varga, 1962). With the extracellular potentials and transmembrane potentials now known, it is easy to calculate the intracellular potentials, and the whole process is repeated.

Using this method, we analyzed the effects of low $[Ca^{2+}]_o$, assuming an enhanced cellular excitability and no chemical synaptic interactions, using first a 10×10 array of neurons (Traub et al., 1985b), and later an array with 2,000 neurons (Dudek and Traub, 1989). Calcium currents were blocked, and the cells were rendered hyperexcitable either by shifting the voltage-dependent rate functions along the voltage axis or by injecting depolarizing currents. With sufficiently high extracellular resistivity, synchronized population spikes occurred, just as they do experimentally (Figure 8.2), with brief negative transients in intracellular recordings referenced to ground. In small networks, three or four action potentials preceded large population spikes, the exact number depending on how similar were the intrinsic properties of the cells. Thus, if all the cells were precisely the same and were subjected to identical shocks, synchrony could occur without any cellular interaction. Essentially, the extracellular medium allows coupling[3] between cellular oscillators that have similar frequencies and so tend to produce coherent group oscillations. We also noted, particularly in large neuronal arrays, that synchrony could disappear – see Figure 4 of Dudek and Traub (1989) – even through cells continued to fire. Although repetitive population spikes do decline experimentally, as seen in Figure 1 of Taylor and Dudek (1984b), there appears also to be a simultaneous decrease in cellular firing.

Our simulations lend support to the concept that extracellular potentials can induce synchrony, but they are not definitive. Several experimental factors need to be further specified. For instance: (i) What is the mechanism of action-potential repolarization in a low-$[Ca^{2+}]_o$ medium? This if of interest because action potentials are normally repolarized, at least in part, by calcium-dependent currents (see Chapter 2). We have emphasized how extracellular currents induced by the inward I_{Na} are important for synchrony, but outward K currents may be important as well, and it is important to know the spatial localization and magnitude of such currents. (ii) How similar are the intrinsic properties of the neurons? This is critical for analyzing quantitatively synchrony induced by relatively weak intercellular forces. (iii) How does extracellular resistivity along axes parallel to the stratum pyramidale compare with the extracellular resistivity perpendicular to the stratum pyramidale? From a simulation point of view, we may note that a neuron now overlies its own extracellular space, an unrealistic approximation that helps to keep down the number of extracellular nodes. A more refined representation of the extracellular space might be appropriate.

Thus far, we have examined field interactions with chemical synapses blocked. Dudek and his colleagues have shown, however, that field effects probably are important during picrotoxin-induced synchronized bursts as well (Dudek et al., 1986; Snow and Dudek, 1984b). The evidence is similar to that for low-$[Ca^{2+}]_o$ bursts. Population spikes are aligned with action potentials in individual cells, and transmembrane depolarizations (intracellular negativities) often lead into the action potentials. Notice that a picrotoxin-induced synchronized burst has something in common with a low-$[Ca^{2+}]_o$ burst. The large excitatory synaptic

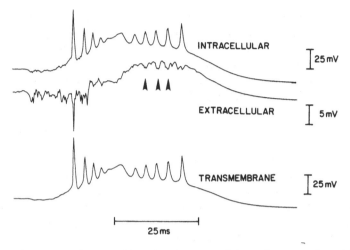

Figure 8.3. Phase-locking of action potentials to sharp transients in the epileptiform field potential occurs during picrotoxin-induced synchronized bursts (Snow and Dudek, 1984b). This phenomenon can be reproduced in the simulation shown here, when an excitatory synaptic network is combined with field-potential interactions, using the methods shown in Figure 8.2. (From Dudek and Traub, 1989, with permission.)

drive (see Chapter 6) during the picrotoxin bursts ensures that all the cells in the population are very excitable and that many of the cells are generating action potentials. One might expect that field effects should be observable. We have shown that field effects might synchronize action potentials during a synchronized burst (Figures 8.3 and 8.4) (Traub et al., 1985a). The technique involves combining the type of synaptic network model described in Chapters 5 and 6 with an extracellular lattice, as illustrated in Figure 8.2. The simulated epileptiform field potential becomes much smoother and more realistic than when field interactions are not included (cf. Figure 6.5). Note that in Figure 8.4 slow dendritic negativities occur during a synchronized burst. This reflects the location of excitatory recurrent synapses in both the apical and basilar dendrites of the model and probably of the slice.

The study of field interactions in the brain may be crucial to an understanding of the cellular mechanisms of epilepsy. Apparently, once initiated, a tonic seizure does not depend on synaptic transmission. How, then, should we view a connection between *interictal spikes* or synchronized bursts (which critically depend on excitatory synapses) and *seizures*? Certainly, an interictal-spike focus has an epidemiological correlation with clinical epilepsy, but is the connection causal, and if so, what mechanisms are involved? The issue is tricky, because in the evaluation of patients for epilepsy surgery one cannot assume that a patient's sei-

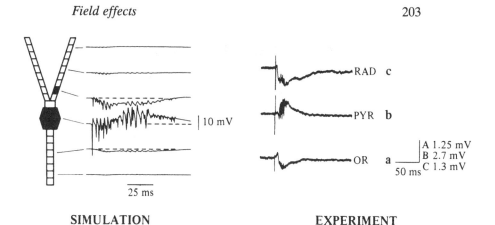

SIMULATION   EXPERIMENT

Figure 8.4. Left: Simulation of extracellular potentials at different dendritic levels in a model that includes both synaptic and field-potential interactions. The somatic field potential resembles experimental records (cf. Figure 3.13) much more than do simulated records when field potentials are not included (e.g., Figure 6.5). (From Traub et al., 1985a, with permission.) Right: Experimental records (rearranged from Swann et al., 1986a, with permission); note the different time scale. In both simulation and experiment there are slow negativities in dendritic layers and a slow positivity in the somatic layer. Excitatory synapses in the model are located in both apical and basilar dendrites (see Figure 4.2).

zures originate from that part of the brain where interictal spikes are most prominent, or where spikes are even detectable. We must at least consider the hypothesis, then, that various brain injuries render cortical tissue susceptible either to developing synchronized bursts (EEG spikes or interictal spikes) or to developing seizures by processes that are partly or completely independent. We must then consider carefully factors that regulate extracellular resistivity (e.g., the volume of the extracellular space) and ionic milieu in trying to understand epileptogenesis (Dietzel et al., 1980, 1982a,b; Heinemann et al., 1986; Traynelis and Dingledine, 1988, 1989a,b; Yaari et al., 1986).

9 Theoretical approaches: mathematical neural networks

The structural features of our hippocampal model are motivated by and largely supported by physiological experiments. In many ways the model works, generating cellular and neuronal population responses that look realistic. Nevertheless, the model is complicated. It involves a number of different parameters, simulations of the model use large amounts of computer time, and there is no obvious way to represent the model in a tractable set of equations. Can we simplify things and make a reduced model that retains "essential features" while gaining in physical or mathematical intuition? (This can be a dangerous game: Essential features may end up being defined as just those features that the reduced model exhibits.)

One approach was discussed briefly in Chapter 7 in the section on chaos: to take one signal generated by the model that represents its average behavior such as the number of pyramidal cells firing as a function of time. We then ask if this output has a small "dimension" (specifically, the correlation dimension). If it does, we might be able to construct a simple system to generate an output indistinguishable from the complex output. Such a system might have less than 15 or 20 variables or "degrees of freedom," as compared with the thousands of variables in the original system. This approach is intriguing (Babloyantz and Destexhe, 1986; Babloyantz et al, 1985). We need to emphasize that the results for the hippocampal model are extremely preliminary. Even if this approach works, we must remember that the average output may be only tenuously connected with the function of the underlying neuronal system. Although there is little direct proof, we imagine that the brain cares which cells are active, not just how many are active.

Another technique meriting consideration involves what we call "mathematical neural networks," a term intended to distinguish a class of abstract models whose goal may or may not be to describe a part of the brain faithfully. These interesting constructs are discussed in the next section.

General perspective[1]

What features do biological neuronal networks of the brain have in common with abstract neural networks? This question is important because abstract neural networks are of interest as physical systems in their own right: They shed light on the nature of certain kinds of computations; and they may have engineering applications (Hopfield and Tank, 1986). They comprise, in common with the brain (i) a large number of "elementary" units, each with comparable complexity (the complexity per unit being small for abstract neural networks, and large for biological networks), (ii) a large number of connections between neurons, or elements, (iii) a dynamical behavior that may not be readily apparent from the properties of the individual elements or of the connections; and (iv) a system with complementary descriptions. Both their dynamic behavior as *physical systems* and their computational behavior as *logical systems* may be described. We have already devoted considerable attention to topics (i)–(iii) for a particular biological neuronal network, the in vitro rodent CA3 region. Topic (iv) remains elusive, because we have no computational interpretation of the physical behavior of the CA3 region as yet. A major hurdle is that we cannot specify the spatiotemporal patterns of input to the CA3 region or the outputs from it. Without his type of experimental information, it is difficult either to formulate or to test a hypothesis on the computations that transform inputs to output.

It may be useful to describe briefly some types of mathematical neural networks that are currently of interest. Our list is, of course, not complete. Indeed, there is now a vast literature on neuronal networks, on computational neuroscience (particularly for vision), and on cognition approached from a network perspective (Churchland and Sejnowski, 1988; Sejnowski, Koch, and Churchland, 1988; Zipser and Andersen, 1988). We shall not even attempt to enter into all of this literature. Rather, we shall describe certain general approaches that have been taken.

The Hopfield model

First we consider a model often denoted the Hopfield model. For the following account we are indebted to the treatment of this subject by Hertz, Krogh, and Palmer (1990). This model is based on treatments of the statistical physics of "spin glasses" (Edwards and Anderson, 1975; Kirkpatrick and Sherrington, 1978), disordered physical systems that have many (locally) stable configurations. The Hopfield model is of interest as a physical system in its own right. It provides an example of how memories can be stored and retrieved in a distributed network of simple elements with local interactions. A body of theory has built up around it; see, for example, the papers of Amit, Gutfreund, and Sompolinsky (1985a,b).

The Hopfield model is a system with N different spins S_i, with $S_i = \pm 1$. In the context of a "neural" network, "$S_i = +1$" is used to mean "neuron i is firing at its maximum rate," and "$S_i = -1$" means "neuron i is firing at its minimum rate." The term "spin" for the S_i reflects the history of this subject, deriving some of its motivation from magnetic systems. Each spin has an interaction with all other spins. These interactions are described by a set of real numbers T_{ij}, $(i,j = 1, \ldots, N)$, and in the Hopfield model it is usually assumed that the T matrix is symmetric, that is, that $T_{ij} = T_{ji}$ for all i and j. One way for the Hopfield model to evolve in time is this: Pick a spin i at random, and calculate the "field" it experiences, called h_i, where $h_i = \sum_{j=1}^{N} T_{ij} S_j$. Then, with probability $1/(1 + e^{-2\beta h_i})$, set $S_i = +1$; otherwise, set $S_i = -1$. (Here, β is a parameter playing the role of inverse temperature.) Now, randomly pick a new spin, and repeat the process. Because of the symmetry of the T matrix, it can be shown that a Hamiltonian, or energy function, exists: $H(S_1, \ldots, S_n) = -\sum_{ij} T_{ij} S_i S_j$. The Hamiltonian is a function associated with each state $\vec{S} = \{S_1, \ldots, S_n\}$ of the system. At zero temperature ($\beta = \infty$), it has the property of being nonincreasing with time; this can be verified directly from the dynamical rule (stated earlier) by checking what happens to the energy when one spin is altered. The Hamiltonian defines the temperature-dependent distribution of states at thermal equilibrium. Specifically, this distribution is the Boltzmann distribution, so that the probability of finding the system in a region R of its phase space is proportional to $\sum_{S \in R} e^{-\beta H(S)}$, where the sum is taken over all states S in the region R, and β is the inverse temperature. Such a system can have multiple stable states or metastable states that can be viewed as memories or "answers." (A stable state or a metastable state is a state such that single spin flips increase H; stable states globally minimize H. At zero temperature, a metastable or stable state can be considered as a fixed point of a dynamical system.) Computation consists in letting the system settle into a metastable or stable state, that is, a local or global minimum of its Hamiltonian, respectively. [To be precise, the *free energy* is minimized (Amit et al., 1985a), but we shall not pursue this.] A system of this sort can be constructed so that at least some of the fixed points are specified in advance, provided one does not try to specify too many fixed points. The way this is done is as follows: Let the desired fixed points be denoted ξ^α, $\alpha = 1, \ldots, r$. The state of spin i for ξ^α is denoted ξ_i^α. In the original Hopfield model, one "encodes" the memories so that the ξ_i^α behave as independent random variables. We construct the desired network by defining the

$$T_{ij} = \frac{1}{N} \sum_{a=1}^{r} \xi_i^a \xi_j^a.$$

To check that a particular ξ^a is stable (i.e., after a small perturbation of ξ^a at zero temperature, the system tends to return to ξ^a), we calculate h_i for $S_i = \xi_i^a$. If h_i has the same sign as ξ_i^a, then ξ^a will tend to be stable (see the preceding dynamical rules). But

$$h_i = \sum_{j=1}^{N} T_{ij} S_j = \frac{1}{N} \sum_{j,\alpha} \xi_i^\alpha \xi_j^\alpha \xi_j^a = \frac{1}{N} \sum_j \xi_i^a (\xi_j^a)^2 + \frac{1}{N} \sum_{j,\alpha \neq a} \xi_i^\alpha \xi_j^\alpha \xi_j^a$$

so

$$h_i = \xi_i^a + \frac{1}{N} \sum_{j,\alpha \neq a} \xi_i^\alpha \xi_j^\alpha \xi_j^a$$

The first term certainly has the same sign as S_i, because it is S_i. If the spins in the different memory states are randomly distributed, the expected value of the second term is zero. The second term will be the sum of $N(r - 1)$ random variables, each of value $\pm 1/N$ with equal probability, and so each with variance $1/N^2$. With N large, the second term will have a Gaussian distribution with variance

$$\frac{N(r - 1)}{N^2} = \frac{r - 1}{N}$$

and standard deviation

$$\sigma = \sqrt{\frac{r - 1}{N}}$$

Thus, if r, the number of memories, is small relative to N, the second term will be small also. It follows that the ξ^α are indeed stable "memories."

An unfortunate side effect of this construction of the T_{ij} is that local energy minima may exist that are not included among the $\{\xi^\alpha\}$; these may be considered "false memories." The spin-glass model behaves as a content-addressable memory. Starting from a state S that is "close" to one of the $\{\xi^\alpha\}$, the system will evolve toward that ξ^α. Unfortunately, the time required for the system to actually reach the particular ξ^α can be long. The argument for this depends not on displaying equations of motion but on demonstrating the existence of pairs of states that are distinct at a large number of sites, but still have energies that are similar.

For the Hamiltonian to exist, the connections must be symmetric, that is, $T_{ij} = T_{ji}$. To see this, suppose that S_i connects to S_j. A Hamiltonian, were it to exist, would have to contain a term with $S_i \times S_j$, so that S_j must influence S_i. Without a Hamiltonian, analytical calculations of the behavior of the system become more complicated.

Variations of Hopfield networks form an active field of study. For example, one can make the connections nonsymmetric. Even in this non-Hamiltonian case, it may be possible to find T_{ij} that make certain predefined spin states stable fixed points in the dynamics. In general, however, complicated trajectories might appear. A general classification of the different dynamical behaviors (periodic orbits, chaotic attractors, and so on) may be difficult.

Even when the "neurons" are not simple spins (equal to ± 1), but rather are simple electrical devices with capacitance, leakage resistance, and a threshold output function, and the connections serve to inject current into the different "neurons," the system still "computes" a local minimun of its energy function. Hopfield and Tank (1986) have shown how a network can be constructed whose energy function is defined cleverly in advance. They give examples of particular energy functions that represent well-known problems in combinatorial optimization, such as the traveling-salesman problem. By evolving onto a local minimum, the network, in effect, finds a "good" (but not generally the optimum) solution of the optimization problem. However, two features of these networks offer points for critical comparison with biological neuronal networks. First, the connections between elements are symmetrical. Second, the energy minima, or fixed points, are states in which some of the neurons are sending their maximal output, while others are sending their minimal output.

Basically, Hopfield networks and their variations suggest that memories are encoded in the long-term equilibrium behavior of a dynamical system. In the case of symmetric connections in the original Hopfield model, $T_{ij} = T_{ji}$, the long-term evolution is defined by a number of fixed points. For more general kinds of dynamical systems, the long-term behavior may be defined by periodic orbits or by one or more chaotic attractors. In the latter case, the memory might be encoded somehow in the geometrical structure of the attractor. The idea that a memory corresponds to the geometry of an equilibrium attractor or fixed point is attractive because of its mathematical elegance, but it should be viewed with caution. It remains unclear that equilibrium behaviors can be reached in the short times that we know it takes for a real brain to recall a memory. Many recognition tasks do in fact take place within hundreds of milliseconds. The equilibrium view might be appropriate, however, in other biological contexts, where, for example, memory does require a long time.

Layered neural networks

Another neural network architecture that may be useful for pattern recognition and other tasks is the layered neural network without feedback (Rumelhart, Hinton, and Williams, 1986). Here, the set of "neurons" is partitioned into k subsets or "layers." Neurons of layer j send their output to some or all of the "neurons" of layer $j + 1$. Layer-1 neurons are input cells, and layer-k neurons are output cells. Layered networks are most interesting when $k > 2$, so that there are intermediate layers of "hidden units." Typically, each connection (say from cell i to cell j) has a weight attached to it, w_{ij}. During a time step of operation, each cell i generates an output S_i, a real number, which it sends equally to all of its followers. Cell j then computes its own S_j, which generally takes the form $f(\Sigma_{i \to j} w_{ij} S_i)$, the sum being taken over all neurons i that send outputs to neuron j. In the actual use of the network for, say, a pattern-recognition task, there are two phases, a learning phase and an operation phase. In the learning phase, one wants to choose all the w_{ij} in some optimal sense. One needs, of course, to define "optimal." Let us define the operation of the network, for a given set of $\{w_{ij}\}$, as a map from the set of states of the input neurons, I, to the set of states of the output neurons, O, so that $N(\{w_{ij}\}) : I \to O$; the notation implies that the map N depends on all of the w_{ij}. Suppose that for each state $s \; \varepsilon \; I$ there is a desired state $t \; \varepsilon \; O$, denoted $t = D(s)$. Suppose further that there is a well-defined numerical measure of how far $D(s)$ is from $N(\{w_{ij}\})(s)$, called $m[D(s), \, N(\{w_{ij}\})(s)]$. We want to choose the w_{ij} so as to minimize the expected value, over all inputs s, weighted with respect to their chances of occurrence, of $m[D(s), \, N(\{w_{ij}\})(s)]$. The back-propagation algorithm, derived from the chain rule of the differential calculus (Rumelhart et al., 1986), applies to this general situation. Although we have tried to specify the performance of the network clearly, in practical situations it may be difficult to specify exactly the measure m, the "desired" output map D for all inputs, and the appropriate probability measure on the set of all inputs. For this reason, much of the work in this field tends to involve simulations. Layered networks have been used to model certain aspects of information processing in the primate visual system (Zipser and Andersen, 1988).

For mathematical neural networks to enhance our comprehension of the behavior of collections of nerve cells in the brain, a comparison of their respective features may be useful. Such a comparison can constrain both the structure and dynamics of a more abstract network model. This has been an important motivation for the techniques and the problems that we address in this book.

Comparison of the CA3 region with mathematical neural networks

Structural comparison. First, the CA3 region does not consist of discrete layers with connections only between layers. Instead, connections contain multiple cycles, and indeed every cell can be expected to lie on multiple cycles (Traub et al., 1984). This feature of the model is supported by the experimental observation that intracellular stimulation of at least one-third of the neurons can lead, when inhibition is blocked, to a synchronized discharge in the entire population (Miles and Wong, 1983). The figures in this book likewise illustrate how stimulation of a single cell can elicit a population burst involving that same cell (Figures 6.12 and 6.13). This cannot happen in a layered network. Another factor suggesting that the CA3 network is not layered is that synchronized waves of firing can propagate across the slice in both directions (Knowles et al., 1987; Miles et al., 1988). Although the hippocampus encodes information, at least in part, by modification of synaptic efficacies, the physical significance of modifying a particular synapse or set of synapses is not clear in a system of complex network topology with multiple reentrant loops.

Second, the recurrent excitatory connections in the hippocampus seem not to be symmetrical. So if cell a monosynaptically excites cell b, cell b need not excite a. In fact, we have never observed reciprocal excitatory connections in 22 monosynaptically connected pairs of cells. Thus, the network does not possess a structural feature of the "classical" Hopfield model necessary for the definition of a Hamiltonian.

Functional comparison. Finally, the CA3 region, at least in vitro, lacks another cardinal feature of (Hamiltonian) spin-glass systems used as models of memory (Hopfield, 1982; Hopfield and Tank, 1986). In such models, a memory corresponds to a fixed point in a dynamical system, wherein each cell is firing at either its maximal or its minimal rate. But the CA3 region, so far as we can determine, does not settle into any equilibrium behavior, consisting of constant firing rates for all of the cells. Thus, there is no fixed point in the CA3 dynamical system. Rather, the system as a whole oscillates, although oscillations may be difficult to recognize in individual cells. Therefore, if memories are encoded in firing patterns of CA3 neurons, the coding scheme appears not to consist in assigning a particular firing rate to each individual neuron. Another important point to consider is the apparent instability[2] of hippocampal networks, at least simulated ones. We showed that exciting 1 cell out of 9,000 during a partially synchronized burst was sufficient to change the composition (although not the mean frequency) of all future partially synchronized bursts. The classical Hopfield model, on the other hand, at least at low temperatures, is stable to perturbations when it is near a "memory"; indeed, this is the whole point of using it as a content-addressable memory.

On the other hand, we remain unclear how to construct an abstract network to represent the CA3 region. We must include some representation of intrinsic currents and synaptic actions of both long and short durations. In contrast, the dynamics of a spin glass do not include the past: Its future evolution depends on the present spins. But in the CA3 region, all collective phenomena seem to depend critically on the way past events, such as slowly relaxing intrinsic or synaptic conductances, are represented in the present. This should be the starting point for a biological (or at least hippocampal) theory of neuronal networks. Progress has been made in this direction (Pytte, Grinstein, and Traub, in press).

Comparison with other oscillatory systems. Although repeated simulations allow us to examine the effects of changing parameters, such as synaptic strengths, we have no analytical theory that provides quantitative results without the simulations. It is well to consider some reasons why the analysis of this system is difficult. Why is it not just another example of a set of coupled oscillators? Systems of coupled oscillators may lend themselves to mathematical analysis provided the coupling is weak, so that the effect of an input to one oscillator from another is to advance or delay its phase (Ermentrout and Kopell, 1984; Kopell and Ermentrout, 1986), an idea that has been applied to the analysis of swimming in lampreys (Cohen, 1987). However, the effect of synaptic inputs, either excitatory or inhibitory, is extremely powerful in the CA3 region, so that under proper conditions one cell can evoke a burst in another, or one inhibitory input can abort a burst that might otherwise occur. The system then has some aspects of a switching network, but the multiplicity of possible states of each neuron, and the long durations of some of the transmitter-induced and intrinsic currents, make it easier to describe the cells with differential equations than as logical devices. We do not yet know what form a proper mathematical analysis of CA3 circuitry will take.

In some very general sense, the CA3 region has features similar to those of systems studied in statistical physics: a large number of elements, each of which interacts with some of the others. But, to put this in context, such systems, even those characterized by just one parameter (e.g., percolation problems on an infinite lattice), can lead to mathematical theories of depth and difficulty (Essam, 1972). One source of the difficulty is that the objects of study are infinite and full of rich structure, and the details are important. For example, an analysis of the distribution of finite cluster sizes, near the critical percolation probability (Kesten, 1982; Stauffer, 1985), requires counting the number of clusters of a given size but having a distinct shape. Combinatorial problems of this sort are quite delicate. The brain problem not only has many more parameters, but inescapably involves time, because the system evolves in time. In addition, there are numerous time constants for each neuron, so formal descriptions of neuronal interactions are difficult. We cannot expect a simple reduction of the problem to a simple system – rather, the problem might go away. The difficulty arises from the size of the system and the randomness, as well as from the complexity of the individual elements and synapses. The Appendix to this chapter suggests that some of the ideas involved in the analysis of time-dependent percolations may still provide useful physical insight. The examples discussed in the Appendix have some general features in common with synchronization occurring in a network of neurons, although the details of the respective systems are, of course, very different.

Appendix: Percolation theory *by Lawrence S. Schulman*[3]

Percolation theory is abstracted from problems of the following sorts.

Groundwater percolation. Rain falls on soil, either porous or not so porous. Does it pass through this soil to underground reservoirs, or does it flow away? One pictures the soil as a collection of stones and the like, with variously distributed small passages for the water. If there are routes of linked passages from the surface to the reservoir, then the water can percolate. Here is an abstract model for this problem: Imagine a three-dimensional lattice built of pipes, a gigantic jungle gym. Between each pair of vertices, each pipe has a faucet that may be open or closed. The flow problem then consists of finding a path of open pipes from one end of the lattice to the other. Suppose that for each faucet we fix its state by making an independent coin flip, using a biased coin such that there is probability p of the faucet being open. Clearly, the larger p, the more likely it will be that flow will be possible; moreover, when flow is possible, the amount of flow will also grow with p.

Forest fire. A tree is struck by lightning. It catches fire. If there is a second tree sufficiently close and if the conditions of moisture, and so forth, are suitable, the fire will spread. Similar conditions govern the possibility of further spreading and will determine whether the original fire is restricted to one tree or a small cluster of trees, or whether it becomes a forestwide conflagration. Again, an abstract model can be made. This time, we use a two-dimensional lattice, each vertex representing a tree. For the line connecting each pair of adjacent vertices, we flip a biased coin and with some probability p color the line red. The red-connected pairs are trees such that if one of them is burning, the other will catch fire as a result. (In a windy forest, one might have separate probabilities for the two directions of potential transmission. This would be *directed percolation*.) For small p, no matter which tree was originally struck by the lightning bolt, the resulting cluster of burnt trees will be small. With increasing p, the likelihood of finding a path of red bonds from one end of the forest to the other increases.

Epidemiology. A sick traveler enters a city that is otherwise free of his disease. He comes in contact with several people, some of whom contract the disease. After a few days, and perhaps before they realize they are ill, these people pass on the disease to some of those with whom they come in contact. The ultimate containment or spread of the disease is again suitable for modeling by percolation (at least if one takes a simplified view of the immune system).

The various factors of degree of contact, state of general health, possible previous immunity, and so on, may be subsumed into a single parameter, p, representing the transmission probability. The progress of the epidemic will then be strongly dependent on this parameter. This system differs from the previous examples in two important ways. First, one would not put the points on a lattice. People move around, and bonds could be drawn between far-flung individuals. Second, the element of time enters because (in the model system we are considering) an individual could be reinfected.

The abstract model for the epidemiological problem is more complicated than the models described, but we shall treat it in detail because it resembles the physiological problems encountered in analyzing the behavior of neuronal networks with recurrent excitatory interconnections. We describe the city C by the list of its N inhabitants: $\{A_1, A_2, \ldots, A_N\}$. To simplify the introduction of time, we imagine that disease transmissions occur in lock step; that is, time is discrete. We assume that the disease is transmissible during the time interval between lock steps (say 1 week) and that we count the number of sick individuals at discrete times. We therefore introduce a variable t that measures time in weeks. Now for the abstract model. We make a copy of the city for every value of t; this gives us sets $C_1, C_2, C_3, \ldots$. Imagine a line drawn from an individual in C_t to some other individual in C_{t+1}. This is illustrated in Figure 9.1 for $N = 3$, $t = 1, 2, 3$. Again, we take a biased coin, and with probability p color each of the bonds red. A red bond between A_1 at $t = 1$ and A_3 at $t = 2$ means this: If A_1 were sick at $t = 1$, then A_3 would be sick at $t = 2$. The parameter p combines the likelihood of two individuals meeting, their respective states of health, and so on. Let A_1 be the sick traveler. Then the disease will be persistent if there is a path of red bonds beginning at $A_1, t = 1$ (when A_1 entered the city), that continues indefinitely (through various individuals) for larger and larger t. Figure 9.2 shows a path that persists for five steps among four individuals. Only the red bonds are shown. Notice that the model allows reinfection of a given individual on successive time steps and infection from more than one source. Variations of the model can be introduced to include effects of immunity.

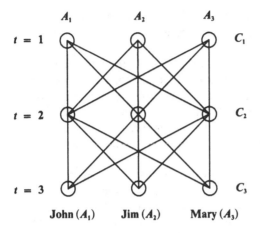

Figure 9.1. Possible bonds between individuals for times (1 → 2) and (2 → 3).

The simplified epidemiological model without immunity was introduced for didactic purposes by Schulman and Seiden (1986), and the disease was given the name "percolitis." In a moment we shall explore quantitative aspects of this model, but for now we want to take up three points that one should consider before getting involved in details. First, what does this have to do with physiology? Second, how good is the model, and are its defects important? Third, because such models are very general and describe other systems in addition to those for which they were invented, what can be learned from anything so general?

The connection with physiology occurs in the following way. In the epidemiological model, the parameter p lumps together a number of factors relating to interpersonal contact, prior disease exposure, and the like. Imagine now that the A_i represent pyramidal neurons, that "having the disease" is interpreted as "is bursting," and that the presence of a red bond represents transmission of bursting from one cell to another. Again, the parameter p lumps together diverse aspects of the topology of the system (whether or not two cells are connected, analogous to A_i meeting A_j) and its functional state (e.g., whether or not the postsynaptic cell is refractory – "immune" – how many inhibitory cells are recruited, and so on). This representation clearly cannot capture all of the richness of the original neuronal system, but might still provide insight into how inhibition can regulate the extent of synchrony in the network. A model of percolitis with immunity might similarly provide insight into oscillatory behavior in neuronal networks.

How good is the model? For the applications with which this contributor (L.S.S.) is familiar, the most important defect in the model concerns the absence of correlations. Consider the eponymous problem, ground-

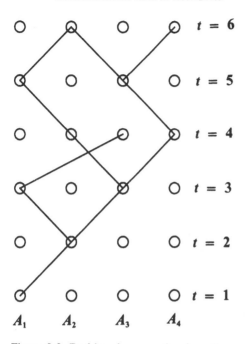

Figure 9.2. Red bonds emanating from the source A_1 at $t = 1$.

water percolation. Suppose the flow can occur both because of spaces between small stones and because of cracks in larger rocks. The cracks may not be randomly distributed, but may have a tendency to cluster near one another. (This is a *positive correlation*. Given a crack through some point $\vec{x}$, the likelihood of a crack through a nearby point $\vec{y}$ is larger than the a priori probability for such a crack had no information about $\vec{x}$ been given.) With clustering of the cracks, it may be easier for the water to find a channel than it would have been had the cracks been randomly distributed. For the epidemiological problem, the city might be divided into groups of people who do not mix much with one another. In such a case, the red bonds should not be distributed homogeneously over all possible pairs (this is analogous to the statistically localized connectivity in the longitudinal hippocampal slice). Clearly, this will have important consequences for the confinement of the disease. Even more, the awareness of the disease may itself modify the validity of the model, as for example, if measures were taken to reduce spread (measures that might reduce p or invalidate the random-bond assumption). For the physiological problem, presumably there is a great deal of structure in the connectivity of the neurons, but that may not be essential for the issue of global bursting or globally synchronized population oscillations. The absorption, however, of synaptic inhibition in an effectively reduced value of p seems more suspect, and one ought perhaps to introduce a more serious modification of the model to treat this.

Finally, can anything useful or interesting be learned from a model that flaunts so blatantly its lack of specificity? That the answer to this question can be yes is one of the achievements of the scientific discipline known as statistical physics. There are subtle phenomena that arise from the collective behavior of many large physical systems. Such phenomena occur broadly and are often independent of the details of the system; nevertheless, their occurrence may not be the least bit obvious. It may be obvious that an epileptiform synchronized event should occur when p is large enough, but it is not so obvious that fluctuation or oscillatory phenomena should be predictable from general principles. The entire topic of *universality* and *critical exponents* provides examples of yet more subtle consequences. We refer the reader to Fisher (1961), Hammersley (1961), Shante and Kirkpatrick (1971), Kesten (1982), Stauffer (1985), and Schulman (in press) for further information on the field, and to Schulman and Seiden (1982, 1986) for an example where these general ideas are sufficient to explain the spiral arms in disk galaxies. Finally, in the detailed discussion to follow, some inkling of the power of the general method may be felt.

We turn to a quantitative treatment of the percolitis problem, both with and without immunity. Recall that we have a city of N people and that t is an integer measuring the number of weeks since the original infected traveler arrived. The effective transmission probability between a pair of individuals is p. For convenience, we define the constant x by $x = pN$. Let $n(t)$ be the number of sick people during week t, and let $\rho(t) = n(t)/N$ be the sick fraction of the population, or the probability that a randomly selected individual is sick. Let us compute the probability that a particular individual is healthy during week $t + 1$. By definition, this is $1 - \rho(t + 1)$. On the other hand, this individual will be healthy only if all transmission "attempts" from the previous week have failed. There have been $n(t)$ such attempts, each with failure probability $1 - p$. Because the attempts are statistically independent, the probability that all disease transmission attempts have failed is $(1 - p)^{n(t)}$. Equating the two expressions for this individual to be healthy, we have

$$1 - \rho(t + 1) = (1 - p)^{n(t)} \tag{1}$$

Using our definitions and rearranging slightly, this becomes

$$\rho(t + 1) = 1 - \left(1 - \frac{x}{N}\right)^{N\rho(t)} = 1 - \left(1 - \frac{x\rho(t)}{N\rho(t)}\right)^{N\rho(t)}$$

Recall that the exponential e^y can be written as the limit for $N \to \infty$ of $(1 + y/N)^N$. It follows that for large N [and $\rho(t)$ bounded away from zero]

$$\rho(t + 1) = 1 - e^{-x\rho(t)} \tag{2}$$

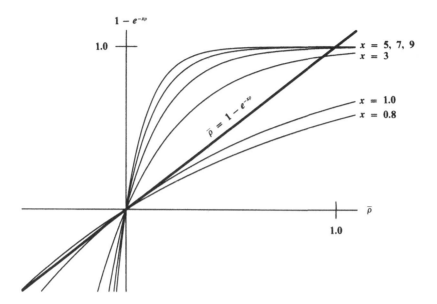

Figure 9.3. Left and right sides of equation (3) plotted as a function of $\bar{\rho}$, for various x.

This is the fundamental law for the average progress of the disease. Our first question is this: Will the disease persist, or will it go away? Suppose $\rho(t)$ tends to some asymptotic value, $\bar{\rho}$, that may or may not be zero. Then equation (2) becomes

$$\bar{\rho} = 1 - e^{-x\bar{\rho}} \tag{3}$$

This is a transcendental equation, which for all x has the solution $\bar{\rho} = 0$. However, there is a second real root that we can discover by plotting the left and right sides of equation (3) as a function of $\bar{\rho}$. This is illustrated in Figure 9.3.

Because $\bar{\rho}$ must be nonnegative to be physically meaningful, it is only for $x > 1$ that the nonzero solution makes sense. Thus, for $x < 1$ (or $p < 1/N$), the disease dies out. This is reasonable: x is the expected number of people that any sick individual may infect at a given time step. If each person infects, on average, less than one other, then the disease should eventually disappear. For $x > 1$, we appear to have two choices, but in fact only the nonzero solution is stable (and hence able to represent an asymptotic value for $\bar{\rho}$). That is, if we start the iteration of $\rho(t)$ with some nonzero value [using equation (2)], and if $x > 1$, the number of sick people will increase until it approaches the positive root $\bar{\rho}$ illustrated in Figure 9.3. We shall not prove this explicitly, although it follows from another calculation that we are about to do. Thus, $\bar{\rho}$ is a function of x (or p). This function is shown in Figure 9.4.

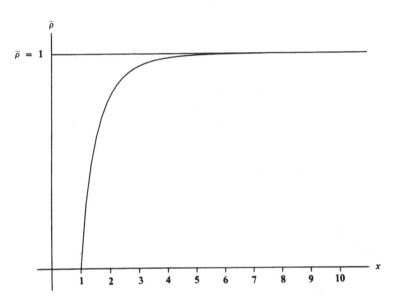

Figure 9.4. Equilibrium value of the fraction of diseased individuals as a function of the transmission probability p, where $x = Np$.

Of interest is the rate at which the system approaches equilibrium. Consider the root $\bar{\rho} = 0$, and consider the asymptotic time dependence of $\rho(t)$ as it approaches zero. Take equation (2) and expand in powers of the (supposed) small $\rho(t)$ to lowest relevant order:

$$\rho(t+1) = 1 - \left[1 - x\rho(t) \quad + \frac{x^2}{2}\rho(t)^2 + \cdots\right] \qquad (4a)$$

$$\cong x\rho(t) \quad - \frac{x^2}{2}\rho(t)^2 \qquad (4b)$$

where terms of order $\rho(t)^3$ are neglected. As $\rho(t) \to 0$, only the first term in equation (4b) need be kept, and we see that successive values of $\rho(t)$ are a factor x smaller (or larger, depending on whether $x < 1$ or $x > 1$) than their predecessors. Once in the small-ρ regime, we have

$$\rho(t) \sim x^t \times \text{constant} \qquad (5)$$

Thus, $\rho(t) \to 0$ precisely when $x < 1$. Defining the positive constant γ by $x = \exp(-\gamma)$, equation (5) becomes

$$\rho(t) = (\text{constant})e^{-\gamma t} \qquad (6)$$

The relaxation is therefore exponential, and γ is the relaxation rate. It follows that for $x > 1$ (i.e., $\gamma < 0$), the zero solution for $\bar{\rho}$ is not stable, and because there is only one other real root, it should be the attractor.[4]

Finally, we come to the question of what happens for $x = 1$ exactly. This is of particular interest because it illustrates the point made earlier about the ability to make rather general statements despite minimal detailed physiological information.

For $x = 1$, it is necessary to keep the second term in equation (4b), for otherwise nothing happens. The equation then reads

$$\rho(t + 1) = \rho(t) - \frac{1}{2} \rho(t)^2 \tag{7}$$

For this iteration rule, $\rho(t)$ goes to zero, but not exponentially. To the leading approximation, the solution to equation (7) is

$$\rho(t) = \frac{2}{t} \tag{8}$$

as can be verified by substitution.[5] By the standards of exponential decay, this is extremely slow. What is happening in our imaginary city is that if several people become ill, it will be quite possible for the disease to spread fairly widely before ultimately fading away. The slow decay of $\rho(t)$ reflects the propensity of the system to sustain large fluctuations. These large fluctuations are the hallmark of what is known in statistical physics terminology as *critical phenomena*. The behavior of the network of CA3 neurons at intermediate strengths of synaptic inhibition may exhibit critical phenomena (see Figures 7.5 and 7.17).

Finally, we shall consider a version of percolitis in which some minor complications have been introduced. First, this will show that the model is flexible enough to allow variation. Second, the particular complications will provide qualitatively new phenomena. Third, something like these phenomena do occur in neurophysiology.

Our first modification is to allow an individual to spread the disease for 2 weeks, not just 1 week. Thus, an apparently well individual has some probability q of transmitting the disease in the week following his illness. By the same logic that was used to derive equation (1), we obtain

$$1 - \rho(t + 1) = (1 - p)^{n(t)} (1 - q)^{n(t-1)} \tag{9}$$

Recalling that $p = x/N$, and defining $q = y/N$, the large-N form of equation (9) is

$$\rho(t + 1) = 1 - e^{-x\rho(t) - y\rho(t-1)} \tag{10}$$

which is a mild extension of equation (2). Our second modification is conceptually richer and is the introduction of *immunity*. We postulate that for the week following a bout of percolitis an individual cannot again fall prey to the disease (even though he can transmit it to others). This is a short-term immunity. It also has a clear analogy with one type of refractory behavior of neurons (but not the long-duration refractoriness produced by $g_{K[Ca]}$). To introduce this effect into our equations, we merely multiply the right-hand side of equation (10) by $[1 - \rho(t)]$. To justify this, imagine the appearance of the graph of the city at time $t + 1$, before we allow for immunity. There are occupied (red) bonds coming from time t and time $t - 1$, each such red bond allowing transmission of the disease. Some of these will not "take," precisely because their targets were sick at time t. The fraction of such failures is $\rho(t)$, because that is the sick fraction of time t. Therefore, to calculate the fraction that will fall ill, we multiply by $1 - \rho(t)$.

We thus find the equation for the time evolution of the expected fraction of sick people for the case of 2-week contagion and 1-week immunity to be

$$\rho(t + 1) = [1 - e^{-x\rho(t) - y\rho(t-1)}][1 - \rho(t)] \qquad (11)$$

For $x + y < 1$, this model shares the properties of the simpler system in that the only equilibrium is $\rho = 0$. For values of $x + y$ greater than 1, there is again a positive solution to equation (11) with $\rho(t - 1) = \rho(t + 1)$, that is, a nonzero disease level. But in contrast to the former situation, that solution may not be stable. For y sufficiently large, the system begins to oscillate. Thus, for $x = 1$ and $y = 0.5$, the system reaches a steady state, with $\rho(t - 1) = \rho(t) = \rho(t + 1) \ldots \cong 0.21826$. However, for $x = 1$ and $y = 3$, the system [starting from $\rho(0) \sim \rho(1) \sim 0.01$] first (in about 50–100 time steps) approaches $\rho \sim 0.45$, but does not quite stabilize there. Successive time steps overshoot or undershoot this value, and the difference from the average slowly grows in time. After another 200 steps, successive time steps have ρ going between 0.25 and 0.67. Finally, perhaps 500 steps later, we find the system completely stabilized and taking successive values 0.2219 and 0.7023 (average 0.462).

For systems that can exist in many possible states, it is helpful to display the preferred state as a function of system parameters. Our "system" so far has three states: $\rho = 0$, $\rho = $ constant > 0, and ρ oscillatory. Our parameters are x and y (both ≥ 0), and what we know so far is that $\rho = 0$ corresponds to $x + y \leq 1$. What we do not yet know is the behavior on the other side of the line $x + y = 1$. For which x and y do we get $\rho = $ constant, and for which is ρ oscillatory? We shall calculate the detailed answer to that question later, but we would like to give our conclusions in graphic form before getting involved in algebra. The answer is that there exists a curve, y as a function of x, such that for (x, y) above that curve we get oscillations, and below it a steady state. This is illustrated in Figure 9.5. Region A is below the line $y = 1 - x$ and represents $\rho = 0$. The curve between regions B and C is that mentioned earlier, a curve that separates the steady rate (region B) from oscillatory behavior. Such a diagram is analogous to solid-liquid-gas phase diagrams in physics. One can easily imagine the usefulness of this kind of diagram (or a higher-dimensional

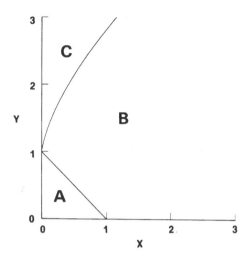

Figure 9.5. Phase diagram for percolitis model with 2-week contagion. In region A $(x + y < 1)$, the only stable solution is $\rho_{xy} = 0$. In region B, a stable solution exists, given by $\rho_{xy}/(1 - \rho_{xy}) = 1 - e^{-(x+y)\rho_{xy}}$. In region C, oscillatory (but not steady-state) solutions exist. The boundary between regions B and C is defined by the equation $y = x + 1/(1 - \rho_{xy})$, where ρ_{xy} is defined by the previous equation.

version) in brain studies. One might have several parameters (e.g., the strengths of different types of synapses) such that as lines (or surfaces or hypersurfaces) are crossed in the parameter space, qualitatively different behaviors occur, perhaps significant changes in oscillation frequencies or epileptiform phenomena.

The actual calculation of the curve separating regions B and C in Figure 9.5 proceeds by taking a putative steady-state value of ρ and checking it for stability under the time-evolution equation, equation (11). A steady-state value of ρ, call it $\bar{\rho}$, must satisfy

$$\bar{\rho} = (1 - \exp[-(x + y)\bar{\rho}])(1 - \bar{\rho}) \qquad (12)$$

Consider a small deviation from this value

$$\rho(t) = \bar{\rho} + \eta(t) \qquad (13)$$

Insert this $\rho(t)$ into equation (11) and expand, keeping only lowest-order terms in $\eta(t)$. This yields

$$\eta(t + 1) = [x\eta(t) + y\eta(t - 1)](1 - 2\bar{\rho}) - \frac{\bar{\rho}}{1 - \bar{\rho}}\eta(t) \qquad (14)$$

This linear homogeneous equation for $\eta(t)$ has a solution of the form

$$\eta(t) = s^t \qquad (15)$$

with s a number, in general complex. The original solution $\bar{\rho}$ will be stable if $|s| < 1$. By substituting equation (15) in (14), we find that s satisfies

$$s^2 = (xs + y)(1 - 2\bar{\rho}) - \frac{\bar{\rho}}{1 - \bar{\rho}} s \tag{16}$$

Clearly, this can be solved for general $\bar{\rho}$, but for our purposes we need only the locus of a particular breakdown in stability, namely, the transition from $\rho(t) \to$ constant to $\rho(t) \to \bar{\rho} +$ (small term changing sign on successive time steps). In terms of $\eta(t)$ and the solution of equation (15), this corresponds to $s = -1$. Inserting $s = -1$ into equation (16) and manipulating terms gives for the breakdown locus

$$y - x = \frac{1}{1 - \bar{\rho}} \tag{17}$$

When one views $\bar{\rho}$ as an implicit function of x and y [as given by equation (12)], equation (17) becomes the equation for the curve separating regions B and C in Figure 9.5.

There is actually quite a bit more information in equation (16) than is displayed in the figure. For values of (x, y) near the curve, one obtains the growth or decay rates of oscillations. For applications, it may also be important to know the values ρ takes when it settles into its oscillatory mode. For our problem, this can be found by taking equation (11) at two successive time steps and defining two unknowns $u = \rho(t - 1) = \rho(t + 1)$ and $v = \rho(t) = \rho(t + 2)$. In general, though, things are not so easy. But one can still get information near the line and within region C. This is done by expanding equation (11) [in $\eta(t)$] to the first nontrivial term beyond the linear. We do not go into this in any detail, being content to apprise the reader of the potential usefulness of these techniques from bifurcation theory (Devaney, 1986; Lichtenberg and Lieberman, 1983).

In the general study of dynamical systems, the appearance of the sort of oscillatory behavior we have just seen is a common and characteristic phenomenon. For example, a similar structure within predator–prey equations has been studied intensively, as, for example, in the work of Schaffer and Kot (1986), and has contributed significantly to the modern study of chaos. There is reason to believe (Babloyantz and Destexhe, 1986; Babloyantz et al., 1985) (see Chapter 7) that these ideas may be of relevance in brain studies as well. In the model CA3 network, there is, of course, a richer structure, with inhibitory cells, spontaneous firing, and so on.

Conclusion

Our primary goals in this book have been two. The first has been to determine if our current experimental data concerning cellular physiology and synaptic connections suffice to account for various types of collective phenomena exhibited by the in vitro CA3 region. The answer here is yes, up to a point. Many details concerning the quantitative electrophysiology of single neurons, the spatial structure of synaptic connections, and the events required to elicit synaptic plasticity remain to be elucidated, as do the implications of such details for population behavior. The second goal has been to obtain insight into the hippocampus as a (perhaps) novel physical system. Is a particular collective behavior analogous to a well-understood physical paradigm, such as a chain reaction or a time-dependent percolation? Or are there, alternatively, interesting new principles at work, perhaps pertinent to basic questions of brain function? Here again, the answer is yes, up to a point. Synchronized bursts in the presence of picrotoxin appear analogous to a chain reaction, and the ideas of percolation have proved helpful intuitively, if not yet quantitatively. Hippocampal physiology and mathematical physics may yet prove to have something to offer each other. It is our view that "conventional" neural network models, layered neural networks, and symmetric spin-glass models are not appropriate for description of the CA3 region of the hippocampus, although modified, more complex "spin models" may well prove to be helpful.

In Chapters 6 and 7 we postulated a two-step model for information processing in the hippocampal CA3 region: An afferent input produces a direct primary response, followed by an overlapping secondary response mediated by recurrent synapses that interconnect the cells; compare the work of Marr (1971). The primary response will be somewhat sensitive to the "state of the system," that is, to the presence of AHP currents in pyramidal cells and the efficacy of the different synapses. The secondary response will be more sensitive to the state of the system, including any ongoing population activity. Although we can estimate the numbers of cells that will participate in secondary responses from system parameters, such as the strength of inhibitory synapses (Chapter 6), it

may be difficult or impossible to predict exactly which cells will participate in a secondary response. As time passes after the afferent stimulus,
there will be less and less relation between the population activity and
the input. The relevant time scale here seems to be in the hundreds of
milliseconds (Chapter 7). Memory models such as LTP focus on modification of the afferent synapses, which will modify the primary purpose.
However, we suggest that changes in local circuits offer still further
possibilities for information storage. Our work suggests that modifications in the strength of the recurrent excitatory synapses between pyramidal cells, the strength of the recurrent excitatory synapses onto inhibitory cells, or the effectiveness of any or all of the different types of
inhibition could induce a variety of behaviors ranging from "gross" synchronized population bursts to subtle alterations in the probability of a
delayed burst in a particular pyramidal cell. In one sense, at least, we
agree with abstract neural modelers. We imagine that memories are
encoded in some distributed fashion across a group of synapses, rather
than in a single synapse. To decode the resulting changes in neuronal
population activities represents a challenge for both experimental and
modeling techniques.

Our model makes it possible and meaningful to pose precise questions
along these lines. As experimental data accrue on the adequate conditions for synapses to change their properties, we can then explore, in
simulations, what consequences for the population as a whole any particular type of synaptic modification will have. The resulting hypotheses
ought then to be verifiable (or falsifiable!).

Notes

Prologue

1 Brain slices have many uses, including the study of cellular physiology, synaptic function and plasticity, morphology, drug effects, and pathologic effects of anoxia and seizures. Perhaps the most important aspect of the hippocampal slice is that synaptic circuitry is retained, so that the slice can generate population activities. Other mammalian preparations that have been used in vivo to study (relatively) isolated neuronal populations include isolated or undercut cortex (Burns, 1950; Burns and Webb, 1979), the deafferented hippocampus (Spencer and Kandel, 1961a), and hippocampal transplants (Buzsáki et al., 1987a). The physiological stage for the hippocampal slice was set by Andersen, Bliss, and Skrede (1971), who noted that physiological responses to pathway stimulation (perforant path, mossy fibers, Schaffer collaterals) were relatively confined to "chips" about 1 mm wide. This is not to say that individual axons are confined to such chips. Another in vitro preparation, retaining much of the normal synaptic organization preserved in an acute slice, is the slice culture (Frotscher and Gähwiler, 1988; Thompson and Gähwiler, 1989a–c). Slice cultures form a single layer of cells, making access to cells easier for intracellular recording, drug iontophoresis, and optical recording. Perfused whole-brain preparations (Llinás and Mühlethaler, 1988; Richerson and Getting, 1987) may be used in the future to study hippocampal physiology.

2 One possible region may prove to be the pyriform cortex (Wilson and Bower, 1989). There is considerable information on the properties of pyriform neurons and on the anatomical arrangement of the synaptic interconnections (Haberly, 1985).

3 There might be exceptions if, for example, a subset of neurons with identical properties is lumped into one model neuron, with synapses between neurons in the subset ignored, and synaptic inputs to neurons in the subset from the outside averaged together in some way. See Getting (1983).

4 There is also another approach to the hippocampus as a neuronal system, based ultimately on the work of Norbert Wiener (1958) on the reconstruction of nonlinear functionals from the response to white noise. We shall not enter into this approach here; the reader is referred to the original papers (Berger et al., 1988a,b; Sclabassi et al., 1988).

Chapter 1

1 The reader is referred to Figure 1.2 for the definition of stratum pyramidale and the other hippocampal strata.

2 In our discussion of hippocampal pathways, we use the traditional term "limbic system," although the limbic system is perhaps not really a system at all (Brodal, 1981). The term "limbic system" was first introduced in 1937 by Papez, who argued that certain interconnected brain structures were critical for "emotional expression," as well as for processing olfactory inputs. We shall use the term "limbic system" in its more anatomical sense to refer to a set of interconnected brain regions that includes (but is not limited to) the pyriform cortex, hippocampus, subicular complex, entorhinal cortex, cingulate cortex, septal nuclei, hypothalamus, and the anterior nuclear group of the thalamus.

3 Hippocampal damage following anoxia/ischemia is not unusual in clinical experience. It may be associated with other lesions, including laminar necrosis of cortex and cell loss in the basal ganglia and cerebellar Purkinje layer. Zola-Morgan et al. (1986) argue that CA1 and the subiculum are in the same vascular territory; ischemia would be unlikely, therefore, to destroy CA1 and leave the subiculum intact. Excitotoxic damage appears more likely: The Schaffer collaterals from CA3 to CA1 (i) do not extend to subiculum and (ii) use N-methyl-D-aspartic acid (NMDA) receptors, which may mediate glutamic-induced cell death (Meldrum et al., 1987; Rothman, 1984, 1986). Because NMDA receptors are not restricted to CA1, however, this concept does not by itself explain why the neuropathology can be so confined.

4 The dichotomy "collective behavior directly imposed from outside" versus "collective behavior emergent with parameters set by outside influences" corresponds roughly to "phasic" versus "tonic" influences from input structures. Such a dichotomy is likely to be much too simple.

5 It is of interest that the behavioral correlates of hippocampal EEG and neocortical EEG are, in general, different; that is, rhythmic waves may appear in the EEG of one structure at times when rhythmicity is not apparent in the other structure. For example, during walking and exploration, the limbic cortex tends to show theta rhythm while the neocortical EEG is "desynchronized." Furthermore, whereas the cellular mechanisms of EEG spikes and sharp waves are likely to be broadly similar in hippocampus and neocortex, such similarity of mechanisms may not necessarily hold for rhythmic EEG waves.

6 In contrast, during an epileptiform synchronized burst, or during a physiological sharp wave, cell firing occurs during a local extracellular positivity in the stratum pyramidale. The extracellular positivity is explained by the outward flow of synaptic currents across the somatic membrane, the excitatory synaptic current sinks being in the dendrites, while inhibitory synaptic currents are (at least relatively) suppressed during the epileptiform event. The situation during theta waves is evidently different.

7 By "type of seizure" we are referring to cellular mechanism, not to the clinical classification of seizure types.

8 Hippocampal sclerosis consists of neuronal loss and gliosis. This lesion in

Sommer's sector (CA1) is correlated with complex partial seizures; the damage need not be confined to Sommer's sector (Brown, 1973). Margerison and Corsellis (1966) examined brain material obtained at autopsy from 55 patients with chronic seizure disorders. Hippocampal sclerosis was found in 36 cases. Pathological changes were found in CA1, in the "end folium" (the hilus of the dentate), or in both; it was found that pathology could be unilateral or bilateral in different combinations. Cell loss was also found in the amygdala. The lesions were most likely to be found in patients whose seizures originated in the temporal lobe (by clinical and/or EEG criteria), but the correlation of neuropathology with seizure origin was not absolute. Thus, with EEG spikes and sharp waves in one temporal lobe, the pathology might be most striking in the other temporal lobe, or the pathology might be bilateral. The mechanisms by which hippocampal sclerosis is produced are not certain. It seems likely that both anoxic damage and seizures themselves could contribute. Interestingly, the hippocampal-sclerosis lesion does not appear to be associated with loss of GABA neurons (Babb et al., 1989).

9 The term "theta" in human EEG simply refers to waves with a frequency of 4–7 Hz. It should not be confused with "theta rhythm," as described in rodents. The latter refers to an EEG rhythm, having defined behavioral concomitants, recorded in the hippocampus and related structures.

10 Indeed, as mentioned earlier, CA3 pyramidal-cell firing is relatively depressed during exploration.

11 Some attempts at construction of a computational model have been made (Zipser, 1985).

Chapter 2

1 These determinations are generally made with sharp electrodes, which may introduce a shunt into the membrane (Clements and Redman, 1989).

2 There is experimental evidence that a part of the DAP is not calcium-dependent (Konnerth, Lux, and Heinemann, 1986b). Simulations suggest that this calcium-independent DAP represents discharge of dendritic membrane capacitance that is charged by inward somatic currents flowing during the Na-dependent action potential (Traub, 1982).

3 Electroresponsiveness of dendrites was suggested some years ago to account for fast prepotentials in hippocampal neurons (Spencer and Kandel, 1961c) and for the partial spikes seen in chromatolytic motoneurons (Kuno and Llinás, 1970; Traub and Llinás, 1977). The phenomenon was demonstrated directly in alligator Purkinje cells (Llinás and Nicholson, 1971) and, since then, in many other types of neurons. Besides hippocampal neurons, examples include inferior olivary cells (Llinás and Yarom, 1981a,b), mammalian Purkinje cells (Llinás and Sugimori, 1980b), and thalamic neurons (Jahnsen and Llinás, 1984a,b).

Chapter 4

1 There are many aspects of modeling single neurons that we shall not consider here. We omit these topics not because they are uninteresting but

because they have not yet proved critical to the problems of collective behavior of most interest to us. Examples are inclusion of the axonal initial segment or a piece of the more distal axon (Dodge and Cooley, 1973; Traub, 1977), presynaptic terminals (Llinás, Steinberg, and Walton, 1976), electrotonic junctions (Traub and Wong, 1983b), dendrodendritic synapses (Shepherd and Brayton, 1979), intracellular calcium distribution (Ahmed and Connor, 1988; Zucker, 1989), dendritic spines (Brown et al., 1988a; Pongracz, 1985; Shepherd et al., 1985; Stratford et al., 1989), and explicit descriptions of NMDA-receptor kinetics (Forsythe and Westbrook, 1988).

2 The precise symmetry condition is as follows. First, define (spatial) "electrotonic coordinates" to mean distance along a dendrite measured in terms of the local space constant. Consider a segment S of the equivalent cylinder that corresponds (in a map such as illustrated in Figure 4.1) to a set of cylindrical segments $S_1, \ldots, S_k$ in the branching dendrite. Call the electrotonic coordinates for the segments $X_1, \ldots, X_k$ $(0 \leq X_i \leq L)$. If synaptic input per unit membrane area to one segment, say the first, is $f(X_1)$, then the synaptic input per unit for each i must be $f(X_i)$.

3 In such an experiment, a steady current, or a current pulse, is injected into the soma through a microelectrode, and the resulting voltage response is recorded. The voltage response reflects the membrane properties and electrotonic architecture of the cell body and dendrites (and, to a lesser extent, the axon). One must be careful not to activate voltage-dependent conductances. One also needs to assume that no significant shunt is being produced by synaptic activity.

4 To see this, note that the probability density for channel closure is $(e^{-t/\tau})/\tau$, $\tau = 23$ ms. The mean channel open time is the expected value of this function, $\int_0^\infty ((te^{-t/\tau})/\tau)dt = \tau$.

5 There are now data on the membrane localizations of high-threshold calcium channels in cultured hippocampal neurons (Jones et al., 1989).There is one issue that the reader may find confusing here: Because the apical dendrites of hippocampal pyramidal cells have a relatively short electrotonic length (about 1.0), a calcium spike anywhere in the tree might be expected to produce a large transient at the soma that perhaps would be indistinguishable from a spike in or near the soma. There are two issues to be considered. First, the term "electrotonic length," when unqualified, refers to the DC electrotonic length in space constants λ, $\lambda = (rR_m/2R_i)^{1/2}$. The frequency-dependent space constant λ_ω is more relevant for the spatial propagation of transient events, and $\lambda_\omega < \lambda$ (see Problem 5 in this chapter). Second, a transient event on a dendritic branch will be attenuated by the impedance "load" of the other branches (Rinzel and Rall, 1974) and so will produce a smaller voltage change at the soma than would the same event occurring simultaneously on all of the branches (at the same electrotonic distance from the soma).

6 Later, when we consider extracellular field effects, it will be necessary to alter this assumption.

7 Units: nF, mV, ms, nA, μS. In contrast to most of the physiological literature, but for ease of mathematical expression, we write membrane potential relative to resting potential, rather than relative to extracellular potential.

Compartment numbers: 1–8 are basilar dendritic cylinder, 9 is soma, 10 is apical branch, 11–19 are one apical cylinder, 20–28 are the other apical cylinder.

8 The M current was included in an earlier version of the model (Traub et al., 1987b).

Chapter 5

1 Some other values for Schaffer-collateral conduction velocity in the literature are as follows: 0.2–0.35 m/s (Andersen et al., 1978); 0.2 m/s (Grinvald et al., 1982); 0.5 m/s (Knowles, Traub, and Strowbridge, 1987); 0.36–0.38 m/s (Tielen, Lopes da Silva, and Mollevanger, 1981). Along the longitudinal axis of the hippocampus, an estimate of 0.38–0.63 m/s was obtained for axon conduction velocity (Bartesaghi, Gessi, and Sperti, 1983).

2 This scaling factor would not be necessary but for edge effects.

3 For clarity, the programming language used for illustrations is more like PL/I than FORTRAN.

Chapter 6

1 Picrotoxin may bind to the Cl^- ionophore (Ticku, Ban, and Olsen, 1978), although other data suggest that its block of GABA-activated Cl^- currents may occur via a distinct action (Yakushiji et al., 1987). Bicuculline blocks GABA-activated currents competitively, whereas penicillin does not, at least not in the millimolar concentrations used in physiological experiments (Yakushiji et al., 1987). Penicillin has been reported to decrease the average duration of the open state of the $GABA_A$-activated Cl^- channel (Mathers, 1987). These compounds are not believed to affect intrinsic membrane properties at the concentrations generally used. An interesting historical reference on the clinically relevant epileptic properties of penicillin is that of Walker, Johnson, and Kollros (1945). Penicillin may block dendritic IPSPs at a lower concentration than that required to block somatic IPSPs (Avoli, 1984).

2 Things are not quite this simple, because there are different types of glutamate receptors with different properties. The late component of pyramidal EPSPs is sometimes voltage-dependent (Miles and Wong, 1986) and may represent an NMDA effect (Dingledine, Hynes, and King, 1986). Both NMDA-dependent and non-NMDA-dependent EPSPs likely are of importance in the synchronized bursts we shall be considering (Dingledine et al., 1986), but we shall not enter into these intricacies here.

3 By coincidence, in the form of epilepsy observed when CA1 is bathed in high-K solutions, a minimum of about 1,500 cells has been estimated as the requirement for synchronized population spikes (Traynelis and Dingledine, 1989b). The mechanism of these CA1 events is not the same as for synchronized bursts in disinhibited CA3 (see Chapter 8).

4 Blocking slow IPSPs in the model has an interesting side effect when $c_i = 0$; that is, once all the cells are firing, they stay firing. The average of 20 continuously active excitatory inputs per cell "overwhelms" the ability of

intrinsic K currents to repolarize the cell. We are not aware whether or not that is the case experimentally.

5 In our first study of propagation of synchronized discharges, we showed that the population wave could travel at the same velocity as the axon conduction velocity provided that sufficiently many cells were stimulated and provided that there were enough connections running throughout the system (Traub et al., 1987a). At that time, no information was available on the conduction velocity of local CA3 recurrent collaterals, although the velocity in Schaffer collaterals was known. At least in the longitudinal slice, the number of global connections appears to be small.

6 Some related studies on the spatial structure of synaptic connections are these: Christian and Dudek (1988a) applied microdrops of glutamate in CA3 in the transverse slice while recording intracellularly. They found a maximal effect of glutamate when the drop was about 200 μ toward the hilus from the recorded cell. They also found evidence of excitatory interactions between CA1 cells, especially in the longitudinal slice (Christian and Dudek, 1988b). Anatomical studies are generally consistent with the notion that excitatory collaterals go farther, on average, than collaterals of inhibitory cells. Thus, Finch et al. (1983) traced CA3 pyramidal-cell axon collaterals up to 1 mm, whereas CA1 interneuron axons spanned about 300 μ in either direction. Somogyi et al. (1983b) observed the total tangential spread of axons of an interneuron cell type to be from 300 to 500 μ. Tamamaki et al. (1984) traced pyramidal-cell axons for more than 4 mm in each hippocampus.

7 CA1 supports a different kind of synchronized activity – field bursts – more readily than does CA3 (Jefferys and Haas, 1982; Snow and Dudek, 1984a, 1986; Taylor and Dudek, 1982; Traynelis and Dingledine, 1988; Yaari, Konnerth and Heinemann, 1986). These events do not depend on synaptic transmission and represent a type of phenomenon different from what we are considering here (see Chapter 8).

8 For example, Thompson and Gähwiler (1989a–c) studied the effects of repetitive mossy-fiber stimulation in slice cultures. That treatment caused a 22% decrease in $g_{IPSP(Cl)}$ and a 2–8-mV depolarizing shift in the equilibrium potential of Cl^- IPSPs, the latter effect possibly being due to an increase in external K^+ concentration (Korn et al., 1987).

9 To confirm this, we repeated the run with $c_i = 3$ nS when slow IPSPs were blocked; 8,998 of the 9,000 pyramidal cells were recruited by stimulating a single cell.

10 Afterdischarges in slices from tetanus-toxin-injected rats have somewhat different properties than picrotoxin afterdischarges: The events occur at a much lower rate, the intervals between secondary bursts are longer, and the events are capable of propagating at velocities up to 0.25 m/s (Jefferys, 1989).

Chapter 7

1 Our model, as discussed later, suggests that "population oscillations" are not oscillations in the strict mathematical sense. Rather, the underlying dynamics appear to be chaotic, even when individual isolated cells are strict oscillators. We hope that this abuse of terminology will not prove confusing.

2 It seems to be a general property of large physical systems in the vicinity of a so-called second-order phase transition that the variance of some feature of the system (e.g., the cluster size in the case of a percolating system) becomes unbounded. It will be interesting to determine if this concept applies in a direct, rather than intuitive, way to hippocampal networks.

3 In our model, all strictly spontaneous activity takes place in pyramidal cells only, as a result of a steady inward current and/or spontaneous EPSPs. It has not been determined for the slice whether or not spontaneous discharges can take place in i cells, although background firing in these cells is certainly observed.

4 Could the small blips in the correlation record be significant? It is difficult to say for sure, but they probably are not. The peaks in waves (upper traces) are at about 50 cells. The expected correlation between two randomly chosen clusters, each of 50 cells, is $(50 \times 50)/9,000$, which is less than 1. On the other hand, typically 200 to 300 cells fire repeatedly during each event. If again the cells were picked randomly, an upper bound for the random correlation would be about $(250 \times 250)/9,000$, or about 7.

5 This method of analysis derives indirectly from a theorem of Takens (1981) concerning the "reconstruction" of a dynamical system involving n variables, $x_1, \ldots, x_n$, from sufficiently long observations of only one of them, say x_1. We are indebted to Ralph Siegel for the following observation: Strictly speaking, Takens's theorem does not apply to our $x(t)$ defined earlier, because $x(t)$ is not one of the variables in the underlying dynamical system, but is rather a function of them. The same technical comment applies to EEG signals.

6 When sufficiently many cells are firing, or when currents flowing in the extracellular space are sufficiently large, then the models of neuronal activity and of extracellular current flow become inseparably coupled; that is, extracellular currents influence neuronal firing, as well as vice versa; see Chapter 8 and Taylor and Dudek (1984a,b) and Traub et al. (1985a,b).

Chapter 8

1 We thank Dr. F. E. Dudek for critical comments on this chapter.

2 We refer in this chapter only to rodent hippocampus, wherein pyramidal cells are arranged in a tight layer, favoring field interactions. In the human hippocampus, particularly in CA1, the layering of pyramidal cells is less prominent, and the role of field effects there is more uncertain than for rodents. Nevertheless, population spikes are recordable in human hippocampus, at least in the dentate gyrus (Masukawa et al., 1988, 1989), suggesting the occurrence of field effects there as well.

3 The coupling is weak for field effects compared with chemical synapses in that one cell has a small influence on any other cell via the extracellular medium. Coherent oscillations occur when a large number of cells are firing more or less together, and then field interactions can lock the cells together. In contrast, a single cell may strongly influence a postsynaptic cell and sometimes drive it to fire.

Chapter 9

1 We thank Geoffrey Grinstein for his important criticisms of this section.
2 By "instability" in this context we refer not to epileptogenesis or to the development of population bursts but rather to the sensitivity of detailed firing patterns to small perturbations; that is, a small amount of noise will influence which cells will fire when, without necessarily having much effect on how many cells will fire in all (see Chapter 7).
3 Dr. Schulman's address: Department of Physics, Clarkson University, Potsdam, NY 13676. The work in this appendix was supported in part by the National Science Foundation.
4 To see this, consider the map $f(\rho) = 1 - e^{-x\rho}$ in a small neighborhood of the nonzero fixed point $\bar{\rho}$, $\bar{\rho} = 1 - e^{-x\bar{\rho}}$. The derivative map is $f'(\rho) = -xe^{-x\rho}$; $\bar{\rho}$ will be a stable fixed point if $|f'(\bar{\rho})| < 1$. Thus, we must have $xe^{-x\bar{\rho}} < 1$, or alternatively, $x(1 - \bar{\rho}) < 1$. To demonstrate this, we solve equation (3) for x,

$$x = \frac{-\log(1 - \bar{\rho})}{\bar{\rho}}$$

whence

$$x(1 - \bar{\rho}) = (1 - 1/\bar{\rho})\log(1 - \bar{\rho}) = \log[(1 - \bar{\rho})^{(1 - 1/\bar{\rho})}] = \frac{-(1-\bar{\rho})}{\bar{\rho}}\log(1 - \bar{\rho})$$

which must be shown to be less than 1 for $0 < \bar{\rho} < 1$. Let $\bar{\rho} = \sin^2\theta$. The problem is equivalent to showing that for $0 < \theta < \pi/2$ we have

$$\frac{\cos^2\theta}{\sin^2\theta} \log(\cos^2\theta) < 1$$

Equivalently, we must demonstrate that $g(\theta) \equiv \log(\cos\theta) + \frac{1}{2}\tan^2\theta > 0$. For $\theta = 0$, $g(0) = 0$. We need only show that $dg/d\theta > 0$ for $0 < \theta < \pi/2$. But

$$\frac{dg}{d\theta} = -\tan\theta + \tan\theta \frac{d}{d\theta}\tan\theta = (\tan\theta)^3 > 0$$

Thus, we know that at the fixed point, $x(1 - \bar{\rho}) < 1$, and hence $|f'(\bar{\rho})| < 1$, so that the fixed point is an attractor: Once the fixed point $\bar{\rho}$ is approached sufficiently closely, further approach will behave as a power of $f'(\rho)$, i.e., exponentially.
5 Thus, the left side of equation (7) is

$$\frac{2}{t+1} = \frac{2}{t}\frac{1}{1 + 1/t} = \frac{2}{t}\left[1 - \frac{1}{t} + O(\frac{1}{t^2})\right]$$

The right side is

$$\frac{2}{t} - \frac{1}{2}\left\{\frac{2}{t}\right\}^2$$

The two sides agree to order $1/t^2$.

References

Abeles, M. (1982a). Role of the cortical neuron. Integrator or coincidence detector. *Israel J. Med Sci.* 18:83–92.

(1982b). *Local Cortical Circuits.* Springer, Berlin.

Adams, P. R., Constanti, A., Brown, D. A., and Clark, R. B. (1982). Intracellular Ca^{2+} activates a fast-voltage sensitive K^+ current in vertebrate sympathetic neurons. *Nature* 296:746–8.

Adams, P. R., and Galvan, M. (1986). Voltage-dependent currents of vertebrate neurons and their role in membrane excitability. In Delgado-Escueta, A. V., Ward, A. A., Jr., Woodbury, D. M., and Porter, R. J., eds., *Advances in Neurology, Vol. 44, Basic Mechanisms of the Epilepsies. Molecular and Cellular Approaches,* pp. 137–70. Raven Press, New York.

Adrian, E. D. (1936). The spread of activity in the cerebral cortex. *J. Physiol.* 88:127–61.

Ahmed, Z., and Connor, J. A. (1988). Calcium regulation by and buffer capacity of molluscan neurons during calcium transients. *Cell Calcium* 9:57–69.

Aldrich, R. W., Jr., Getting, P. A., and Thompson, S. H. (1979). Inactivation of delayed outward current in molluscan neurone somata. *J. Physiol.* 291:507–30.

Alger, B. E., and Nicoll, R. A. (1980a). Epileptiform burst afterhyperpolarization: calcium-dependent potassium potential in hippocampal CA1 pyramidal cells. *Science* 210:1122–4.

(1980b). Spontaneous inhibitory post-synaptic potentials in hippocampus: mechanism for tonic inhibition. *Brain Res.* 200:195–200.

(1982a). Feed-forward dendritic inhibition in rat hippocampal pyramidal cells studied *in vitro. J. Physiol.* 328:105–23.

(1982b). Pharmacological evidence for two kinds of GABA receptor on rat hippocampal pyramidal cells studied *in vitro. J. Physiol.* 328:125–41.

Alger, B. E., and Williamson, A. (1988). A transient calcium-dependent potassium component of the epileptiform burst after-hyperpolarization in rat hippocampus. *J. Physiol.* 399:191–205.

Alonso, A., and Garcia-Austt, E. (1987a). Neuronal sources of theta rhythm in the entorhinal cortex of the rat. I. Laminar distribution of theta field potentials. *Exp. Brain Res.* 67:493–500.

(1987b). Neuronal sources of theta rhythm in the entorhinal cortex of the rat. II. Phase relations between unit discharges and theta field potentials. *Exp. Brain Res.* 67:502–9.

Alonso, A., Gaztelu, J. M., Buño, W., Jr., and Garcia-Austt, E. (1987). Cross-correlation analysis of septohippocampal neurons during θ-rhythm. *Brain Res.* 413:135–46.

Alonso, A., and Köhler, C. (1982). Evidence for separate projections of hippocampal pyramidal and non-pyramidal neurons to different parts of the septum in the rat brain. *Neurosci. Lett.* 31:209–14.

(1984). A study of the reciprocal connections between the septum and the entorhinal area using anterograde and retrograde axonal transport methods in the rat brain. *J. Comp. Neurol.* 225:327–43.

Altafullah, I., and Halgren, E. (1988). Focal medial temporal lobe spike-wave complexes evoked by a memory task. *Epilepsia* 29:8–13.

Alvarez-Royo, P., Mesches, M., Allen, J., Saltzmann, W., Squire, L. R., and Zola-Morgan, S. (1988). Independence of memory functions and emotional behavior: separate contributions of the hippocampal formation and the amygdala. *Soc. Neurosci. Abstr.* 14:1043.

Amaral, D. G. (1986). Amygdalohippocampal and amygdalocortical projections in the primate brain. *Adv. Exp. Med. Biol.* 203:3–17.

Amaral, D. G., and Kurz, J. (1985). An analysis of the origins of the cholinergic and noncholinergic septal projections to the hippocampal formation of the rat. *J. Comp. Neurol.* 240:37–59.

Amaral, D. G., and Witter, M. P. (1989). The three-dimensional organization of the hippocampal formation: a review of anatomical data. *Neuroscience* 31:571–91.

Amit, D. J., Gutfreund, H., and Sompolinsky, H. (1985a). Spin-glass models of neural networks. *Phys. Rev. A* 32:1007–18.

(1985b). Storing infinite numbers of patterns in a spin-glass model of neural networks. *Phys. Rev. Lett.* 55:1530–3.

Andersen, P., Bliss, T. V. P., and Skrede, K. K. (1971). Lamellar organization of hippocampal excitatory pathways. *Exp. Brain Res.* 13:222–38.

Andersen, P., Eccles, J. C., and Løyning, Y. (1963). Recurrent inhibition in the hippocampus with identification of the inhibitory cell and its synapses. *Nature* 198:540–2.

Andersen, P., Silfvenius, H., Sundberg, S., Sveen, O., and Wigström, H. (1978). Functional characteristics of unmyelinated fibres in the hippocampal cortex. *Brain Res.* 144:11–18.

Anderson, W. W., Swartzwelder, H. S., and Wilson, W. A. (1987). The NMDA receptor antagonist 2-amino-5-phosphonovalerate blocks stimulus train-induced epileptogenesis but not epileptiform bursting in the rat hippocampal slice. *J. Neurophysiol.* 57:1–21.

Andrade, R., Malenka, R. C., and Nicoll, R. A. (1986). A G protein couples serotonin and GABA$_B$ receptor to the same channels in hippocampus. *Science* 234:1261–5.

Andrade, R., and Nicoll, R. A. (1987). Pharmacologically distinct actions of serotonin on single pyramidal neurones of the rat hippocampus recorded *in vitro*. *J. Physiol.* 394:99–124.

Andrew, R. D., Taylor, C. P., Snow, R. W., and Dudek, F. E. (1982). Coupling in rat hippocampal slices: dye transfer between CA1 pyramidal cells. *Brain Res. Bull.* 8:211–22.

Angelides, K. J., Elmer, L. W., Loftus, D., and Elson, E. (1988). Distribution and lateral mobility of voltage-dependent sodium channels in neurons. *J. Cell Biol.* 106:1911–25.

Aram, J. A., and Wong, R. K. S. (1989). Synchronization of inhibitory potentials in the neocortex is resistant to excitatory amino acid blockers. *Soc. Neurosci. Abstr.* 15:339.

Arieli, A., and Grinvald, A. (1988). Dynamic patterns of on-going coherent activity in neuronal assemblies revealed by real-time optical imaging in cat cortex. *Soc. Neurosci. Abstr.* 14:1122.

Arnolds, D. E. A. T., Lopes da Silva, F. H., Aitink, J. W., Kamp, A., and Boejinga, P. (1980). The spectral properties of hippocampal EEG related to behavior in man. *Electroenceph. Clin. Neurophysiol.* 50:324–8.

Ascher, P., and Nowak, L. (1988). Quisqualate and kainate activated channels in mouse central neurones in culture. *J. Physiol.* 399:227–45.

Ashcroft, F. M., and Stanfield, P. R. (1981). Calcium dependence of the inaction of calcium currents in skeletal muscle fibers of an insect. *Science* 213:224–6.

Ashwood, T. J., Collingridge, G. L., Herron, C. E., and Wheal, H. V. (1987). Voltage-clamp analysis of somatic gamma-aminobutyric acid responses in adult rat hippocampal neurones *in vitro*. *J. Physiol.* 384:27–37.

Atwood, H. L., and Wojtowicz, J. M. (1986). Short-term and long-term plasticity and physiological differentiation of crustacean motor synapses. *Intern. Rev. Neurobiol.* 28:275–362.

Auer, R. N., Jensen, M. L., and Whishaw, I. Q. (1989). Neurobehavioral deficit due to ischemic brain damage limited to half of the CA1 sector of the hippocampus. *J. Neurosci.* 9:1641–7.

Avoli, M. (1984). Penicillin induced hyperexcitability in the in vitro hippocampal slice can be unrelated to impairment of somatic inhibition. *Brain Res.* 323:154–8.

Avoli, M., Gloor, P., Kostopoulos, G., and Gotman, J. (1983). An analysis of penicillin-induced generalized spike and wave discharges using simultaneous recordings of cortical and thalamic single neurons. *J. Neurophysiol.* 50:819–37.

Babb, T. L., Pretorius, J. K., Kupfer, W. R., Crandall, P. H. (1989). Glutamate decarboxylase-immunoreactive neurons are preserved in human epileptic hippocampus. *J. Neurosci.* 9:2562–74.

Babloyantz, A., and Destexhe, A. (1986). Low-dimensional chaos in an instance of epilepsy. *Proc. Natl. Acad. Sci. U.S.A.* 83:3513–17.

Babloyantz, A., Salazar, J. M., and Nicolis, C. (1985). Evidence of chaotic dynamics of brain activity during the sleep cycle. *Phys. Lett.* 111A:152–6.

Baisden, R. H., Woodruff, M. L., and Hoover, D. B. (1984). Cholinergic and non-cholinergic septohippocampal projections: a double-label horseradish peroxidase-acetylcholinesterase study in the rabbit. *Brain Res.* 290:146–51.

Barker, J. L., and Harrison, N. L. (1988). Outward rectification of inhibitory postsynaptic currents in cultured rat hippocampal neurones. *J. Physiol.* 403:41–55.

Barrionuevo, G., Kelso, S. R., Johnston, D., and Brown, T. H. (1986). Conductance mechanism responsible for long-term potentiation in monosynaptic and isolated excitatory synaptic inputs to hippocampus. *J. Neurophysiol.* 55:540–50.

Bartesaghi, R., Gessi, T., and Sperti, L. (1983). Interlamellar transfer of impulses in the hippocampal formation. *Exper. Neurol.* 82:550–67.

Bekkers, J. M., and Stevens, C. F. (1989). NMDA and non-NMDA receptors are colocalized at individual excitatory synapses in cultured rat hippocampus. *Nature* 341:230–3.

Benardo, L. S., Masukawa, L. M., and Prince, D. A. (1982). Electrophysiology of isolated hippocampal pyramidal dendrites. *J. Neurosci.* 2:1614–22.

Benardo, L. S., and Prince, D. A. (1982). Cholinergic pharmacology of mammalian hippocampal pyramidal cells. *Neuroscience* 7:1703–12.

Ben-Ari, Y., Krnjevic, K., and Reinhardt, W. (1980). Lability of synaptic inhibition of hippocampal pyramidal cells. *J. Physiol.* 298:36P–7P.

Bennett, M. R., Jones, P., and Lavidis, N. A. (1986). The probability of quantal secretion along visualised terminal branches at amphibian (*Bufo marinus*) neuromuscular synapses. *J. Physiol.* 379:257–74.

Berger, T. W., Eriksson, J. L., Ciarolla, D. A., and Sclabassi, R. J. (1988a). Nonlinear systems analysis of the hippocampal perforant path–dentate projection. II. Effects of random impulse train stimulation. *J. Neurophysiol.* 60:1077–94.

(1988b). Nonlinear systems analysis of the hippocampal perforant path–dentate projection. III. Comparison of random train and paired impulse stimulation. *J. Neurophysiol.* 60:1077–94.

Berger, T. W., Swanson, G. W., Milner, T. A., Lynch, G. S., and Thompson, R. F. (1980). Reciprocal anatomical connections between hippocampus and subiculum in the rabbit: evidence for subicular innervation of regio superior. *Brain Res.* 183:265–76.

Blake, J. F., Brown, M. W., and Collingridge, G. L. (1988). CNQX blocks acidic amino acid induced depolarizations and synaptic components mediated by non-NMDA receptors in rat hippocampal slices. *Neurosci. Lett.* 89:182–6.

Bland, B. H., Andersen, P., Ganes, T., and Sveen, O. (1980). Automated analysis of rhythmicity of physiologically identified hippocampal formation neurons. *Exp. Brain Res.* 38:205–19.

Bland, B. H., Seto, M., and Rowntree, C. I. (1983). The relation of multiple hippocampal theta cell discharge rates to slow wave theta frequency. *Physiol. Behav.* 31:111–17.

Bland, S. K., and Bland, B. H. (1986). Medial septal modulation of hippocampal theta cell discharges. *Brain Res.* 375:102–16.

Borst, J. G. G., Leung, L.-W. S., and MacFabe, D. F. (1987). Electrical activity of the cingulate cortex. II. Cholinergic modulation. *Brain Res.* 407:81–93.

Boss, B. D., Peterson, G. M., and Cowan, W. M. (1985). On the number of neurons in the dentate gyrus of the rat. *Brain Res.* 338:144–50.

Boss, B. D., Turlejski, K., Stanfield, B. B., and Cowan, W. M. (1987). On the numbers of neurons in fields CA1 and CA3 of the hippocampus of Sprague-Dawley and Wistar rats. *Brain Res.* 406:280–7.

Braak, H. (1974). On the structure of the human archicortex. I. The cornu Ammonis. A Golgi and pigment architectonic study. *Cell Tissue Res.* 152:349–83.

Brace, H. M., Jefferys, J. G. R., and Mellanby, J. (1985). Long-term changes in hippocampal physiology and learning ability of rats after intrahippocampal tetanus toxin. *J. Physiol.* 368:343–57.

Braitenberg, V. (1978). Cortical architectonics: general and areal. In Brazier, M. A. B., and Petsche, H., eds., *Architectonics of the Cerebral Cortex,* pp. 443–65. Raven, New York.

Breese, C. R., Hampson, R. E., and Deadwyler, S. A. (1989). Hippocampal place cells: stereotypy and plasticity. *J. Neurosci.* 9:1097–111.

Brehm, P., and Eckert, R. (1978). Calcium entry leads to inactivation of calcium channel in *Paramecium. Science* 202:1203–6.

Brehm, P., Eckert, R., and Tillotson, D. (1980). Calcium-mediated inactivation of calcium current in *Paramecium. J. Physiol.* 306:193–203.

Brenner, R. P., and Atkinson, R. (1982). Generalized paroxysmal fast activity: electroencephalographic and clinical features. *Ann. Neurol.* 11:386–90.

Bridgman, P. A., Malamut, B. L., Sperling, M. R., Saykin, A. J., and O'Connor, M. J. (1989). Memory during subclinical seizures. *Neurology* 39:853–6.

Brierley, J. B., and Cooper, J. E. (1962). Cerebral complications of hypotensive anaesthesia in healthy adult. *J. Neurol. Neurosurg. Psychiatry* 25:24–30.

Brodal, A. (1981). *Neurological Anatomy in Relation to Clinical Medicine.* Oxford University Press, 1981.

Brown, A. G., and Noble, R. (1982). Connections between hair follicle afferent fibres and spinocervical tract neurons in the cat: the synthesis of receptive fields. *J. Physiol.* 323:77–91.

Brown, A. M., Morimoto, K., Tsuda, Y., and Wilson, D. L. (1981a). Calcium current-dependent and voltage-dependent inactivation of calcium channels in *Helix aspersa. J. Physiol.* 320:193–218.

Brown, D. A., and Griffith, W. H. (1983a). Calcium-activated outward current in voltage-clamped hippocampal neurones of the guinea-pig. *J. Physiol.* 337:287–301.

   (1983b). Persistent slow inward calcium current in voltage-clamped hippocampal neurones of the guinea-pig. *J. Physiol.* 337:303–20.

Brown, M. W., and Cassell, M. D. (1980). Estimates of the number of neurones in the human hippocampus. *J. Physiol.* 301:58P–9P.

Brown, S., and Schäfer, E. A. (1888). An investigation into the functions of the occipital and temporal lobes of the monkey's brain. *Phil. Trans. Roy. Soc. Lond.* 179B:303–27.

Brown, T. H., Chang, V. C., Ganong, A. H., Keenan, C. L., and Kelso, S. R. (1988a). Biophysical properties of dendrites and spines that may control the induction and expression of long term synaptic potentiation. In Landfield, P. W., and Deadwyler, S. A., eds., *Long-Term Potentiation: From Biophysics to Behavior,* pp. 201–64. A. R. Liss, New York.

238   *References*

Brown, T. H., Chapman, P. F., Kairiss, E. W., and Keenan, C. L. (1988b). Long-term synaptic potentiation. *Science* 242:724–8.

Brown, T. H., Fricke, R. A., and Perkel, D. A. (1981b). Passive electrical constants in three classes of hippocampal neurons. *J. Neurophysiol.* 46:812–27.

Brown, T. H., and Johnston, D. (1983). Voltage-clamp analysis of mossy fiber synaptic input to hippocampal neurons. *J. Neurophysiol.* 50:487–507.

Brown, T. H., Wong. R. K. S., and Prince, D. A. (1979). Spontaneous miniature synaptic potentials in hippocampal neurons. *Brain Res.* 177:194–9.

Brown, W. J. (1973). Structural substrates of seizure foci in the human temporal lobe. In Brazier, M. A. B., ed., *Epilepsy. Its Phenomenon in Man,* pp. 339–74. Academic Press, New York.

Buckle, P. J., and Haas, H. L. (1982). Enhancement of synaptic transmission by 4-aminopyridine in hippocampal slices of the rat. *J. Physiol.* 326:109–22.

Bullock, T. H., McClune, M. C., and Buzsáki, G. (1988). Distribution of coherence of micro-EEG in the hippocampus of the rat asleep and awake. *Soc. Neurosci. Abstr.* 14:127.

Buño, W., Jr., Garcia-Sanchez, J. L., Garcia-Austt, E. (1978). Reset of hippocampal rhythmical activities by afferent stimulation. *Brain Res. Bull.* 3:21–8.

Buño, W., Jr., and Velluti, J. C. (1977). Relationships of hippocampal theta cycles with bar pressing during self-stimulation. *Physiol. Behav.* 19:615–21.

Burns, B. D. (1950). Some properties of the cat's isolated cerebral cortex. *J. Physiol.* 111:50–68.

Burns, B. D., and Webb, A. C. (1979). The correlation between discharge times of neighbouring neurons in isolated cerebral cortex. *Proc. Roy. Soc. Lond. B* 203:347–60.

Buzsáki, G. (1984). Long-term changes of hippocampal sharp-waves following high frequency afferent activation. *Brain Res.* 300:179–82.

(1985). Electroanatomy of the hippocampal rhythmic slow activity (RSA) in the behaving rat. In Buzsáki, G., and Vanderwolf, C., eds., *Electrical Activity of the Archicortex,* pp. 143–64. Akadémiai Kiadó, Budapest.

(1986). Hippocampal sharp waves: their origin and significance. *Brain Res.* 398:242–52.

(1989). Two-stage model of memory trace formation: a role for "noisy" brain states. *Neuroscience* 31:551–70.

Buzsáki, G., Bickford, R. G., Ryan, L. J., Young, S., Prohaska, O., Mandel, R. J., and Gage, F. H. (1989a). Multisite recording of brain field potentials and unit activity in freely moving rats. *J. Neurosci. Meth.* 28:209–17.

Buzsáki, G., Czopf, J., Kondákor, I., Björklund, A., and Gage, F. H. (1987a). Cellular activity of intracerebrally transplanted fetal hippocampus during behavior. *Neuroscience* 22:871–83.

Buzsáki, G., Czopf, J., Kondákor, I., and Kellényi, L. (1986). Laminar distribution of hippocampal rhythmic slow activity (RSA) in the behaving rat: current-source density analysis. Effects of urethane and atropine. *Brain Res.* 365:125–37.

Buzsáki, G., and Eidelberg, E. (1982). Convergence of associational and commissural pathways on CA1 pyramidal cells of the rat hippocampus. *Brain Res.* 237:283–96.

(1983). Phase relations of hippocampal projection cells and interneurons to theta activity in the anesthetized rat. *Brain Res.* 266:334–9.

Buzsáki, G., Gage, F. H., Czopf, J., and Björklund, A. (1987b). Restoration of rhythmic slow activity (theta) in the subcortically denervated hippocampus by fetal CNS transplants. *Brain Res.* 400:334–48.

Buzsáki, G., Grastyán, E., Tveritskaya, I. N., and Czopf, J. (1979). Hippocampal evoked potentials and EEG changes during classical conditioning in the rat. *Electroenceph. Clin. Neurophysiol.* 47:67–74.

Buzsáki, G., Grastyán, E., Czopf, J., Kellényi, L., and Prohaska, O. (1981). Changes in neuronal transmission in the rat hippocampus during behavior. *Brain Res.* 225:234–47.

Buzsáki, G., Leung, L.-W. S., and Vanderwolf, C. H. (1983). Cellular bases of hippocampal EEG in the behaving rat. *Brain Res. Rev.* 6:139–71.

Buzsáki, G., Ponomareff, G., Bayardo, F., Ruiz, R., and Gage, F. H. (1989b). Neuronal activity in the subcortically denervated hippocampus: a chronic model for epilepsy. *Neuroscience* 28:527–38.

Buzsáki, G., Rappelsberger, P., and Kellényi, L. (1985). Depth profiles of hippocampal rhythmic slow activity ('theta rhythm') depend on behaviour. *Electroenceph. Clin. Neurophysiol.* 61:77–88.

Calabresi, P., Benedetti, M., Mercuri, N. B., and Bernardi, G. (1989). Selective depression of synaptic transmission by tetanus toxin: a comparative study on hippocampal and neostriatal slices. *Neuroscience* 30:663–70.

Carbone, E., and Lux, H. D. (1984). A low voltage-activated, fully inactivating Ca channel in vertebrate sensory neurones. *Nature* 310:501–2.

Carpenter, G. A., and Grossberg, S. (1987). Discovering order in chaos: stable self-organization of neural recognition codes. *Ann. N.Y. Acad. Sci.* 504:33–51.

Carslaw, H. S., and Jaeger, J. C. (1959). *Conduction of Heat in Solids,* 2nd ed., Oxford University Press.

Case Records of the Massachusetts General Hospital. (1988). Case 39-1988. *N. Engl. J. Med.* 319:849–60.

Cassell, M. D., and Brown, M. W. (1977). Cell counts of the stratum pyramidale of the hippocampus of the rat. *Life Sci.* 21:1187–91.

Cavado, C., and Reinoso-Suárez, F. (1988). Connections of the prefrontal cortex with the hippocampal formation in the cat and macaque monkey. *Soc. Neurosci. Abstr.* 14:858.

Chagnac-Amitai, Y., and Connors, B. W. (1989). Synchronized excitation and inhibition driven by intrinsically bursting neurons in neocortex. *J. Neurophysiol.* 62:1149–62.

Chamberlin, N. L., and Dingledine, R. (1988). GABAergic inhibition and the induction of spontaneous epileptiform activity by low chloride and high potassium in the hippocampal slice. *Brain Res.* 445:12–18.

(1989). Control of epileptiform burst rate by CA3 hippocampal cell afterhyperpolarizations in vitro. *Brain Res.* 492:337–46.

Chamberlin, N. L., Traub, R. D., and Dingledine, R. (1990). Role of EPSPs in initiation of spontaneous synchronized burst-firing in rat hippocampal neurons bathed in high potassium. *J. Neurophysiol.* 64:1000–1008.

Chan, C. Y., Hounsgaard, J., and Midtgaard, J. (1989). Excitatory synaptic responses in turtle cerebellar Purkinje cells. *J. Physiol.* 409:143–56.

Chen, Q. X., Kay, A. R., Stelzer, A., and Wong, R. K. S. (1990). $GABA_A$-receptor function is regulated by phosph ylation in acutely dissociated guinea-pig hippocampal neurones. *J. Physiol.* 420:207–22.

Chesnut, T. J., and Swann, J. W. (1988). Epileptiform activity induced by 4-aminopyridine in immature hippocampus. *Epil. Res.* 2:187–95.

Christian, E. P., and Dudek, F. E. (1988a). Characteristics of local excitatory circuits studied with glutamate microapplication in the CA3 area of rat hippocampal slices. *J. Neurophysiol.* 59:90–109.

(1988b). Electrophysiological evidence from glutamate microapplications for local excitatory circuits in the CA1 area of rat hippocampal slices. *J. Neurophysiol.* 59:110–23.

Chronister, R. B., and DeFrance, J. F. (1979). Organization of projection neurons of the hippocampus. *Exp. Neurol.* 66:509–23.

Chronister, R. B., Sikes, R. W., and White, L. E., Jr. (1976). The septo-hippocampal system: significance of the subiculum. In DeFrance, J. F., ed., *The Septal Nuclei*, pp. 115–32. Plenum Press, New York.

Churchland, P. S., and Sejnowski, T. J. (1988). Perspectives on cognitive neuroscience. *Science* 242:741–5.

Claiborne, B. J., Amaral, D. G., and Cowan, W. M. (1986). A light and electron microscopic analysis of the mossy fibers of the rat dentate gyrus. *J. Compar. Neurol.* 246:435–58.

Clements, J. D., Forsythe, I. D., and Redman, S. J. (1987). Presynaptic inhibition of synaptic potentials evoked in cat spinal motoneurones by impulses in single group Ia axons. *J. Physiol.* 383:153–69.

Clements, J. D., and Redman, S. J. (1989). Cable properties of cat spinal motorneurons measured by combining voltage clamp, current clamp and intracellular staining. *J. Physiol.* 409:63–87.

Cohen, A. H. (1987). Effects of oscillator frequency on phase-locking in the lamprey central pattern generator. *J. Neurosci. Meth.* 21:113–25.

Cole, A. E., and Nicoll, R. A. (1984). Characterization of a slow cholinergic post-synaptic potential recorded *in vitro* from rat hippocampal pyramidal cells. *J. Physiol.* 352:173–88.

Colino, A., and Halliwell, J. V. (1987). Differential modulation of three separate K-conductances in hippocampal CA1 neurons by serotonin. *Nature* 328:73–7.

Collingridge, G. L., Gage, P. W., and Robertson, B. (1984). Inhibitory post-synaptic currents in rat hippocampal CA1 neurones. *J. Physiol.* 356:551–64.

Collingridge, G. L., Kehl, S. J., and McLennan, H. (1983a). The antagonism of amino acid-induced excitation of rat hippocampal CA1 neurones in vitro. *J. Physiol.* 334:19–31.

(1983b). Excitatory amino acids in synaptic transmission in the Schaffer collateral-commissural pathway of the rat hippocampus. *J. Physiol.* 334:33–46.

Colmers, W. F., Lukowiak, K., and Pittman, Q. J. (1987). Presynaptic action of neuropeptide Y in area CA1 of the rat hippocampal slice. *J. Physiol.* 383:285–99.

Connor, J. A., Wadman, W. J., Hockberger, P. E., and Wong, R. K. S. (1988). Sustained dendritic gradients of Ca^{2+} induced by excitatory amino acids in hippocampal neurons. *Science* 241:339–41.

Connors, B. W. (1984). Initiation of synchronized neuronal bursting in neocortex. *Nature* 310:685–7.

Cook, T. M., and Crutcher, K. A. (1985). Extensive target cell loss during development results in mossy fibers in the regio superior (CA1) of the rat hippocampal formation. *Dev. Brain Res.* 21:19–30.

Corsellis, J. A. N., Goldberg, G. J., and Norton, A. R. (1968). "Limbic encephalitis" and its association with carcinoma. *Brain* 91:481–96.

Cotman, C. W., Flatman, J. A., Ganong, A. H., and Perkins, M. N. (1986). Effects of excitatory amino acid antagonists on evoked and spontaneous excitatory potentials in guinea-pig hippocampus. *J. Physiol.* 378:403–15.

Creutzfeldt, O., and Houchin, J. (1974). Neuronal basis of EEG waves. In Creutzfeldt, O., ed., *Handbook of Electroencephalography and Clinical Neurophysiology, Vol. 2C*, pp. 5–55. Elsevier, Amsterdam.

Creutzfeldt, O., Watanabe, S., and Lux, H. D. (1966). Relations between EEG phenomena and potentials of single cortical cells. I. Evoked responses after thalamic and epicortical stimulation. *Electroenceph. Clin. Neurophysiol.* 20:1–18.

Crunelli, V., Forda, S., and Kelly, J. S. (1983). Blockade of amino acid-induced depolarizations and inhibition of excitatory postsynaptic potentials in rat dentate gyrus. *J. Physiol.* 341:627–40.

Crutcher, K. A., Madison, R., and Davis, J. N. (1981). A study of the rat septohippocampal pathway using anterograde transport of horseradish peroxidase. *Neuroscience* 6:1961–73.

Cull-Candy, S. G., and Usowicz, M. M. (1987). Multiple conductance channels activated by excitatory amino acids in cerebellar neurones. *Nature* 325:525–8.

Currie, S., Heathfield, K. W. G., Henson, R. A., and Scott, D. F. (1971). Clinical course and prognosis of temporal lobe epilepsy. A survey of 666 patients. *Brain* 94:173–90.

Curtis, D. R., Duggan, A. W., Felix, D., Johnston, G. A. R., and McLennan, H. (1971). Antagonism between bicuculline and GABA in the cat brain. *Brain Res.* 33:57–73.

Daly, D. D. (1979). Use of the EEG for diagnosis and evaluation of epileptic seizures and nonepileptic episodic disorders. In Klass, D. W., and Daly, D. D., eds., *Current Practice of Clinical Electroencephalography*, pp. 221–68. Raven Press, New York.

Daniel, J. W., and Moore, R. E. (1978). *Computation and Theory in Ordinary Differential Equations*. Freeman, San Francisco.

Davis, H. P., Tribuna, J., Pulsinelli, W. A., and Volpe, B. T. (1986). Reference and working memory of rats following hippocampal damage induced by transient forebrain ischemia. *Physiol. Behav.* 37:387–92.

Deisz, R. A., and Prince, D. A. (1989). Frequency-dependent depression of inhibition in guinea-pig neocortex *in vitro* by $GABA_B$ receptor feed-back on GABA release. *J. Physiol.* 412:513–41.

del Castillo, J., and Katz, B. (1954). Quantal components of the end-plate potential. *J. Physiol.* 124:560–73.

Delgado-Escueta, A. V., Ward, A. A., Jr., Woodbury, D. M., and Porter, R. J. eds. (1986). *Advances in Neurology, Vol. 44, Basic Mechanisms of the Epilepsies. Molecular and Cellular Approaches.* Raven Press, New York.

Delmar, M., Jalife, J., and Michaels, D. C. (1986). Effects of changes in excitability and intercellular coupling on synchronization in the rabbit sino-atrial node. *J. Physiol.* 370:127–50.

Destrade, C., and Ott, T. (1980). Blockade of high frequency rhythmical slow activity by intrahippocampal injection of a glutamic acid antagonist. *Neurosci. Lett.* 18:73–8.

Devaney, R. L. (1986). *An Introduction to Chaotic Dynamical Systems.* W. A. Benjamin, Menlo Park, Calif.

Devinsky, O., Kelley, K., Porter, R. J., and Theodore, W. H. (1988). Clinical and electroencephalographic features of simple partial seizures. *Neurology* 38:1347–52.

Dichter, M., Herman, C., and Selzer, M. (1973). Penicillin epilepsy in isolated islands of hippocampus. *Electroenceph. Clin. Neurophysiol.* 34:631–8.

Dichter, M., and Spencer, W. A. (1969a). Penicillin-induced interictal discharges from the cat hippocampus. I. Characteristics and topographical features. *J. Neurophysiol.* 32:649–62.

(1969b). Penicillin-induced interictal discharges from the cat hippocampus. II. Mechanisms underlying origin and restriction. *J. Neurophysiol.* 32:663–87.

Dickinson, P. S., and Marder, E. (1989). Peptidergic modulation of a multi-oscillator system in the lobster. I. Activation of the cardiac sac motor pattern by the neuropeptides proctolin and red pigment-concentrating hormone. *J. Neurophysiol.* 61:833–44.

Dickinson, P. S., Mecsas, C., and Marder, E. (1990). Neuropeptide fusion of two motor-pattern generator circuits. *Nature* 344:155–8.

Dietz, S., Frotscher, M., and Abt, K. (1987). Quantitative Untersuchungen zur schichtenspezifischen Verteilung von Neuronen im Hippocampus des Meerschweinchens. *Verh. Anat. Ges.* 81:883–4.

Dietzel, I., Heinemann, U., Hofmeier, G., and Lux, H. D. (1980). Transient changes in the size of the extracellular space in the sensorimotor cortex of cats in relation to stimulus-induced changes in potassium concentration. *Exp. Brain Res.* 40:432–9.

(1982a). Stimulus-induced changes in extracellular Na^+ and Cl^- concentration in relation to changes in the size of the extracellular space. *Exp. Brain Res.* 46:73–84.

(1982b). Changes in the extracellular volume in the cerebral cortex of cats in relation to stimulus induced epileptiform afterdischarges. In Klee, M. R., Lux, H. D., and Speckmann, E.-J., eds., *Physiology and Pharmacology of Epileptogenic Phenomena*, pp. 5–12. Raven Press, New York.

Dietzel, I., Heinemann, U., Lux, H. D. (1989). Relations between slow extracellular potential changes, glial potassium buffering, and electrolyte and cellular volume changes during neuronal hyperactivity in cat brain. *Glia* 2:25–44.

Dingledine, R., and Gjerstad, L. (1979). Penicillin blocks hippocampal IPSPs, unmasking prolonged EPSPs. *Brain Res.* 168:205–9.

(1980). Reduced inhibition during epileptiform activity in the in vitro hippocampal slice. *J. Physiol.* 305:297–313.

Dingledine, R., Hynes, M. A., and King, G. L. (1986). Involvement of N-methyl-D-aspartate receptors in epileptiform bursting in the rat hippocampal slice. *J. Physiol.* 380:175–189.

Dingledine, R., Roth, A. A., and King, G. L. (1987). Synaptic control of pyramidal cell activation in the hippocampal slice preparation in the rat. *Neuroscience* 22:553–61.

Dodge, F. A., Jr., and Cooley, J. W. (1973). Action potential of the motoneuron. *IBM J. Res. Dev.* 17:219–29.

Domann, R., Dorn, T., and Witte, O. W. (1989). $GABA_A$- and $GABA_B$-dependent IPSPs following penicillin-induced paroxysmal depolarizations in the hippocampal slice. *Soc. Neurosci. Abstr.* 15:340.

Dudek, F. E., Snow, R. W., and Taylor, C. P. (1986). Role of electrical interactions in synchronization of epileptiform bursts. In Delgado-Escueta, A. V., Ward, A. A., Jr., Woodbury, D. M., and Porter, R. J., eds., *Advances in Neurology, Vol. 44, Basic Mechanisms of the Epilepsies. Molecular and Cellular Approaches*, pp. 593-617. Raven Press, New York.

Dudek, F. E., and Traub, R. D. (1989). Local synaptic and electrical interactions in hippocampus: experimental data and computer simulations. In Byrne, J. H., and Berry, W. O., eds., *Neural Models of Plasticity*, pp. 378-402. Academic Press, San Diego.

Durand, D. (1984). The somatic shunt cable model for neurons. *Biophys. J.* 46:645–53.

Dutar, P., Lamour, Y., and Jobert, A. (1985). Septohippocampal neurons in the rat: an in vivo intracellular study. *Brain Res.* 340:135–42.

Dutar, P., and Nicoll, R. A. (1988). A physiological role for $GABA_B$ receptors in the central nervous system. *Nature* 332:156–8.

Eckhorn, R., Bauer, R., Jordan, W., Brosch, M., Kruse, W., Munk, M., and Reitboek, H. J. (1988). Coherent oscillations: a mechanism of feature linking in the visual cortex? Multiple electrode and correlation analyses in the cat. *Biol. Cybern.* 60:121–30.

Eckmann, J.-P., And Ruelle, D. (1985). Ergodic theory of chaos and strange attractors. *Rev. Mod. Phys.* 57:617–56.

Edwards, F. A., Konnerth, A., Sakmann, B., and Takahashi, T. (1989). A thin slice preparation for patch clamp recordings from neurones of the mammalian central nervous system. *Pflüg. Arch.* 414:600–12.

Edwards, S. F., and Anderson, P. W. (1975). Theory of spin glasses. *J. Phys. F* 5:965–74.

Eichenbaum, H., and Cohen, N. J. (1988). Representation in the hippocampus: what do hippocampal neurons code? *Trends Neurosci.* 11:244–8.

Eichenbaum, H., Wiener, S. I., Shapiro, M. L., and Cohen, N. J. (1989). The organization of spatial coding in the hippocampus: a study of neural ensemble activity. *J. Neurosci.* 9:2764–75.

Erdös, P., and Rényi, A. (1960). On the evolution of random graphs. *Publ. Math. Instit. Hungar. Acad. Sci.* 5:17–61.

Ermentrout, G. B., and Kopell, N. (1984). Frequency plateaus in a chain of weakly coupled oscillators. I. *SIAM J. Math. Anal.* 15:215–37.

Essam, J. W. (1972). Percolation and cluster size. In Domb, C., and Green, M. S., eds., *Phase Transitions and Critical Phenomena, Vol. 2*, pp. 197–270. Academic Press, London.

Faber, D. S., and Korn, H. (1980). Single-shot channel activation accounts for duration of inhibitory postsynaptic potentials in a central neuron. *Science* 208:612–15.

(1982). Transmission at a central inhibitory synpase. I. Magnitude of unitary postsynaptic conductance change and kinetics of channel activation. *J. Neurophysiol.* 48:654–78.

(1989). Electrical field effects: their relevance in central neural networks. *Physiol. Rev.* 69:821–63.

Feldman, J. L., and Ellenberger, H. H. (1988). Central coordination of respiratory and cardiovascular control in mammals. *Ann. Rev. Physiol.* 50:593–606.

Finch, D. M., Nowlin, N. L., and Babb, T. L. (1983). Demonstration of axonal projection of neurons in the rat hippocampus and subiculum by intracellular injection of HRP. *Brain Res.* 271:201–16.

Finch, D. M., Wong, E. E., Derian, E. L., and Babb. T. L. (1986). Neurophysiology of limbic system pathways in the rat: projections from the subicular complex and hippocampus to the entorhinal cortex. *Brain Res.* 397:205–13.

Fisher, C. M., and Adams, R. D. (1964). Transient global amnesia. *Acta Neurol. Scand.* 40(Suppl. 9):1–83.

Fisher, M. E. (1961). Critical probabilities for cluster size and percolation problems. *J. Math. Phys.* 2:620–7.

Fisher, R. S., and Alger, B. E. (1984). Electrophysiological mechanisms of kainic acid-induced epileptiform activity in the rat hippocampal slice. *J. Neurosci.* 4:1312–23.

Fisher, R. S., and Prince, D. A. (1977a). Spike-wave rhythms in cat cortex induced by parenteral penicillin. I. Electroencephalographic features. *Electroenceph. Clin. Neurophysiol.* 42:608–24.

(1977b). Spike-wave rhythms in cat cortex induced by parenteral penicillin. II. Cellular features. *Electroenceph. Clin. Neurophysiol.* 42:625–39.

Forsythe, I. D., and Westbrook, G. L. (1988). Slow excitatory postsynaptic currents mediated by N-methyl-D-aspartate receptors on cultured mouse central neurones. *J. Physiol.* 396:515–33.

Fox, S. E., Wolfson, S., and Ranck, J. B., Jr. (1986). Hippocampal theta rhythm and the firing of neurons in walking and urethane anesthetized rats. *Exp. Brain Res.* 62:495–508.

Franck, J. E., and Schwartzkroin, P. A. (1985). Do kainate-lesioned hippocampi become epileptogenic? *Brain Res.* 329:309–13.

Frankenhaeuser, B. (1962). Potassium permeability in myelinated nerve fibres of *Xenopus laevis. J. Physiol.* 160:54–61.

Frankenhaeuser, B., and Hodgkin, A. L. (1957). The action of calcium on the electrical properties of squid axons. *J. Physiol.* 137:218–44.

Freeman, W. J. (1979). Nonlinear dynamics of paleocortex manifested in the olfactory EEG. *Biol. Cybern.* 35:21–37.

French, C. R., and Gage, P. W. (1985). A threshold sodium current in pyramidal cells in rat hippocampus. *Neurosci. Lett.* 56:289–93.

Freund, T. F., and Antal, M. (1988). GABA-containing neurons in the septum control inhibitory interneurons in the hippocampus. *Nature* 336:170–3.

Fricke, R. A., and Prince, D. A. (1984). Electrophysiology of dentate gyrus granule cells. *J. Neurophysiol.* 51:195–209.

Friedlander, M. J., Sayer, R. J., and Redman, S. J. (1988). Synaptic transmission between individual CA3 and CA1 neurons in the hippocampus. *Soc. Neurosci. Abstr.* 14:18.

Friedman, H. R., and Goldman-Rakic, P. S. (1988). Activation of the hippocampus and dentate gyrus by working-memory: a 2-deoxyglucose study of behaving rhesus monkeys. *J. Neurosci.* 8:4693–706.

Frotscher, M. (1985). Mossy fibres form synapses with identified pyramidal basket cells in the CA3 region of the guinea-pig hippocampus: a combined Golgi-electron microscope study. *J. Neurocytol.* 14:245–59.

(1989). Mossy fiber synapses on glutamate decarboxylase-immunoreactive neurons: evidence for feed-forward inhibition in the CA3 region of the hippocampus. *Exp. Brain Res.* 75:441–5.

Frotscher, M., and Gähwiler, B. H. (1988). Synaptic organization of intracellularly stained CA3 pyramidal neurons in slice cultures of rat hippocampus. *Neuroscience* 24:541–51.

Frotscher, M., Kugler, P., Misgeld, U., and Zilles, K. (1988). *Neurotransmission in the Hippocampus.* Springer, Berlin.

Frotscher, M., and Zimmer, J. (1983). Lesion-induced mossy fibers to the molecular layer of the rat fascia dentata: identification of postsynaptic granule cells by the Golgi-EM technique. *J. Comp. Neurol.* 215:299–311.

Fung, S. J., Boxer, P. A., Morales, F. R., and Chase, M. H. (1982). Hyperpolarizing membrane responses induced in lumbar motoneurons by stimulation of the nucleus reticularis pontis oralis during active sleep. *Brain Res.* 248:267–73.

Gabbott, P. L. A., Martin, K. A. C., and Whitteridge, D. (1987). Connections between pyramidal neurons in layer 5 of cat visual cortex (area 17). *J. Compar. Neurol.* 259:364–81.

Gabrieli, J. D. E., Cohen, N. J., and Corkin, S. (1988). The impaired learning of semantic knowledge following bilateral medial temporal-lobe resection. *Brain Cogn.* 7:157–77.

Gähwiler, B. H. (1981). Morphological differentiation of nerve cells in thin organotypic cultures derived from rat hippocampus and cerebellum. *Proc. Roy. Soc. Lond. B* 211:287–90.

Gähwiler, B. H., and Brown, D. A. (1985a). Functional innervation of cultured hippocampal neurones by cholinergic afferents from co-cultured septal explants. *Nature* 313:577–9.

(1985b). GABA$_B$-receptor-activated K$^+$ current in voltage-clamped CA$_3$ pyramidal cells in hippocampal cultures. *Proc. Natl. Acad. Sci. U.S.A.* 82:1558–62.

Gamrani, H., Onteniente, B., Seguela, P., Geffard, M., and Calas, A. (1986). Gamma-aminobutyric acid-immunoreactivity in the rat hippocampus. A light and electron microscopic study with anti-GABA antibodies. *Brain Res.* 364:30–8.

Garbarg, M., Barbin, G., Feger, J., and Schwartz, J. C. (1974). Histaminergic pathway in rat brain: evidence by lesions of the medial forebrain bundle. *Science* 186:833–4.

Gastaut, H. (1970). Clinical and electroencephalographical classification of epileptic seizures. *Epilepsia* 11:102–13.

Gastaut, H., and Tassinari, C. A. (1975). Ictal discharges in different types of seizures. In Gastaut, H., and Tassinari, C. A., eds., *Handbook of Electroencephalography and Clinical Neurophysiology, Vol. 13, Part A, Epilepsies,* pp. 20–45. Elsevier, Amsterdam.

Gaztelu, J. M., and Buño, W., Jr. (1982). Septo-hippocampal relationships during EEG theta rhythm. *Electroenceph. Clin. Neurophysiol.* 54:375–87.

Getting, P. A. (1983). Mechanisms of pattern generation underlying swimming in *Tritonia*. II. Network reconstruction. *J. Neurophysiol.* 49:1017–35.

Getting, P. A., and Dekin, M. S. (1985a). Mechanisms of pattern generation underlying swimming in *Tritonia*. IV. Gating of central pattern generator. *J. Neurophysiol.* 53:466–80.

(1985b). *Tritonia* swimming. A model system for integration within rhythmic motor systems. In Selverston, A. I., ed., *Model Neural Networks and Behavior,* pp. 3–20. Plenum Press, New York.

Gilbert, C.D., and Wiesel, T. N. (1983). Clustered intrinsic connections in the cat visual cortex. *J. Neurosci.* 3:1116–33.

Ginsborg, B. L. (1973). Electrical changes in the membrane in junctional transmission. *Biochim. Biophys. Acta* 300:289–317.

Goldenberg, G., Wimmer, A., and Maly, J. (1983). Amnesic syndrome with a unilateral thalamic lesion: a case report. *J. Neurol.* 229:79–86.

Goldensohn, E. S., and Purpura, D. P. (1963). Intracellular potentials of cortical neurons during focal epileptogenic discharges. *Science* 139:840–2.

Gottlieb, D. I., and Cowan, W. M. (1973). Autoradiographic study of the commissural and ipsilateral association connections of the hippocampus and dentate gyrus of the rat. I. The commissural connections. *J. Compar. Neurol.* 149:393–442.

Grantyn, R., Shapovalov, A. I., and Shiriaev, B. I. (1984a). Tracing of frog sensory-motor synapses by intracellular injection of horseradish peroxidase. *J. Physiol.* 349:441–58.

(1984b). Relation between structural and release parameters at the frog sensory-motor synapse. *J. Physiol.* 349:459–74.

Grassberger, P., and Procaccia, I. (1983). Measuring the strangeness of strange attractors. *Physica* 9D:189–208.

Grastyán, E., Karmos, G., Vereczkey, L., Martin, J., and Kellényi, L. (1965). Hypothalamic motivational processes as reflected by their hippocampal electrical correlates. *Science* 149:91–3.

Gray, C. M., and Singer, W. (1989). Stimulus-specific neuronal oscillations in orientation columns of cat visual cortex. *Proc. Natl. Acad. Sci. U.S.A.* 86:1698–702.

Gray, R., and Johnston, D. (1985). Rectification of single GABA-gated chloride channels in adult hippocampal neurons. *J. Neurophysiol.* 54:134–42.

(1987). Noradrenaline and β-adrenoceptor agonists increase activity of voltage-dependent calcium channels in hippocampal neurons. *Nature* 327:620–2.

Greenamyre, J. T., Olson, J. M., Penney, J. B., Jr., and Young, A. B. (1985). Autoradiographic characterization of N-methyl-D-aspartate-, glutamate- and kainate-sensitive glutamate binding sites. *J. Pharmacol. Exp. Ther.* 233:254–63.

Griffith, W. H. (1988). Membrane properties of cell types within guinea pig basal forebrain nuclei in vitro. *J. Neurophysiol.* 59:1590–612.

Griffith, W. H., and Matthews, R. T. (1986). Electrophysiology of AChE-positive neurons in basal forebrain slices. *Neurosci. Lett. 71:169–74.*

Grinvald, A. (1985). Real-time optical mapping of neuronal activity: from single growth cones to the intact mammalian brain. *Ann. Rev. Neurosci.* 8:263–305.

Grinvald, A., Manker, A., and Segal, M. (1982). Visualization of the spread of electrical activity in rat hippocampal slices by voltage-sensitive optical probes. *J. Physiol.* 33:269–91.

Grinvald, A., Ross, W. N., and Farber, I. (1981). Simultaneous optical measurements of electrical activity from multiple sites on processes of cultured neurons. *Proc. Natl. Acad. Sci. U.S.A.* 78:3245–9.

Gritti, I., Mariotti, M., and Mancia, M. (1987). Limbic and brainstem afferents to thalamic mediodorsal nucleus: a horseradish peroxidase study. *Neurosci. Lett.* 76:345–50.

Gustafsson, B., Galvan, M., Grafe, P., and Wigström, H. (1982). A transient outward current in a mammalian central neurone blocked by 4-aminopyridine. *Nature* 299:252–4.

Gustafsson, B., and Wigström, H. (1988). Physiological mechanisms underlying long-term potentiation. *Trends Neurosci.* 11:156–62.

Gutnick, M. J., Connors, B. W., and Prince, D. A. (1982). Mechanisms of neocortical epileptogenesis in vitro. *J. Neurophysiol.* 48:1321–35.

Guy, N., and Ropert, N. (1990). Serotonin facilitates GABAergic inhibition on hippocampal CA1 neurones in vitro. *J. Physiol.* 423:94P.

Haas, D. C., and Ross, G. S. (1986). Transient global amnesia triggered by mild head trauma. *Brain* 109:251–7.

Haas, H. L. (1982). Cholinergic disinhibition in hippocampal slices of the rat. *Brain Res.* 233:200–4.

Haas, H. L., and Jefferys, J. G. R. (1984). Low-calcium field burst discharges of CA1 pyramidal neurones in rat hippocampal slices. *J. Physiol.* 354:185–201.

Haas, H. L., and Konnerth, A. (1983). Histamine and noradrenaline decrease calcium-activated potassium conductance in hippocampal pyramidal cells. *Nature* 302:432–4.

Haberly, L. B. (1985). Neuronal circuitry in olfactory cortex: anatomy and functional implications. *Chem. Senses* 10:219–38.

Hablitz, J. J. (1984). Picrotoxin-induced epileptiform activity in the hippocampus: role of endogenous versus synaptic factors. *J. Neurophysiol.* 51:1011–27.

Hablitz, J. J., and Johnston, D. (1981). Endogenous nature of spontaneous bursting in a hippocampal pyramidal neurons. *Cell. Molec. Neurobiol.* 1:325–334.

Hablitz, J. J., and Thalmann, R. H. (1987). Conductance changes underlying a late synaptic hyperpolarization in hippocampal CA3 neurons. *J. Neurophysiol.* 58:160–79.

Halgren, E. (1982). Mental phenomena induced by stimulation in the limbic system. *Human Neurobiol.* 1:251–60.

Halgren, E., Babb, T. L., and Crandall, P. H. (1978). Human hippocampal formation EEG desynchronizes during attentiveness and movement. *Electroenceph. Clin. Neurophysiol.* 44:778–81.

Halgren, E., Smith, M. E., and Stapleton, J. M. (1985). Hippocampal field-potentials evoked by repeated vs. nonrepeated words. In Buzsáki, G., and Vanderwolf, C., eds., *Electrical Activity of the Archicortex*, pp. 67–81. Akadémiai Kiadó, Budapest.

Halgren, E., and Wilson, C. L. (1985). Recall deficits produced by afterdischarges in the human hippocampal formation and amygdala. *Electroenceph. Clin. Neurophysiol.* 61:375–80.

Halliwell, J. V., and Adams, P. R. (1982). Voltage-clamp analysis of muscarinic excitation in hippocampal neurons. *Brain Res.* 250:71–92.

Hammersley, J. M. (1961). Comparison of atom and bond percolation processes. *J. Math. Phys.* 2:728–33.

Heath, R. G. (1972). Pleasure and brain activity in man. *J. Nerv. Ment. Dis.* 154:3–18.

Heinemann, U., Konnerth, A., Pumain, R., and Wadman, W. J. (1986). Extracellular calcium and potassium concentration changes in chronic epileptic brain tissue. In Delgado-Escueta, A. V., Ward, A. A., Jr., Woodbury, D. M., and Porter, R. J., eds., *Advances in Neurology, Vol. 44, Basic Mechanisms of the Epilepsies. Molecular and Cellular Approaches*, pp. 641–61. Raven Press, New York.

Heinzel, H.-G. (1988a). Gastric mill activity in the lobster. I. Spontaneous modes of chewing. *J. Neurophysiol.* 59:528–50.

(1988b). Gastric mill activity in the lobster. II. Proctolin and octopamine initiate and modulate chewing. *J. Neurophysiol.* 59:551–65.

Heinzel, H.-G., and Selverston, A. I. (1988). Gastric mill activity in the lobster. III. Effects of proctolin on the isolated central pattern generator. *J. Neurophysiol.* 59:566–85.

Heit, G., Smith, M. E., and Halgren, E. (1988). Neural encoding of individual words and faces by the human hippocampus and amygdala. *Nature* 333:773–5.

Henson, R. A., Hoffman, H. L., and Urich, H. (1965). Encephalomyelitis with carcinoma. *Brain* 88:449–63.

Hertz, J., Krogh, A., and Palmer, R. G. (1990). *Introduction to the Theory of Neural Networks*. Addison-Wesley, Reading, Mass.

Hoch, D. B., and Dingledine, R. (1986). GABAergic neurons in rat hippocampal culture. *Dev. Brain Res.* 25:53–64.

Hodgkin, A. L., and Huxley, A. F. (1952a). Currents carried by sodium and potassium ions through the membrane of the giant axon of *Loligo*. *J. Physiol.* 116:449–72.

(1952b). The components of membrane conductance in the giant axon of *Loligo*. *J. Physiol.* 116:473–96.

(1952c). The dual effect of membrane potential on sodium conductance in the giant axon of *Loligo*. *J. Physiol.* 116:497–506.

(1952d). A quantitative description of membrane current and its application to conduction and excitation in nerve. *J. Physiol.* 117:500–44.

Hoffman, W. H., and Haberly, L. B. (1989). Bursting induces persistent all-or-none EPSPs by an NMDA-dependent process in piriform cortex. *J. Neurosci.* 9:206–15.

Honoré, T., Davies, S. N., Drejer, J., Fletcher, E. J., Jacobsen, P., Lodge, D., and Nielsen, F. E. (1988). Quinoxalinediones: potent competitive non-NMDA glutamate receptor antagonists. *Science* 241:701–3.

Hopfield, J. J. (1982). Neural networks and physical systems with emergent collective computational abilities. *Proc. Natl. Acad. Sci. U.S.A.* 79:2554–8.

Hopfield, J. J., and Tank, D. W. (1986). Computing with neural circuits: a model. *Science* 233:625–33.

Horel, J. A. (1978). The neuroanatomy of amnesia. *Brain* 101:403–45.

Horton, H., and Levitt, P. (1986). Developmental studies with a specific cell surface marker for limbic system neurons. *Prog. Dev. Biol.* A:111–13.

Hotson, J. R., and Prince, D. A. (1980). A calcium-activated hyperpolarization follows repetitive firing in hippocampal neurons. *J. Neurophysiol.* 43:409–19.

Hotson, J. R., Prince, D. A., and Schwartzkroin, P. A. (1979). Anomalous inward rectification in hippocampal neurons. *J. Neurophysiol.* 42:889–95.

Huguenard, J. R., Hamill, O. P., and Prince, D. A. (1989). Sodium channels in dendrites of rat cortical pyramidal neurons. *Proc. Natl. Acad. Sci. U.S.A.* 86:2473–7.

Hume, R. I., and Purves, D. (1983). Apportionment of the terminals from single pre-ganglionic axons to target neurones in the rabbit ciliary ganglion. *J. Physiol.* 338:259–75.

Humphrey, D. R. (1968). Re-analysis of the antidromic cortical response. II. On the contribution of cell discharge and PSPs to the evoked potentials. *Electroenceph. Clin. Neurophysiol.* 25:421–42.

Huxley, A. F. (1959). Ion movements during nerve activity. *Ann. N.Y. Acad. Sci.* 81:221–46.

Insausti, R., and Amaral, D. G. (1988). Distribution of cortical projections the monkey entorhinal cortex: an autoradiographic study. *Soc. Neurosci. Abstr.* 14:858.

Ishizuka, N., Krzemieniewska, K., and Amaral, D. G. (1986). Organization of pyramidal cell axonal collaterals in field CA3 of the rat hippocampus. *Soc. Neurosci. Abstr.* 12:1254.

Ishizuka, N., Weber, J., and Amaral, D. G. (1990). Organization of intrahippocampal projections originating from CA3 pyramidal cells in the rat. *J. Comp. Neurol.* 295:580–623.

Isokawa-Akesson, M., Wilson, C. L., and Babb, T. L. (1987). Diversity in periodic pattern of firing in human hippocampal neurons. *Exper. Neurol.* 98:137–51.

Ives, A. E., and Jefferys, J. G. R. (1990). Synchronization of epileptiform bursts induced by 4-aminopyridine in the in-vitro hippocampal slice preparation. *Neurosci. Lett.* 112:239–45.

Jahnsen, H. (1980). The action of 5-hydroxytryptamine on neuronal membranes and synaptic transmission in area CA1 of the hippocampus in vitro. *Brain Res.* 197:83–94.

Jahnsen, H., and Llinás, R. (1984a). Electrophysiological properties of guinea-pig thalamic neurones: an *in vitro* study. *J. Physiol.* 349:205–26.

(1984b). Ionic basis for the electroresponsiveness and oscillatory properties of guinea-pig thalamic neurones *in vitro*. *J. Physiol.* 349:227–47.

Jalife, J. (1984). Mutual entrainment and electrical coupling as mechanisms for synchronous firing of rabbit sino-atrial pace-maker cells. *J. Physiol.* 356:221–43.

Jankowska, E., and Roberts, W. J. (1972). Synaptic action of single interneurones mediating Ia inhibition of motoneurones. *J. Physiol.* 222:623–42.

Jefferys, J. G. R. (1981). Influence of electric fields on the excitability of granule cells in guinea-pig hippocampal slices. *J. Physiol.* 319:143–52.

(1984). Current flow through hippocampal slices. *Soc. Neurosci. Abstr.* 10:1074.

(1989). Chronic epileptic foci in vitro in hippocampal slices from rats with the tetanus toxin epileptic syndrome. *J. Neurophysiol.* 62:458–68.

(1990). Basic mechanisms of focal epilepsies. *Exper. Physiol.* 75:127–62.

Jefferys, J. G. R., and Haas, H. L. (1982). Synchronized bursting of CA1 hippocampal pyramidal cells in the absence of synaptic transmission. *Nature* 300:448–50.

Jefferys, J. G. R., and Williams, S. F. (1987). Physiological and behavioural consequences of seizures induced in the rat by intrahippocampal tetanus toxin. *Brain* 110:517–32.

(1989). Intrahippocampal cholera toxin, but not its B subunit, induces a subacute epileptic focus in rats: an *in vitro* study. *J. Physiol.* 413:1–36.

Jensen, M. S., and Yaari, Y. (1988). The relationship between interictal and ictal paroxysms in an in vitro model of focal hippocampal epilepsy. *Ann. Neurol.* 24:591–8.

Johnson, J. W., and Ascher, P. (1987). Glycine potentiates the NMDA response in cultured mouse brain neurons. *Nature* 325:529–31.

Johnston, D. (1981). Passive cable properties of hippocampal CA3 pyramidal neurons. *Cell. Molec. Neurobiol.* 1:41–55.

Johnston, D., and Brown, T. H. (1981). Giant synaptic potential hypothesis for epileptiform activity. *Science* 211:294–7.

(1983). Interpretation of voltage-clamp measurements in hippocampal neurons. *J. Neurophysiol.* 50:464–86.

(1984). Mechanisms of neuronal burst generation. In Schwartzkroin, P. A., and Wheal, H., eds., *Electrophysiology of Epilepsy*, pp. 277–301. Academic Press, New York.

Johnston, D., Hablitz, J. J., and Wilson, W. A. (1980). Voltage clamp discloses slow inward current in hippocampal burst-firing neurones. *Nature* 286:391–3.

Jones, O. T., Kunze, D. L., and Angelides, K. J. (1989). Localization and mobility of ω-conotoxin-sensitive Ca^{2+} channels in hippocampal CA1 neurons. *Science* 244:1189–93.

Kandel, E. R., and Spencer, W. A. (1961a). Excitation and inhibition of single pyramidal cells during hippocampal seizure. *Exper. Neurol.* 4:162–79.

(1961b). Electrophysiology of hippocampal neurons. II. Afterpotentials and repetitive firing. *J. Neurophysiol.* 24:243–59.

Kass, I. S., and Lipton, P. (1982). Mechanisms involved in irreversible anoxic damage to the in vitro rat hippocampal slice. *J. Physiol.* 332:459–72.

Katz, B. (1969). *The Release of Neural Transmitter Substances.* Liverpool University Press.

Katz, B., and Miledi, R. (1968). The role of calcium in neuromuscular facilitation. *J. Physiol.* 199:729–41.

Kawaguchi, Y., and Hama, K. (1987). Two subtypes of non-pyramidal cells in rat hippocampal formation identified by intracellular recording and HRP injection. *Brain Res.* 411:190–5.

(1988). Physiological heterogeneity of nonpyramidal cells in rat hippocampal CA1 region. *Exp. Brain Res.* 72:494–502.

Kay, A. R., Miles, R., and Wong, R. K. S. (1986). Intracellular fluoride alters the kinetic properties of calcium currents facilitating the investigation of synaptic events in hippocampal neurons. *J. Neurosci.* 6:2915–20.

Kay, A. R., and Wong, R. K. S. (1986). Isolation of neurons suitable for patch-clamping from adult mammalian central nervous systems. *J. Neurosci. Meth.* 16:227–38.

(1987). Calcium current activation kinetics in isolated pyramidal neurones of the CA1 region of the mature guinea-pig hippocampus. *J. Physiol.* 392:603–16.

Kehl, S. J., and McLennan, H. (1985a). An electrophysiological characterization of inhibitions and postsynaptic potentials in rat hippocampal CA3 neurones in vitro. *Exp. Brain Res.* 60:299–308.

(1985b). A pharmacological characterization of chloride- and potassium-dependent inhibitions in the CA3 region of the rat hippocampus in vitro. *Exp. Brain Res.* 60:309–17.

Kerr, D. I. B., Ong, J., Prager, R. H., Gynther, B. D., and Curtis, D. R. (1987). Phaclofen: a peripheral and central baclofen antagonist. *Brain Res.* 405:150–4.

Kesten, H. (1982). *Percolation Theory for Mathematicians.* Birkhäuser, Boston.

Kirkpatrick, S., and Sherrington, D. (1978). Infinite-ranged models of spin-glasses. *Phys. Rev. B* 17:4384–403.

Kisvarday, Z. F., Martin, K. A. C., Freund, T. F., Magloczky, Z., Whitteridge, D., and Somogyi, P. (1986). Synaptic targets of HRP filled layer III pyramidal cells in the cat striate cortex. *Exp. Brain Res.* 64:541–52.

Kisvarday, Z. F., Martin, K. A. C., Friedlander, M. J., and Somogyi, P. (1987). Evidence for interlaminar inhibitory circuits in the striate cortex of the cat. *J. Compar. Neurol.* 260:1–19.

Kisvarday, Z. F., Martin, K. A. C., Whitteridge, D., and Somogyi, P. (1985). Synaptic connections of intracellularly filled clutch cells: a small type of basket cell in the visual cortex of the cat. *J. Compar. Neurol.* 241:111–37.

Klüver, H. (1951). Functional differences between the occipital and temporal lobes. With special reference to the interrelations of behavior and extracerebral mechanisms. In Jeffress, L. A., ed., *Cerebral Mechanisms in Behavior. The Hixon Symposium,* pp. 147–82. Wiley, New York.

Knowles, W. D., Schneiderman, J. H., Wheal, H. V., Stafstrom, C. E., and Schwartzkroin, P. A. (1984). Hyperpolarizing potentials in guinea pig hippocampal CA3 neurons. *Cell. Molec. Neurobiol.* 4:207–30.

Knowles, W. D., and Schwartzkroin, P. A. (1981a). Local circuit synaptic interactions in hippocampal brain slices. *J. Neurosci.* 1:318–22.

(1981b). Axonal ramifications of hippocampal CA1 pyramidal cells. *J. Neurosci.* 1:1236–41.

Knowles, W. D., Traub, R. D., and Strowbridge, B. W. (1987). The initiation and spread of epileptiform bursts in the *in vitro* hippocampal slice. *Neuroscience* 21:441–55.

Köhler, C., Chan-Palay, V., and Wu, J.-Y. (1984). Septal neurons containing glutamic acid decarboxylase immunoreactivity project to the hippocampal region in the rat brain. *Anat. Embryol.* 169:41–4.

Komisaruk, B. R. (1970). Synchrony between limbic system theta activity and rhythmical behavior in rats. *J. Compar. Physiol. Psychol.* 70:482–92.

Konnerth, A., Heinemann, U., and Yaari, Y. (1984). Slow transmission of neural activity in hippocampal area CA1 in absence of active chemical synapses. *Nature* 307:69–71.

(1986a). Nonsynaptic epileptogenesis in the mammalian hippocampus in vitro. I. Development of seizurelike activity in low extracellular calcium. *J. Neurophysiol.* 56:409–23.

Konnerth, A., Lux, H. D., and Heinemann, U. (1986b). Ionic properties of burst generation in hippocampal pyramidal cell somata "in vitro." *Exp. Brain Res.* S14:368–74.

Konnerth, A., Takahashi, T., Edwards, F., and Sakmann, B. (1988). Single channel and synaptic currents recorded in neurons of mammalian brain and spinal cord slices. *Soc. Neurosci. Abstr.* 14:1046.

Konopacki, J., MacIver, M. B., Bland, B. H., and Roth, S. H. (1987). Carbachol-induced EEG "theta" activity in hippocampal brain slices. *Brain Res.* 405:196–8.

Kopell, N., and Ermentrout, G. B. (1986). Symmetry and phaselocking in chains of weakly coupled oscillators. *Comm. Pure Appl. Math.* 39:623–60.

Korn, H., and Faber, D. S. (1987). Regulation and significance of probabilistic release mechanisms at central synapses. In Edelman, G., Gall, C., and Cowan, W. M., eds., *Synaptic Function,* pp. 57–108. Wiley, New York.

Korn, H., Faber, D. S., and Triller, A. (1986). Probabilistic determination of synaptic strength. *J. Neurophysiol.* 55:402–21.

Korn, H., Mallet, A., Triller, A., and Faber, D. S. (1982). Transmission at a central synapse. II. Quantal description of release with a physical correlate for binomial *n. J. Neurophysiol.* 48:679–707.

Korn, S. J., Giacchino, J. L., Chamberlin, N. L., and Dingledine, R. (1987).

Epileptiform burst activity induced by potassium in the hippocampus and its regulation by GABA-mediated inhibition. *J. Neurophysiol.* 57:325–40.

Kosaka, T. (1980). The axon initial segment as a synaptic site: ultrastructure and synaptology of the initial segment of the pyramidal cell in the rat hippocampus (CA3 region). *J. Neurocytol.* 9:861–82.

(1983). Gap junctions between non-pyramidal cell dendrites in the rat hippocampus (CA1 and CA3 regions). *Brain Res.* 271:157–61.

Kostyuk, P. G., Krishtal, O. S., and Pidoplichko, V. I. (1981). Calcium inward current and related charge movements in the membrane of snail neurones. *J. Physiol.* 310:403–21.

Kramis, R., Vanderwolf, C. H., and Bland, B. H. (1975). Two types of hippocampal rhythmical slow activity (RSA) in both the rabbit and the rat: relations to behavior and effects of atropine, diethyl ether, urethane and pentobarbital. *Exper. Neurol.* 49:58–85.

Kritchevsky, M., Squire, L. R., and Zouzounis, J. A. (1988). Transient global amnesia: characterization of anterograde and retrograde amnesia. *Neurology* 38:213–19.

Krnjevic, K., Morris, M. E., and Ropert, N. (1986). Changes in free calcium ion concentration recorded inside hippocampal pyramidal cells in situ. *Brain Res.* 374:1–11.

Kuno, M., and Llinás, R. (1970). Enhancement of synaptic transmission by dendritic potentials in chromatolyzed motoneurones of the cat. *J. Physiol.* 210:807–21.

Kuperstein, M., Eichenbaum, H., Van De Mark, T. (1986). Neural group properties in the rat hippocampus during theta rhythm. *Exp. Brain Res.* 61:438–42.

Lacaille, J.-C., Mueller, A. L., Kunkel, D. D., and Schwartzkroin, P. A. (1987). Local circuit interactions between oriens/alveus interneurons and CA1 pyramidal cells in hippocampal slices: electrophysiology and morphology. *J. Neurosci.* 7:1979–93.

Lacaille, J.-C., and Schwartzkroin, P. A. (1988a). Stratum lacunosum-moleculare interneurons of hippocampal CA1 region. I. Intracellular response characteristics, synaptic responses, and morphology. *J. Neurosci.* 8:1400–10.

(1988b). Stratum lacunosum-moleculare interneurons of hippocampal CA1 region. II. Intrasomatic and intradendritic recordings of local circuit synaptic interactions. *J. Neurosci.* 8:1411–24.

Lamour, Y., Dutar, P., and Jobert, A. (1984). Septo-hippocampal and other medial septum–diagonal band neurons: electrophysiological and pharmacological properties. *Brain Res.* 309:227–39.

Lancaster, B., and Adams, P. R. (1986). Calcium-dependent current generating the afterhyperpolarization of hippocampal neurons. *J. Neurophysiol.* 55:1268–82.

Lancaster, B., and Nicoll, R. A. (1987). Properties of two calcium-activated hyperpolarizations in rat hippocampal neurones. *J. Physiol.* 389:187–203.

Lancaster, B., and Wheal, H. V. (1984). The synaptically evoked late hyperpolarization in hippocampal CA1 pyramidal cells is resistant to intracellular EGTA. *Neuroscience* 12:267–75.

Land, B. R., Harris, W. V., Salpeter, E. E., and Salpeter, M. M. (1984). Diffusion and binding constants for acetylcholine derived from the falling phase of miniature endplate currents. *Proc. Natl. Acad. Sci. U.S.A.* 81:1594–8.

Lanthorn, T. H., Storm, J., and Andersen, P. (1984). Current-to-frequency transduction in CA1 hippocampal pyramidal cells: slow prepotentials dominate the primary range firing. *Exp. Brain Res.* 53:431–43.

Laurberg, S. (1979). Commissural and intrinsic connections of the rat hippocampus. *J. Compar. Neurol.* 184:685–708.

Lebovitz, R. M., Dichter, M., and Spencer, W. A. (1971). Recurrent excitation in the CA3 region of cat hippocampus. *Int. J. Neurosci.* 2:99–108.

Lehky, S. R., and Sejnowski, T. J. (1988). Network model of shape-from-shading: neural function arises from both receptive and projective fields. *Nature* 333:452–4.

Lerma, J., Herreras, O., Munoz, D., and Solis, J. M. (1985). Interactions between hippocampal penicillin spikes and theta rhythm. *Electroenceph. Clin. Neurophysiol.* 54:782–806.

Leung, L.-W. S. (1980). Behavior-dependent evoked potentials in the hippocampal CA1 region of the rat. I. Correlation with behavior and EEG. *Brain Res.* 198:95–117.

(1982). Nonlinear feedback model of neuronal populations in hippocampal CA1 region. *J. Neurophysiol.* 47:845–68.

(1984). Model of gradual phase shift of theta rhythm in the rat. *J. Neurophysiol.* 52:1051–65.

Leung, L.-W. S., and Borst, J. G. G. (1987). Electrical activity of the cingulate cortex. I. Generating mechanisms and relations to behavior. *Brain Res.* 407:68–80.

Leung, L.-W. S., and Yim, C. Y. (1986). Intracellular records of theta rhythm in hippocampal CA1 cells of the rat. *Brain Res.* 367:323–7.

(1988). Membrane potential oscillations in hippocampal neurons in vitro induced by carbachol or depolarizing currents. *Neurosci. Res. Comm.* 2:159–67.

Levine, S. (1960). Anoxic-ischemic encephalopathy in rats. *Am. J. Pathol.* 36:1–17.

Levitt, P. (1984). A monoclonal antibody to limbic system neurons. *Science* 223:299–301.

Lichtenberg, A. J., and Lieberman, M. A. (1983). *Regular and Stochastic Motion.* Springer, New York.

Lichtman, J. W. (1980). On the predominantly single innervation of submandibular ganglion cells in the rat. *J. Physiol.* 302:121–30.

Lin, J. W., and Faber, D. S. (1988). Synaptic transmission mediated by single club endings on the goldfish Mauthner cell. I. Characteristics of electrotonic and chemical postsynaptic potentials. *J. Neurosci.* 8:1302–12.

Linsker, R. (1988). Self-organization in a perceptual network. *Computer* 21:105–17.

Llano, I., Marty, A., Johnson, J. W., Ascher, P., and Gähwiler, B. H. (1988). Patch-clamp recording of amino acid-activated responses in "organotypic" slice cultures. *Proc. Natl. Acad. Sci. U.S.A.* 85:3221–5.

Llinás, R. (1988). The intrinsic electrophysiological properties of mammalian neurons: insights into central nervous system function. *Science* 242:1654–64.

Llinás, R., and Mühlethaler, M. (1988). Electrophysiology of guinea-pig cerebellar nuclear cells in the *in vitro* brain stem–cerebellar preparation. *J. Physiol.* 404:241–58.

Llinás, R., and Nicholson, C. (1971). Electrophysiological properties of dendrites and somata in alligator Purkinje cells. *J. Neurophysiol.* 34:532–51.

(1975). Calcium role in depolarization secretion coupling: an aequorin study in squid giant synapse. *Proc. Natl. Acad. Sci. U.S.A.* 72:790–4.

Llinás, R., Steinberg, I. Z., and Walton, K. (1976). Presynaptic calcium currents and their relation to synaptic transmission: voltage clamp study in squid giant synapse and theoretical model for the calcium gate. *Proc. Natl. Acad. Sci. U.S.A.* 73:2918–22.

Llinás, R., and Sugimori, M. (1980a). Electrophysiological properties of *in vitro* Purkinje cell somata in mammalian cerebellar slices. *J. Physiol.* 305:171–95.

(1980b). Electrophysiological properties of *in vitro* Purkinje cell dendrites in mammalian cerebellar slices. *J. Physiol.* 305:197–213.

Llinás, R., and Yarom, Y. (1981a). Electrophysiology of mammalian inferior olivary neurones *in vitro*. Different types of voltage-dependent ionic conductances. *J. Physiol.* 315:569–84.

(1981b). Properties and distribution of ionic conductances generating electroresponsiveness of mammalian inferior olivary neurones *in vitro*. *J. Physiol.* 315:569–84.

Lopes da Silva, F. H., Groenewegen, H. J., Holsheimer, J., Room, P., Witter, M. P., van Groen, T., and Wadman, W. J. (1985). The hippocampus as a set of partially overlapping segments with a topographically organized system of inputs and outputs: the entorhinal cortex as a sensory gate, the medial septum as a gain-setting system and the ventral striatum as a motor interface. In Buzsáki, G., and Vanderwolf, C., eds., *Electrical Activity of the Archicortex*, pp. 83–106. Akadémiai Kiadó, Budapest.

López-Barneo, J., Alvarez de Toledo, G., and Yarom, Y. (1985). Electrophysiological properties of guinea pig septal neurons *in vitro*. *Brain Res.* 347:358–62.

Lorente de Nó, R. (1934). Studies on the structure of the cerebral cortex. II. Continuation of the study of the Ammonic system. *J. Psychol. Neurol.* 46:113–77.

(1938). Analysis of the activity of the chains of internuncial neurons. *J. Neurophysiol.* 1:207–44.

McCarren, M., and Alger, B. E. (1985). Use-dependent depression of IPSPs in rat hippocampal pyramidal cells *in vitro*. *J. Neurophysiol.* 53:557–71.

McCormick, D. A., and Prince, D. A. (1985). Two types of muscarinic response to acetylcholine in mammalian cortical neurons. *Proc. Natl. Acad. Sci. U.S.A.* 82:6344–8.

(1986). Mechanisms of action of acetylcholine in the guinea-pig cerebral cortex *in vitro*. *J. Physiol.* 375:169–94.

McCormick, D. A., and Williamson, A. (1989). Convergence and divergence of neurotransmitter action in human cerebral cortex. *Proc. Natl. Acad. Sci. U.S.A.* 86:8098–102.

McIntyre, D. C., and Racine, R. J. (1986). Kindling mechanisms: current progress on an experimental epilepsy model. *Prog. Neurobiol.* 27:1–12.

McIntyre, D. C., and Wong, R. K. S. (1986). Cellular and synaptic properties of amygdala-kindled pyriform cortex *in vitro. J. Neurophysiol.* 55:1295–307.

MaLachlan, E. M. (1978). The statistics of transmitter release at chemical synapses. *Intern. Rev. Physiol.* 17:49–117.

McNamara, J. O., Bonhaus, D. W., Shin, C., Crain, B. J., Gellman, R. L., and Giacchino, J. L. (1984). The kindling model of epilepsy: a critical review. *CRC Critical Rev. Clin. Neurobiol.* 1:341–91.

McNaughton, B. L., Barnes, C. A., and Andersen, P. (1981). Synaptic efficacy and EPSP summation in granule cells of rat fascia dentata studied *in vitro. J. Neurophysiol.* 46:952–66.

MacVicar, B. A., and Dudek, F. E. (1980a). Local synaptic circuits in rat hippocampus: interactions between pyramidal cells. *Brain Res.* 184:220–3.

(1980b). Dye-coupling between CA3 pyramidal cells in slices of rat hippocampus. *Brain Res.* 196:494–7.

(1981). Electrotonic coupling between pyramidal cells: a direct demonstration in rat hippocampal slices. *Science* 213:782–5.

(1982). Electrotonic coupling between granule cells of the rat dentate gyrus: physiological and anatomical evidence. *J. Neurophysiol.* 47:579–92.

MacVicar, B. A., Ropert, N., and Krnjevic, K. (1982). Dye-coupling between pyramidal cells of rat hippocampus in vivo. *Brain Res.* 238:239–44.

MacVicar, B. A., and Tse, F. W. (1989). Local neuronal circuitry underlying cholinergic rhythmical slow activity in CA3 area of rat hippocampal slices. *J. Physiol.* 417:197–212.

Madison, D. V., and Nicoll, R. A. (1982). Noradrenaline blocks accommodation of pyramidal cell discharge in the hippocampus. *Nature* 299:636–8.

(1984). Control of the repetitive discharge of rat CA1 pyramidal neurones *in vitro. J. Physiol.* 354:319–31.

(1986a). Actions of noradrenaline recorded intracellularly in rat hippocampal CA1 pyramidal neurones *in vitro. J. Physiol.* 372:221–44.

(1986b). Cyclic adenosine 3′,5′-monophosphate mediates β-receptor actions of noradrenaline in rat hippocampal pyramidal cells. *J. Physiol.* 372:245–59.

Maldonado, H. M., Delgado-Escueta, A. V., Walsh, G. O., Swartz, B. E., and Rand, R. W. (1988). Complex partial seizures of hippocampal and amygdalar origin. *Epilepsia* 29:420–33.

Malenka, R. C., Kauer, J. A., Zucker, R. S., and Nicoll, R. A. (1988). Postsynaptic calcium is sufficient for potentiation of hippocampal synaptic transmission. *Science* 242:81–4.

Malisch, R., and Ott, T. (1982). Rhythmical slow wave electroencephalographic activity elicited by hippocampal injection of muscarinic agents in the rat. *Neurosci. Lett.* 28:113–18.

Margerison, J. H., and Corsellis, J. A. N. (1966). Epilepsy and the temporal lobes. *Brain* 89:499–530.

Marr, D. (1971). Simple memory: a theory for archicortex. *Phil. Trans. Roy. Soc. Lond. B.* 262:23–81.

Martin, K. A. C. (1988). From single cells to simple circuits in the cerebral cortex. *Quart. J. Exp. Physiol.* 73:637–702.

Martin, K. A. C., and Whitteridge, D. (1984). Form, function and intracortical projections of spiny neurones in the striate visual cortex of the cat. *J. Physiol.* 353:463–504.

Mason, A. J. R., Nicoll, A., Stratford, K. J., and Blakemore, C. (1989). Synaptic transmission between individual neurons in rat visual cortex. *Soc. Neurosci. Abstr.* 15:257.

Masukawa, L. M., Benardo, L. S., and Prince, D. A. (1982). Variations in electrophysiological properties of hippocampal neurons in different subfields. *Brain Res.* 242:341–4.

Masukawa, L. M., Higashima, M., Kim, J., and Spencer, D. (1988). Involvement of the NMDA receptor in abnormal discharges present in hippocampal brain slices from epileptic patients. *Soc. Neurosci. Abstr.* 14:238.

(1989). Epileptiform discharges evoked in hippocampal brain slices from epileptic patients. *Brain Res.* 493:168–74.

Masukawa, L. M., and Prince, D. A. (1982). Enkephalin inhibition of inhibitory input to CA1 and CA3 pyramidal neurons in the hippocampus. *Brain Res.* 249:271–80.

(1984). Synaptic control of excitability in isolated dendrites of hippocampal neurons. *J. Neurosci.* 4:217–27.

Mathers, D. A. (1987). The GABA$_A$ receptor: new insights from single-channel recording. *Synapse* 1:96–101.

Matsumoto, H., and Ajmone-Marsan, C. (1964a). Cortical cellular phenomena in experimental epilepsy: interictal manifestations. *Exper. Neurol.* 9:286–304.

(1964b). Cortical cellular phenomena in experimental epilepsy: ictal manifestations. *Exper. Neurol.* 9:305–26.

Matteoli, M., Haimann, C., Torri-Tarelli, F., Polak, J. M., Ceccarelli, B., and de Camilli, P. (1988). Differential effect of α-latrotoxin on exocytosis from small synaptic vesicles and from large dense core vesicles containing calcitonin gene related peptide at the frog neuromuscular junction. *Proc. Natl. Acad. Sci. U.S.A.* 85:7366–70.

Matthews, D. A., Salvaterra, P. M., Crawford, G. D., Houser, C. R., and Vaughn, J. E. (1987). An immunocytochemical study of choline acetyltransferase-containing neurons and axon terminals in normal and partially deafferented hippocampal formation. *Brain Res.* 402:30–43.

Mayer, M. L., Westbrook, G. L., and Guthrie, P. B. (1984). Voltage-dependent block by Mg^{2+} of NMDA responses in spinal cord neurones. *Nature* 309:261–3.

Mayeux, R. (1979). Sexual intercourse and transient global amnesia. *N. Engl. J. Med.* 300:864.

Meibach, R. C., and Siegel, A. (1977a). Efferent connections of the hippocampal formation in the rat. *Brain Res.* 124:197–224.

(1977b). Efferent connections of the septal area in the rat: an analysis utilizing retrograde and anterograde transport methods. *Brain Res.* 119:1–20.

Meldrum, B. S., Evans, M. C., Swan, J. H., and Simon, R. P. (1987). Protection against hypoxic/ischaemic brain damage with excitatory amino acid antagonists. *Med. Biol.* 65:153–7.

Mendell, L. M., and Henneman, E. (1971). Terminals of single Ia fibers: location, density and distribution within a pool of 300 homonymous motoneurons. *J. Neurophysiol.* 34:171–87.

Mesher, R. A., and Schwartzkroin, P. A. (1980). Can CA3 epileptiform burst discharge induce bursting in normal CA1 hippocampal neurons? *Brain Res.* 183:472–6.

Meyers, D. E. R., and Barker, J. L. (1989). Whole-cell patch-clamp analysis of voltage dependent calcium conductances in cultured embryonic rat hippocampal neurons. *J. Neurophysiol.* 61:467–77.

Miles, R. (1988). Plasticity of recurrent excitatory synapses between CA3 hippocampal pyramidal cells. *Soc. Neurosci. Abstr.* 14:19.

(1990). Synaptic excitation of inhibitory cells by single CA3 hippocampal pyramidal cells of the guinea-pig *in vitro. J. Physiol.*, 428:61–77.

Miles, R., Traub, R. D., and Wong, R. K. S. (1988). Spread of synchronous firing in longitudinal slices from the CA3 region of the hippocampus. *J. Neurophysiol.* 60:1481–96.

Miles, R., and Wong, R. K. S. (1983). Single neurones can initiate synchronized population discharge in the hippocampus. *Nature* 306:371–3.

(1984). Unitary inhibitory synaptic potentials in the guinea-pig hippocampus *in vitro. J. Physiol.* 356:97–113.

(1986). Excitatory synaptic interactions between CA3 neurones in the guinea-pig hippocampus. *J. Physiol.* 373:397–418.

(1987a). Inhibitory control of local excitatory circuits in the guinea-pig hippocampus. *J. Physiol.* 388:611–29.

(1987b). Latent synaptic pathways revealed after tetanic stimulation in the hippocampus. *Nature* 329:724–6.

Miles, R., Wong, R. K. S., and Traub, R. D. (1984). Synchronized afterdischarges in the hippocampus: contribution of local synaptic interaction. *Neuroscience* 12:1179–89.

Misgeld, U., and Frotscher, M. (1986). Postsynaptic-GABAergic inhibition of non-pyramidal neurons in the guinea-pig hippocampus. *Neuroscience* 19:193–206.

Mishkin, M. (1978). Memory in monkeys severely impaired by combined but not by separate removal of amygdala and hippocampus. *Nature* 273:297–8.

Mitchell, S. J., and Ranck, J. B., Jr. (1980). Generation of theta rhythm in medial entorhinal cortex of freely moving rats. *Brain Res.* 189:49–66.

Miyakawa, H., Lev-Ram, V., and Ross, W. N. (1988). Synaptically evoked calcium transients in the dendrites of cerebellar Purkinje cells in vitro. *Soc. Neurosci. Abstr.* 14:759.

Mizukawa, K., McGeer, P. L., Tago, H., Peng, J. H., McGeer, E. G., and Kimura, H. (1986). The cholinergic system of the human hindbrain studied by choline acetyltransferase immunohistochemistry and acetylcholinesterase histochemistry. *Brain Res.* 379:39–55.

Mizumori, S. J. Y., McNaughton, B. L., Barnes, C. A., and Fox, K. B. (1989). Preserved spatial coding in hippocampal CA1 pyramidal cells during reversible suppression of CA3c output: evidence for pattern completion in hippocampus. *J. Neurosci.* 9:3915–28.

Mody, I., Lambert, J. D., and Heinemann, U. (1987). Low extracellular magnesium induces epileptiform activity and spreading depression in rat hippocampal slices. *J. Neurophysiol.* 57:869–88.

Mogul, D. J., and Fox, A. P. (1989). Multiple calcium channel types exist in acutely isolated guinea pig hippocampal neurons from the CA3 region. *Soc. Neurosci. Abstr.* 15:823.

Monaghan, D. T., and Cotman, C. W. (1985). Distribution of *N*-methyl-D-aspartate-sensitive L-[³H]glutamate-binding sites in rat brain. *J. Neurosci.* 5:2909–19.

Montoya, C. P., and Sainsbury, R. S. (1985). The effects of entorhinal cortex lesions on type 1 and type 2 theta. *Physiol. Behav.* 35:121–6.

Morris, R. G. M., Anderson, E., Lynch, G. S., and Baudry, M. (1986). Selective impairment of learning and blockade of long-term potentiation by an *N*-methyl-D-aspartate receptor antagonist, AP5. *Nature* 319:774–6.

Morris, R. G. M., Garrud, P., Rawlins, J. N. P., and O'Keefe, J. (1982). Place navigation impaired in rats with hippocampal lesions. *Nature* 297:681–3.

Mühlethaler, M., Dreifuss, J. J., and Gähwiler, B. H. (1982). Vasopressin excites hippocampal neurones. *Nature* 296:749.

Mulle, C., Steriade, M., and Deschênes, M. (1985). Absence of spindle oscillations in the cat anterior thalamic nuclei. *Brain Res.* 334:169–71.

Muller, R. U., and Kubie, J. L. (1987). The effects of changes in the environment on the spatial firing of hippocampal complex-spike cells. *J. Neurosci.* 7:1951–68.

Muller, R. U., Kubie, J. L., and Ranck, J. B., Jr. (1987). Spatial firing patterns of hippocampal complex-spike cells in a fixed environment. *J. Neurosci.* 7:1935–50.

Nadler, J. V., Perry, B. W., and Cotman, C. W. (1980). Selective reinnervation of hippocampal area CA1 and the fascia dentata after destruction of CA3-CA4 afferents with kainic acid. *Brain Res.* 182:1–9.

Nadler, J. V., Vaca, K. W., White, W. F., Lynch, G. S., and Cotman, C. W. (1976). Aspartate and glutamate as possible transmitters of excitatory hippocampal afferents. *Nature* 260:538–40.

Neuman, R. S., Cherubini, E., and Ben-Ari, Y. (1987). Network bursts triggered by single cell stimulation in the rat hippocampus. *Soc. Neurosci. Abstr.* 13:765.

(1989). Endogenous and network bursts induced by *N*-methyl-D-aspartate and magnesium-free medium in the CA3 region of the hippocampal slice. *Neuroscience* 28:393–9.

Newberry, N. R., and Nicoll, R. A. (1984). A bicuculline-resistant inhibitory post-synaptic potential in rat hippocampal pyramidal cells *in vitro*. *J. Physiol.* 348:239–54.

(1985). Comparison of the action of baclofen with γ-aminobutyric acid on rat hippocampal cells *in vitro*. *J. Physiol.* 360:161–85.

Nicoll, R. A. (1988). The coupling of neurotransmitter receptors to ion channels in the brain. *Science* 241:545–51.

Nilsson, O. G., Shapiro, M. L., Gage, F. L., Olton, D. S., and Björklund, A. (1987). Spatial learning and memory following fimbria-fornix transection and grafting of fetal septal neurons to the hippocampus. *Exp. Brain Res.* 67:195–215.

Norman, R. S. (1972). Cable theory for finite-length dendritic cylinders with initial and boundary conditions. *Biophys. J.* 12:25–45.

Nowak, L., Bregestovski, P., Ascher, P., Herbert, A., and Prochiantz, A. (1984). Magnesium gates glutamate-activated channels in mouse central neurones. *Nature* 307:462–5.

Numann, R., and Wong, R. K. S. (1984). Voltage-clamp study on GABA response desensitization in single pyramidal cells dissociated from the hippocampus of adult guinea pigs. *Neurosci. Lett.* 47:289–94.

Numann, R. E., Wadman, W. J., and Wong, R. K. S. (1987). Outward currents of single hippocampal cells obtained from the adult guinea-pig. *J. Physiol.* 393:331–53.

Nuñez, A., Garcia-Austt, E., and Buño, W., Jr. (1987). Intracellular theta rhythm generation in identified hippocampal pyramids. *Brain Res.* 416:289–300.

Nunzi, M. G., Gorio, A., Milan, F., Freund, T. F., Somogyi, P., and Smith, A. D. (1985). Cholecystokinin immunoreactive cells form symmetrical synaptic contacts with pyramidal and non-pyramidal neurons in the hippocampus. *J. Compar. Neurol.* 237:485–505.

Ogata, N., and Ueno, S. (1976). Mode of activation of pyramidal neurons by mossy fiber stimulation in thin hippocampal slices *in vitro. Exper. Neurol.* 53:567–84.

O'Keefe, J. (1979). A review of the hippocampal place cells. *Prog. Neurobiol.* 13:419–39.

O'Keefe, J., and Nadel, L. (1978). *The Hippocampus as a Cognitive Man.* Clarendon Press, Oxford.

Olesen, J., and Jurgensen, M. B. (1986). Leao's spreading depression in the hippocampus explains transient global amnesia. A hypothesis. *Acta Neurol. Scand.* 73:219–20.

Onodera, H., Sato, G., and Kogure, K. (1986). Lesions to Schaffer collaterals prevent ischemic death of CA1 pyramidal cells. *Neurosci. Lett.* 68:169–74.

Onteniente, B., Tago, H., Kimura, H., and Maeda, T. (1986). Distribution of γ-aminobutyric acid-immunoreactive neurons in the septal region of the rat brain. *J. Compar. Neurol.* 248:422–30.

Ott, E. (1981). Strange attractors and chaotic motions of dynamical systems. *Rev. Mod. Phys.* 53:655–71.

Owen, D. G., Segal, M., and Barker, J. L. (1984). A Ca-dependent Cl⁻ conductance is present in cultured mouse spinal neurones. *Nature* 311:567–70.

Panual, P., Revuelta, A. V., Cheney, D. L., Wu, J.-Y., and Costa, E. (1984). An immunohistochemical study on the location of GABAergic neurons in the rat septum. *J. Compar. Neurol.* 222:69–80.

Papez, J. W. (1937). A proposed mechanism of emotion. *Arch. Neurol. Psychiat.* 38:725–43.

Parkinson, J. K., Murray, E. A., and Mishkin, M. (1988). A selective mnemonic role for the hippocampus in monkeys: memory for the location of objects. *J. Neurosci.* 8:4159–67.

Paxinos, G., and Watson, G. (1986). *The Rat Brain in Stereotaxic Coordinates.* Academic Press, Sydney.

Pedley, T. A., and Traub, R. D. (1985). Physiology of epilepsy. In Swash, M., and Kennard, C., eds., *Scientific Basis of Clinical Neurology,* pp. 320–46. Churchill Livingstone, London.

—— (1990). Physiological basis of the EEG. In Daly, D. D., and Pedley, T. A., eds., *Current Practice of Clinical Electroencephalography,* 2nd ed., pp. 107–37. Raven Press, New York.

Peng, Y.-y., and Frank, E. (1989a). Activation of GABA$_B$ receptors causes presynaptic inhibition at synapses between muscle spindle afferents and motoneurons in the spinal cord of bullfrogs. *J. Neurosci.* 9:1502–15.

—— (1989b). Activation of GABA$_A$ receptors causes presynaptic and postsynaptic inhibition at synapses between muscle spindle afferents and motoneurons in the spinal cord of bullfrogs. *J. Neurosci.* 9:1516–22.

Petsche, H., Gogolak, G., and Van Zwieten, P. A. (1965). Rhythmicity of septal cell discharges at various levels of reticular excitation. *Electroenceph. Clin. Neurophysiol.* 19:25–33.

Petsche, H., and Stumpf, C. (1960). Topographic and toposcopic study of origin and spread of the reticular synchronizing arousal pattern in the rabbit. *Electroenceph. Clin. Neurophysiol.* 12:589–600.

Petsche, H., Stumpf, C., and Gogolak, G. (1962). Significance of the rabbit's septum as a relay station between the midbrain and the hippocampus. I. The control of hippocampus arousal activity by septum cells. *Electroenceph. Clin. Neurophysiol.* 14:202–11.

Pitler, T. A., and Landfield, P. W. (1987). Probable Ca^{2+}-mediated inactivation of Ca$^{2\&}$-mediated currents in mammalian brain neurons. *Brain Res.* 410:147–53.

Plonsey, R. (1969). Volume conductor fields of action currents. *Biophys. J.* 4:317–28.

Pongracz, F. (1985). The function of dendritic spines: a theoretical study. *Neuroscience* 15:933–46.

Poolos, N. P., Mauk, M. D., and Kocsis, J. D. (1987). Activity-evoked increases in extracellular potassium modulate presynaptic excitability in the CA1 region of the hippocampus. *J. Neurophysiol.* 58:404–16.

Prince, D. A. (1968). The depolarization shift in "epileptic" neurons. *Exper. Neurol.* 21:467–85.

Prince, D. A., and Wilder, B. J. (1967). Conrol mechanisms in cortical epileptogenic foci. *Arch Neurol.* 16:194–202.

Proust, M. (1927). *Remembrance of Things Past,* 2 vols., translated from the French by C. K. Scott Moncrieff and A. Mayor. Random House, New York.

Pun, R. Y. K., Neal, E. A., Guthrie, P. B., and Nelson, P. G. (1986). Active and inactive central synapses in cell culture. *J. Neurophysiol.* 56:1242–56.

Pytte, E., Grinstein, G., and Traub, R. D. (in press). Cellular automaton models of the CA3 region of the hippocampus.

Raisman, G. (1966). The connexions of the septum. *Brain* 89:317–48.

Rall, W. (1962a). Theory of physiological properties of dendrites. *Ann. N.Y. Acad. Sci.* 96:1071–92.

(1962b). Electrophysiology of a dendritic neuron model. *Biophys. J.* 2:145–67.

(1967). Distinguishing theoretical synaptic potentials computed for different soma-dendritic distributions of synaptic input. *J. Neurophysiol.* 30:1138–68.

(1969a). Time constants and electrotonic length of membrane cylinders and neurons. *Biophys. J.* 9:1483–508.

(1969b). Distributions of potential in cylindrical coordinates and time constants for a membrane cylinder. *Biophys. J.* 9:1509–41.

Rall, W., and Rinzel, J. (1973). Branch input resistance and steady attenuation for input to one branch of a dendritic neuron model. *Biophys. J.* 13:648–88.

Redman, S., and Walmsley, B. (1983). Amplitude fluctuations in synaptic potentials evoked in cat spinal motoneurones at identified group Ia synapses. *J. Physiol.* 343:117–33.

Reece, L. J., and Schwartzkroin, P. A. (1988). Effect of cholinergic agonists on lacunosum-moleculare interneurons in rat hippocampus. *Soc. Neurosci. Abstr.* 14:246.

Reitz, J. R., and Milford, F. J. (1960). *Foundations of Electromagnetic Theory.* Addison-Wesley, Reading, Mass.

Ribak, C. E., and Seress, L. (1983). Five types of basket cell in the hippocampal dentate gyrus: a combined Golgi and electron microscopic study. *J. Neurocytol.* 12:577–97.

Ribak, C. E., Seress, L., and Amaral, D. G. (1985). The development, ultrastructure and synaptic connections of the mossy cells of the dentate gyrus. *J. Neurocytol.* 14:835–57.

Ribak, C. E., Seress, L., Peterson, G. M., Seroogy, K. B., Fallon, J. H., and Schmued, L. C. (1986). A GABAergic inhibitory component within the hippocampal commissural pathway. *J. Neurosci.* 6:3492–8.

Ribak, C. E., Vaughn, J. E., and Saito, K. (1978). Immunocytochemical localization of glutamic acid decarboxylase in neuronal somata following colchicine inhibition of axonal transport. *Brain Res.* 140:315–32.

Richerson, G. B., and Getting, P. A. (1987). Maintenance of complex neural function during perfusion of the mammalian brain. *Brain Res.* 409:128–32.

Rinzel, J., and Rall, W. (1974). Transient response in a dendritic neuron model for current injected at one branch. *Biophys. J.* 14:759–90.

Roberts, G. W., Woodhams, P. L., Polak, J. M., and Crow, T. J. (1984). Distribution of neuropeptides in the limbic system of the rat: the hippocampus. *Neuroscience* 11:35–77.

Rolls, E. T., Miyashita, Y., Cahusac, P. M. B., Kesner, R. P., Niki, H., Feigenbaum, J. D., and Bach, L. (1989). Hippocampal neurons in the monkey with activity related to the place in which a stimulus is shown. *J. Neurosci.* 9:1835–45.

Ropert, N. (1988). Inhibitory action of serotonin in CA1 hippocampal neurons *in vitro*. *Neuroscience* 26:69–81.

Ropert, N., Miles, R., and Korn, H. (1990). Characteristics of miniature inhibitory postsynaptic currents in CA1 pyramidal neurones of rat hippocampus. *J. Physiol.* 428:707–22.

Rose, G., Diamond, D., and Lynch, G. S. (1983). Dentate granule cells in the rat hippocampal formation have the behavioral characteristics of theta neurons. *Brain Res.* 266:29–37.

Rosene, D. L., and Van Hoesen, G. W. (1977). Hippocampal efferents reach widespread areas of cerebral cortex and amygdala in the rhesus monkey. *Science* 198:315–17.

——— (1987). The hippocampal formation of the primate brain. In Jones, E. G., and Peters, A., eds., *Cerebral Cortex, Vol. 6, Further Aspects of Cortical Function, Including Hippocampus,* pp. 345–456. Plenum Press, New York.

Ross, W. N. Arechiga, H., and Nicholls, J. G. (1987). Optical recording of calcium and voltage transients following impulses in identified leech neurons in culture. *J. Neurosci.* 7:3877–87.

Ross, W. N., and Werman, R. (1987). Mapping calcium transients in the dendrites of Purkinje cells from the guinea-pig cerebellum *in vitro. J. Physiol.* 389:319–36.

Rothman, S. M. (1984). Selective release of excitatory amino acid neurotransmitter mediates anoxic neuronal death. *J. Neurosci.* 4:1884–91.

——— (1986). Glutamate and anoxic neuronal death *in vitro. Adv. Exp. Med. Biol.* 203:687–95.

Rothwell, J. C., Obeso, J. A., and Marsden, C. D. (1986). Electrophysiology of somatosensory reflex myoclonus. In Fahn, S., Marsden, C. D., and Van Woert, M., eds., *Advances in Neurology, Vol. 43, Myoclonus.* pp. 385–98. Raven Press, New York.

Rudell, A. P., and Fox, S. E. (1984). Hippocampal excitability related to the phase of the theta rhythm in urethanized rats. *Brain Res.* 294:350–3.

Rudell, A. P., Fox, S. E., and Ranck, J. B., Jr. (1980). Hippocampal excitability phase-locked to the theta rhythm in walking rats. *Exper. Neurol.* 68:87–96.

Rumelhart, D. E., Hinton, G. E., and Williams, R. J. (1986). Learning internal representations by error propagation. In Rumelhart, D. E., McClelland, J. L., and PDP Research Group, eds., *Parallel Distributed Processing, Vol. 1,* pp. 318–62. M.I.T. Press, Cambridge, Mass.

Rutecki, P. A., Lebeda, F. J., and Johnston, D. (1985). Epileptiform activity induced by changes in extracellular potassium in hippocampus. *J. Neurophysiol.* 54:1363–74.

——— (1987). 4-Aminopyridine produces epileptiform activity in hippocampus and enhances synaptic excitation and inhibition. *J. Neurophysiol.* 57:1911–24.

Sagar, H. J., and Oxbury, J. M. (1987). Hippocampal neuron loss in temporal lobe epilepsy: correlation with early childhood convulsions. *Ann. Neurol.* 22:334–40.

Sah, P., Gibb, A. J., and Gage, P. W. (1988). The sodium current underlying action potentials in guinea pig hippocampal CA1 neurons. *J. Gen. Physiol.* 91:373–98.

Sainsbury, R. S. (1985). Type 2 theta in the guinea pig and the cat. In Buzsáki, G., and Vanderwolf, C. H., eds., *Electrical Activity of the Archicortex,* pp. 11–22. Akadémiai Kiadó, Budapest.

Sakmann, B., Edwards, F., Konnerth, A., and Takahashi, T. (1989). Patch clamp techniques used for studying synaptic transmission in slices of mammalian brain. *Quart. J. Exp. Physiol.* 74:1107–18.

Sawa, M., Kaji, S., and Usuki, K. (1965). Intracellular phenomena in electrically induced seizures. *Electroenceph. Clin. Neurophysiol.* 19:248–55.

Sawa, M., Maruyama, N., and Kaji, S. (1963). Intracellular potential during electrically induced seizures. *Electroenceph. Clin. Neurophysiol.* 15:209–20.

Sawa, M., Nakamura, K., and Naito, H. (1968). Intracellular phenomena and spread of epileptic seizure discharges. *Electroenceph. Clin. Neurophysiol.* 24:146–54.

Sayer, R. J., Friedlander, M. J., and Redman, S. J. (1988). Synaptic transmission between individual CA3 and CA1 neurons in the hippocampus. *Soc. Neurosci. Abstr.* 14:18.

(1990). The time course and amplitude of EPSPs evoked at synapses between pairs of CA3/CA1 neurons in the hippocampal slice. *J. Neurosci.* 10:826–36.

Sayer, R. J., Redman, S. J., and Andersen, P. (1989). Amplitude fluctuations in small EPSPs recorded from CA1 pyramidal cells in the guinea pig hippocampal slice. *J. Neurosci.* 9:840–56.

Schaffer, W. M., and Kot, M. (1986). Differential systems in ecology and epidemiology. In Holden, A. V., ed., *Chaos,* pp. 158–78. Princeton University Press.

Scharfman, H. E., and Schwartzkroin, P. A. (1988a). Selective depression of GABA-mediated IPSPs by somatostatin in area CA1 of rabbit hippocampal slices. *Soc. Neurosci. Abstr.* 14:115.

(1988b). Electrophysiology of morphologically identified mossy cells of the dentate hilus recorded in guinea pig hippocampal slices. *J. Neurosci.* 8:3812–21.

Schlander, M., and Frotscher, M. (1986). Non-pyramidal neurons in the guinea pig hippocampus. A combined Golgi-electron microscope study. *Anat. Embryol.* 174:35–47.

Schneiderman, J. H. (1986). Low concentrations of penicillin reveal rhythmic, synchronous synaptic potentials in hippocampal slice. *Brain Res.* 398:231–41.

(1988). Power spectral analysis of rhythmic field potentials in hippocampal slice: a model of the EEG? *Soc. Neurosci. Abstr.* 14:128.

Schneiderman, J. H., Arnold, D., and Advani, A. (1989). Power spectral analysis of spontaneous field potentials in hippocampal slice. *Neurosci. Lett.* 103:39–43.

Schulman, L. S. (in preparation). *When Things Grow Many.*

Schulman, L. S., and Seiden, P. E. (1982). Percolation analysis of stochastic models of galactic evolution. *J. Stat. Phys.* 27:83–118.

(1986). Percolation and galaxies. *Science* 233:425–31.

Schüz, A., and Munster, A. (1985). Synaptic density on the axonal tree of a pyramidal cell in the motor cortex of a mouse. *Neuroscience* 15:33–9.

Schwartzkroin, P. A. (1978). Secondary range rhythmic spiking in hippocampal neurons. *Brain Res.* 149:247–50.

Schwartzkroin, P. A., and Haglund, M. M. (1986). Spontaneous rhythmic synchronous activity in epileptic human and normal monkey temporal lobe. *Epilepsia* 27:523–33.

Schwartzkroin, P. A., and Knowles, W. D. (1984). Intracellular study of human epileptic cortex: *in vitro* maintenance of epileptiform activity. *Science* 223:709–12.

Schwartzkroin, P. A., and Kunkel, D. D. (1985). Morphology of identified interneurons in the CA1 region of guinea-pig hippocampus. *J. Compar. Neurol.* 232:505–18.

Schwartzkroin, P. A., and Mathers, L. H. (1978). Physiological and morphological identification of a nonpyramidal hippocampal cell type. *Brain Res.* 157:1–10.

Schwartzkroin, P. A., and Mueller, A. L. (1987). Electrophysiology of hippocampal neurons. In Jones, E. G., and Peters, A., eds., *Cerebral Cortex, Vol. 6, Further Aspects of Cortical Function, Including Hippocampus*, pp. 295–343. Plenum Press, New York.

Schwartzkroin, P. A., and Pedley, T. A. (1979). Slow depolarizing potentials in "epileptic" neurons. *Epilepsia* 20:267–77.

Schwartzkroin, P. A., and Prince, D. A. (1977). Penicillin-induced epileptiform activity in the hippocampal *in vitro* preparation. *Ann. Neurol.* 1:463–9.

(1978). Cellular and field potential properties of epileptogenic hippocampal slices. *Brain Res.* 147:117–30.

(1980a). Changes in excitatory and inhibitory synaptic potentials leading to epileptogenic activity. *Brain Res.* 183:61–76.

(1980b). Effects of TEA on hippocampal neurons. *Brain Res.* 185:169–81.

Schwartzkroin, P. A., and Slawsky, M. (1977). Probable calcium spikes in hippocampal neurons. *Brain Res.* 135:157–61.

Schwartzkroin, P. A., and Stafstrom, C. E. (1980). Effects of EGTA on the calcium-activated afterhyperpolarization in hippocampal CA3 cells. *Science* 210:1125–6.

Schwerdtfeger, W. K. (1986). Afferent fibers from the septum terminate on gamma-aminobutyric acid (GABA-) interneurons and granule cells in the area dentata of the rat. *Experientia* 42:392–4.

Sclabassi, R. J., Eriksson, J. L., Port, R. L., Robinson, G. B., and Berger, T. W. (1988). Nonlinear systems analysis of the hippocampal perforant path–dentate projection. I. Theoretical and interpretational considerations. *J. Neurophysiol.* 60:1066–76.

Scott, J. G., and Mendell, L. M. (1976). Individual EPSPs produced by single triceps surae Ia afferent fibers in homonymous and heteronymous motoneurons. *J. Neurophysiol.* 39:679–92.

Scoville, W. B., and Milner, B. (1957). Loss of recent memory after bilateral hippocampal lesions. *J. Neurol. Neurosurg. Psychiatry* 20:11–21.

Segal, M. (1977). Afferents to the entorhinal cortex of the rat studied by the method of retrograde transport of horseradish peroxidase. *Exper. Neurol.* 57:750–765.

(1980). The action of serotonin in the rat hippocampal slice preparation. *J. Physiol.* 303:423–39.

(1982). Multiple actions of acetylcholine at a muscarinic receptor studied in the rat hippocampal slice. *Brain Res.* 246:77–87.

(1983). Rat hippocampal neurons in culture: responses to electrical and chemical stimuli. *J. Neurophysiol.* 50:1249–64.

(1984). Rat hippocampal neurons in culture: properties of GABA-activated Cl⁻-activated ion conductance. *J. Neurophysiol.* 51:500–15.

(1985). Electrophysiological actions of acetylcholine in the hippocampus. In Buzsáki, G., and Vanderwolf, C. H., eds., *Electrical Activity of the Archicortex*, pp. 205–16. Akadémiai Kiadó, Budapest.

(1986). Properties of rat medial septal neurones recorded *in vitro*. *J. Physiol.* 379:309–30.

(1987). Repetitive inhibitory postsynaptic potentials evoked by 4-aminopyridine in hippocampal neurons in vitro. *Brain Res.* 414:285–93.

Segal, M., and Barker, J. L. (1984a). Rat hippocampal neurons in culture: potassium conductances. *J. Neurophysiol.* 51:1409–33.

(1984b). Rat hippocampal neurons in culture: properties of GABA-activated Cl⁻ ion conductance. *J. Neurophysiol.* 51:500–15.

(1984c). Rat hippocampal neurons in culture: voltage-clamp analysis of inhibitory synaptic connections. *J. Neurophysiol.* 52:469–87.

(1986). Rat hippocampal neurons in culture: Ca^{2+} and Ca^{2+}-dependent K^+ conductances. *J. Neurophysiol.* 55:751–66.

Segal, M., Rogawski, M. A., and Barker, J. L. (1984). A transient potassium conductance regulates the excitability of cultured hippocampal and spinal neurons. *J. Neurosci.* 4:604–9.

Segev, I., Fleshman, J. W., Miller, J. P., and Bunow, B. (1985). Modeling the electrical behavior of anatomically complex neurons using a network analysis program: passive membrane. *Biol. Cybern.* 53:27–40.

Sejnowski, T. J., Koch, C., and Churchland, P. (1988). Computational neuroscience. *Science* 241:1299–306.

Seltzer, B., and Pandya, D. N. (1976). Some cortical projections to the parahippocampal area in the rhesus monkey. *Exper. Neurol.* 50:146–60.

Semba, K., and Komisaruk, B. R. (1978). Phase of the theta wave in relation to different limb movements in awake rats. *Electroenceph. Clin. Neurophysiol.* 44:61–71.

Seress, L., and Ribak, C. E. (1985). A combined Golgi-electron microscopic study of non-pyramidal neurons in the CA1 area of the hippocampus. *J. Neurocytol.* 14:717–30.

Shante, V. K. S., and Kirkpatrick, S. (1971). An introduction to percolation theory. *Adv. Phys.* 20:325–57.

Shepherd, G. M., and Brayton, R. K. (1979). Computer simulation of a dendrodendritic synaptic circuit for self- and lateral-inhibition in the olfactory bulb. *Brain Res.* 175:377–82.

Shepherd, G. M., Brayton, R. K., Miller, J. P., Segev, I., Rinzel, J., and Rall, W. (1985). Signal enhancement in distal cortical dendrites by means of interactions between active dendritic spines. *Proc. Natl. Acad. Sci. U.S.A* 82:2192–5.

Shewmon, D. A., and Erwin, R. J. (1988). Focal spike-induced cerebral dysfunction is related to the after-coming slow wave. *Ann. Neurol.* 23:131–7.

Shorvon, S. D. (1986). Classification of epilepsy. In Asbury, A. K., McKhann, G. M., and McDonald, W. I., eds., *Diseases of the Nervous System, Vol. II*, pp. 970–81. Saunders, Philadelphia.

Shuping, J. R., Rollinson, R. D., and Toole, J. F. (1980a). Transient global amnesia. *Ann. Neurol.* 7:281–5.

Shuping, J. R., Toole, J. F., and Alexander, E., Jr. (1980b). Transient global amnesia due to glioma in the dominant hemisphere. *Neurology* 30:88–90.

Sloviter, R. S. (1983). "Epileptic" brain damage in rats induced by sustained electrical stimulation of the perforant path. I. Acute electrophysiological and light microscopic studies. *Brain Res. Bull.* 10:675–97.

(1989). Calcium-binding protein (Calbindin – D_{28k}) and parvalbumin immunocytochemistry: localization in the rat hippocampus with specific reference to the selective vulnerability of hippocampal neurons to seizure activity. *J. Compar. Neurol.* 280:183–96.

Sloviter, R. S., and Nilaver, G. (1987). Immunocytochemical localization of GABA-, cholecystokinin-, vasoactive intestinal polypeptide-, and somatostatin-like immunoreactivity in the area dentata and hippocampus of the rat. *J. Compar. Neurol.* 256:42–60.

Smith, K. L., Turner, J., and Swann, J. W. (1988). Paired intracellular recordings reveal mono- and polysynaptic excitatory interactions in immature hippocampus. *Soc. Neurosci. Abstr.* 14:883.

Smith, M. L. (1988). Recall of spatial location by the amnesic patient H.M. *Brain Cogn.* 7:178–83.

Snow, R. W., and Dudek, F. E. (1984a). Synchronous epileptiform bursts without chemical transmission in CA2, CA3 and dentate areas of the hippocampus. *Brain Res.* 298:382–5.

(1984b). Electrical fields directly contribute to action potential synchronization during convulsant-induced epileptiform bursts. *Brain Res.* 323:114–18.

(1986). Evidence for neuronal interactions by electrical field effects in the CA3 and dentate regions of rat hippocampal slices. *Brain Res.* 367:292–5.

Snow, R. W., Taylor, C. P., and Dudek, F. E. (1983). Electrophysiological and optical changes in slices of rat hippocampus during spreading depression. *J. Neurophysiol.* 50:561–72.

Soltesz, I., Haby, M., Leresche, N., and Crunelli, V. (1988). The $GABA_B$ antagonist phaclofen inhibits the late K^+-dependent IPSP in cat and rat thalamic and hippocampal neurones. *Brain Res.* 448:351–4.

Somjen, G. G., Aitken, P. G., Giacchino, J. L., and McNamara, J. O. (1985). Sustained potential shifts and paroxysmal discharges in hippocampal formation. *J. Neurophysiol.* 53:1079–97.

Somjen, G. G., and Giacchino, J. L. (1985). Potassium and calcium concentrations in interstitial fluid of hippocampal formation during paroxysmal responses. *J. Neurophysiol.* 53:1098–108.

Somogyi, P., Freund, T. F., and Cowey, A. (1982). The axo-axonic interneuron in the cerebral cortex of the rat, cat, and monkey. *Neuroscience* 7:2577–608.

Somogyi, P., Kisvarday, Z. F., Martin, K. A. C., and Whitteridge, D. (1983a). Synaptic connections of morphologically identified and physiologically characterised large basket cells in the striate cortex of cat. *Neuroscience* 10:261–94.

Somogyi, P., Nunzi, M. G., Gorio, A., and Smith, A. D. (1983b). A new type of specific interneuron in the monkey hippocampus forming synapses exclusively with the axon initial segments of pyramidal cells. *Brain Res.* 259:137–42.

Somogyi, P., Smith, A. D., Nunzi, M. G., Gorio, A., Takagi, H., and Wu, J. Y. (1983c). Glutamate decarboxylase immunoreactivity in the hippocampus of the cat: distribution of immunoreactive synaptic terminals with special reference to the axon initial segment of pyramidal neurons. *J. Neurosci.* 3:1450–68.

Spencer, W. A., and Kandel, E. R. (1961a). Hippocampal neuron responses to selective activation of recurrent collaterals of hippocampofugal axons. *Exper. Neurol.* 4:149–61.

 (1961b). Electrophysiology of hippocampal neurons. III. Firing level and time constant. *J. Neurophysiol.* 24:260–71.

 (1961c). Electrophysiology of hippocampal neurons. IV. Fast prepotentials. *J. Neurophysiol.* 24:272–85.

Squire, L. R. (1986). Mechanisms of memory. *Science* 232:1612–19.

Squire, L. R., Shimamura, A. P., and Amaral, D. G. (1989). Memory and the hippocampus. In Byrne, J. H. and Berry, W. O., eds., *Neural Models of Plasticity,* pp. 208–39. Academic Press, San Diego.

Stasheff, S. F., Anderson, W. W., Clark, S., and Wilson, W. A. (1989). NMDA antagonists differentiate epileptogenesis from seizure expression in an in vitro model. *Science* 245:648–51.

Stasheff, S. F., Bragdon, A. C., and Wilson, W. A. (1985). Induction of epileptiform activity in hippocampal slices by trains of electrical stimuli. *Brain Res.* 344:296–302.

Stauffer, D. (1985). *Introduction to Percolation Theory.* Taylor & Francis, London.

Stelzer, A., Kay, A., and Wong, R. K. S. (1988). $GABA_A$ receptor function in hippocampal cells is maintained by phosphorylation factors. *Science* 241:339–41.

Stelzer, A., Slater, N. T., and ten Bruggencate, G. (1987). Activation of NMDA receptors blocks GABAergic inhibition in an *in vitro* model of epilepsy. *Nature* 326:698–701.

Stelzer, A., and Wong, R. K. S. (1989). $GABA_A$ responses in hippocampal neurons are potentiated by glutamate. *Nature* 337:170–3.

Stephan, H. (1983). Evolutionary trends in limbic structures. *Neurosci. Biobehav. Rev.* 7:367–74.

Steriade, M., Domich, L., Oakson, G., and Deschênes, M. (1987). The deafferented reticular thalamic nucleus generates spindle rhythmicity. *J. Neurophysiol.* 57:260–73.

Steriade, M., and Llinás, R. R. (1988). The functional states of the thalamus and the associated neuronal interplay. *Physiol. Rev.* 68:649–742.

Steriade, M., Paré, D., Datta, S., Oakson, G., and Curro Dossi, R. (1989). Different classes of PGO-on neurons in pedunculopontine and laterodorsal tegmental brainstem cholinergic nuclei. *Soc. Neurosci. Abstr.* 15:452.

Steward, O., and Scoville, S. A. (1976). Cells of origin of entorhinal cortical afferents to the hippocampus and fascia dentata of the rat. *J. Compar. Neurol.* 169:347–70.

Stewart, M., and Fox, S. E. (1988). Microiontophoretic atropine eliminates firing of hippocampal theta cells. *Soc. Neurosci. Abstr.* 14:127.

(1989). Two populations of rhythmically bursting neurons in rat medial septum are revealed by atropine. *J. Neurophysiol.* 61:982–93.

Storm, J. (1987). Action potential repolarization and a fast after-hyperpolarization in rat hippocampal pyramidal cells. *J. Physiol.* 385:733–59.

(1988). Temporal integration by a slowly inactivating K^+ current in hippocampal neurons. *Nature* 336:379–81.

(1989). An after-hyperpolarization of medium duration in rat hippocampal pyramidal cells. *J. Physiol.* 409:171–90.

Stratford, K., Mason, A., Larkman, A., Major, G., and Jack, J. (1989). The modelling of pyramidal neurones in the visual cortex. In Durbin, R., Miall, C., and Mitchison, G., eds., *The Computing Neuron,* pp. 296–321. Addison-Wesley, Reading, Mass.

Strowbridge, B. W., and Shepherd, G. M. (1988). Muscarinic excitation of inhibitory circuits in neocortical slices. *Soc. Neurosci. Abstr.* 14:904.

Sutula, T. P., Xiao-Xian, H., Cavazos, J., and Scott, G. (1988). Synaptic reorganization in the hippocampus induced by abnormal functional activity. *Science* 239:1147–50.

Suzuki, S. S., and Smith, G. K. (1985). Single-cell activity and synchronous bursting in the rat hippocampus during waking behavior and sleep. *Exper. Neurol.* 89:71–89.

(1987). Spontaneous EEG spikes in the normal hippocampus. I. Behavioral correlates, laminar profiles and bilateral synchrony. *Electroenceph. Clin. Neurophysiol.* 67:348–59.

(1988a). Spontaneous EEG spikes in the normal hippocampus. II. Relations to synchronous burst discharges. *Electroenceph. Clin. Neurophysiol.* 69:532–40.

(1988b). Spontaneous EEG spikes in the normal hippocampus. III. Relations to evoked potentials. *Electroenceph. Clin. Neurophysiol.* 69:541–9.

(1988c). Spontaneous EEG spikes in the normal hippocampus. IV. Effects of medial septum and entorhinal cortex lesions. *Electroenceph. Clin. Neurophysiol.* 70:73–83.

(1988d). Spontaneous EEG spikes in the normal hippocampus. V. Effects of ether, urethane, pentobarbital, atropine, diazepam and bicuculline. *Electroenceph. Clin. Neurophysiol.* 70:84–95.

Swann, J. W., and Brady, R. J. (1984). Penicillin-induced epileptogenesis in immature rat CA3 hippocampal cells. *Dev. Brain Res.* 314:243–54.

Swann, J. W., Brady, R. J., Friedman, R. J., and Smith, E. J. (1986a). The dendritic origins of penicillin-induced epileptogenesis in CA3 hippocampal pyramidal cells. *J. Neurophysiol.* 56:1718–38.

Swann, J. W., Brady, R. J., Smith, K. L., and Pierson, M. G. (1988). Synaptic mechanisms of focal epileptogenesis in the immature nervous system. In Swann, J., and Messer, A., eds., *Disorders of the Developing*

Nervous System: Changing Views of Their Origins, Diagnoses and Treatments, pp. 19–49. A. R. Liss, New York.

Swann, J. W., Smith, K. L., and Brady, R. J. (1986b). Extracellular K⁺ accumulation during penicillin-induced epileptogenesis in the CA3 region of immature rat hippocampus. *Dev. Brain Res.* 30:243–55.

Swanson, L. W., and Cowan, W. M. (1977). An autoradiographic study of the organization of the efferent connections of the hippocampal formation in the rat. *J. Compar. Neurol.* 172:49–84.

Swanson, L. W., Wyss, J. M., and Cowan, W. M. (1978). An autoradiographic study of the organization of intrahippocampal association pathways in the rat. *J. Compar. Neurol.* 181:681–716.

Swartzwelder, H. S., Lewis, D. V., Anderson, W. W., and Wilson, W. A. (1987). Seizure-like events in brain slices: suppression by interictal activity. *Brain Res.* 410:362–6.

Takens, F. (1981). Detecting strange attractors in turbulence. In Rand, D. A., and Young, L.-S., eds., *Lecture Notes in Mathematics, Vol. 898: Dynamical Systems and Turbulence, Warwick, 1980,* pp. 366–81. Springer, New York.

Tamamaki, N., Abe, K., and Nojyo, Y. (1988). Three-dimensional analysis of the whole axonal arbors originating from single CA2 pyramidal neurons in the rat hippocampus with the aid of a computer graphic technique. *Brain Res.* 452:255–72.

Tamamaki, N., Watanabe, K., and Nojyo, Y. (1984). A whole image of the hippocampal pyramidal neuron revealed by intracellular pressure-injection of horseradish peroxidase. *Brain Res.* 307:336–40.

Tang, C.-M., Dichter, M., and Morad, M. (1989). Quisqualate activates a rapidly inactivating high conductance ionic channel in hippocampal neurons. *Science* 243:1474–7.

Tasker, J. G., and Dudek, F. E. (1989). The effects of osmolality on synchronous bursting in the absence of chemical synaptic transmission in hippocampal slices. *Soc. Neurosci. Abstr.* 15:701.

Tauck, D. L., and Nadler, J. V. (1985). Evidence of functional mossy fiber sprouting in hippocampal formation of kainic acid-treated rats. *J. Neurosci.* 5:1016–22.

Taylor, C. P., and Dudek, F. E. (1982). Synchronous neural afterdischarges in rat hippocampal slices without active chemical synapses. *Science* 218:810–12.

(1984a). Excitation of hippocampal pyramidal cells by an electrical field effect. *J. Neurophysiol.* 52:126–42.

(1984b). Synchronization without active chemical synapses during hippocampal afterdischarges. *J. Neurophysiol.* 52:143–55.

Thalmann, R. H. (1984). Reversal properties of an EGTA-resistant late hyperpolarization that follows synaptic stimulation of hippocampal neurons. *Neurosci. Lett.* 46:103–8.

(1988). Evidence that guanosine triphosphate (GTP)-binding proteins control a synaptic response in brain: effect of pertussis toxin and GTPᵧS on the late inhibitory postsynaptic potential of hippocampal CA3 neurons. *J. Neurosci.* 8:4589–602.

Theodore, W. H., Porter, R. J., and Penry, J. K. (1983). Complex partial seizures: clinical characteristics and differential diagnosis. *Neurology* 33:1115–21.

Thompson, S. M., and Gähwiler, B. H. (1989a). Activity-dependent disinhibition. I. Repetitive stimulation reduces both IPSP driving force and conductance in the hippocampus *in vitro. J. Neurophysiol.* 61:501–11.

(1989b). Activity-dependent disinhibition. II. Effects of extracellular potassium, furosemide, and membrane potential on E_{Cl^-} in hippocampal CA3 neurons. *J. Neurophysiol.* 61:512–23.

(1989c). Activity-dependent disinhibition. III. Desensitization and $GABA_B$ receptor-mediated presynaptic inhibition in the hippocampus *in vitro. J. Neurophysiol.* 61:524–33.

Ticku, M. K., Ban, M., and Olsen, R. W. (1978). Binding of [^{3}II]α-dihydropicrotoxinin, a γ-aminobutyric acid synaptic antagonist, to rat brain membranes. *Molec. Pharacol.* 14:391–402.

Tielen, A. M., Lopes da Silva, F. H., and Mollevanger, W. J. (1981). Differential conduction velocities in perforant path fibres in guinea pig. *Exp. Brain Res.* 42:231–3.

Tielen, A. M., van Leeuwen, F. W., and Lopes da Silva, F. H. (1982). The localization of leucine-enkephalin immunoreactivity within the guinea pig hippocampus. *Exp. Brain Res.* 48:288–95.

Tömböl, T., Babosa, M., and Somogyi, C. (1979). Interneurons: an electron microscopic study of the cat's hippocampal formation. *Acta Morphol. Acad. Sci. Hung.* 27:297–313.

Tömböl, T., Somogyi, G., and Hajdu, F. (1978). Golgi study on cat hippocampal formation. *Anat. Embryol.* 153:331–50.

Tracey, D. J., and Walmsley, B. (1984). Synaptic inputs from identified muscle afferents to neurones of the dorsal spinocerebellar tract in rats. *J. Physiol.* 350:599–614.

Tranchina, D., and Nicholson, C. (1986). A model for the polarization of neurons by extrinsically applied electric fields. *Biophys. J.* 50:1139–56.

Traub, R. D. (1977). Motorneurons of different geometry and the size principle. *Biol. Cybern.* 25:163–76.

(1982). Simulation of intrinsic bursting in CA3 hippocampal neurons. *Neuroscience* 7:1233–42.

(1983). Cellular mechanisms underlying the inhibitory surround of penicillin epileptogenic foci. *Brain Res.* 261:277–84.

Traub, R. D., and Dingledine, R. (1990). Model of synchronized epileptiform bursts induced by high potassium in the CA3 region of the rat hippocampal slice: role of spontaneous EPSPs in initiation. *J. Neurophysiol.* 64:1009–1018.

Traub, R. D., Dudek, F. E., Snow, R. W., and Knowles, W. D. (1985a). Computer simulations indicate that electrical field effects contribute to the shape of the epileptiform field potential. *Neuroscience* 15:947–58.

Traub, R. D., Dudek, F. E., Taylor, C. P., and Knowles, W. W. (1985b). Simulation of hippocampal afterdischarges synchronized by electrical interactions. *Neuroscience* 14:1033–8.

Traub, R. D., Knowles, W. D., Miles, R., and Wong, R. K. S. (1984). Synchronized afterdischarges in the hippocampus: simulation studies of the cellular mechanism. *Neuroscience* 12:1191–200.

(1987a). Models of the cellular mechanism underlying propagation of epileptiform activity in the CA2-CA3 region of the hippocampal slice. *Neuroscience* 21:457–70.

Traub, R., and Llinás, R. (1977). The spatial distribution of ionic conductances in normal and axotomized motorneurons. *Neuroscience* 2:829–49.

(1979). Hippocampal pyramidal cells: significance of dendritic ionic conductances for neuronal function and epileptogenesis. *J. Neurophysiol.* 42:476–96.

Traub, R. D., Miles, R., and Wong, R. K. S. (1987b). Models of synchronized hippocampal bursts in the presence of inhibition. I. Single population events. *J. Neurophysiol.* 58:739–51.

(1988). Large scale simulations of the hippocampus. *IEEE Engineering in Medicine and Biology* 7:31–8.

(1989). Model of the origin of rhythmic population oscillations in the hippocampal slice. *Science* 243:1319–25.

Traub, R. D., Miles, R., Wong, R. K. S., Schulman, L. S., and Schneiderman, J. H. (1987c). Models of synchronized hippocampal bursts in the presence of inhibition. Ongoing spontaneous population events. *J. Neurophysiol.* 58:752–64.

Traub, R. D., and Pedley, T. A. (1981). Virus-induced electrotonic coupling: hypothesis on the mechanism of periodic EEG discharges in Creutzfeldt-Jakob disease. *Ann. Neurol.* 10:405–10.

Traub, R. D., and Wong, R. K. S. (1982). Cellular mechanism of neuronal synchronization in epilepsy. *Science* 216:745–7.

(1983a). Synchronized burst discharge in disinhibited hippocampal slice. II. Model of cellular mechanism. *J. Neurophysiol.* 49:459–71.

(1983b). Synaptic mechanisms underlying interictal spike initiation in a hippocampal network. *Neurology* 33:257–66.

Traub, R. D., Wong, R. K. S., and Miles, R. (1990). A model of the CA3 hippocampal pyramidal cell based on voltage-clamp data. *Soc. Neurosci. Abstr.* 16:1297.

Traynelis, S. F., and Dingledine, R. (1988). Potassium-induced spontaneous electrographic seizures in the rat hippocampal slice. *J. Neurophysiol.* 59:259–76.

(1989a). Role of extracellular space in hyperosmotic suppression of potassium-induced electrographic seizures. *J. Neurophysiol.* 61:927–38.

(1989b). Modification of potassium-induced interictal bursts and electrographic seizures by divalent cations. *Neurosci. Lett.* 98:194–9.

Trojaborg, W. (1968). Changes in spike foci in children. In Kellaway, P., and Petersén, I., eds., *Clinical Electroencephalography in Children*, pp. 213–26. Grune & Stratton, New York.

Turner, D. A. (1984a). Segmental cable evaluation of somatic transients in hippocampal neurons (CA1, CA3, and dentate). *Biophys. J.* 46:73–84.

(1984b). Conductance transients onto dendritic spines in a segmental cable model of hippocampal neurons. *Biophys. J.* 46:85–96.

(1988). Waveform and amplitude characteristics of evoked responses to dendritic stimulation of CA1 guinea-pig pyramidal cells. *J. Physiol.* 395:419–39.

Turner, D. A., and Schwartzkroin, P. A. (1980). Steady-state electrotonic analysis of intracellularly stained hippocampal neurons. *J. Neurophysiol.* 44:184–99.

—— (1983). Electrical characteristics of dendrites and dendritic spines in intracellularly-stained CA3 and dentate neurons. *J. Neurosci.* 3:2381–94.

—— (1984). Passive electrotonic structure and dendritic properties of hippocampal neurons. In Dingledine, R., ed., *Brain Slices*, pp. 25–50. Plenum Press, New York.

Valentino, R. J., and Dingledine, R. (1981). Presynaptic inhibitory effect of acetylcholine in the hippocampus. *J. Neurosci.* 1:784–92.

Vanderwolf, C. H., and Leung, L.-W. S. (1983). Hippocampal rhythmical slow activity: a brief history and the effects of entorhinal lesions and phencyclidine. In Seifert, W., ed., *Neurobiology of the Hippocampus*, pp. 225–302. Academic Press, London.

Vanderwolf, C. H., Leung, L.-W. S., and Cooley, R. K. (1985). Pathways through cingulate, neo- and entorhinal cortices mediate atropine-resistant hippocampal rhythmical slow activity. *Brain Res.* 347:58–73.

Van Hoesen, G. W., Rosene, D. L., and Mesulam, M.-M. (1979). Subicular input from temporal cortex in the rhesus monkey. *Science* 205:608–10.

Varga, R. S. (1962). *Matrix Iterative Analysis.* Prentice-Hall, Englewood Cliffs, N.J.

Vertes, R. P. (1982). Brain stem generation of the hippocampal EEG. *Prog. Neurobiol.* 19:159–86.

—— (1985). Brainstem-septohippocampal circuits controlling the hippocampal EEG. In Buzsáki, G., and Vanderwolf, C. H., eds., *Electrical Activity of the Archicortex*, pp. 33–45. Akadémiai Kiadó, Budapest.

Victor, M., Adams, R. D., and Collins, G. H. (1973). *The Wernicke-Korsakoff Syndrome.* Davis, Philadelphia.

Vincent, S. R., and McGeer, E. G. (1981). A substance P projection to the hippocampus. *Brain Res.* 215:349–51.

Vinogradova, O. S., Brazhnik, E. S., Karanov, A. M., and Zhadina, S. D. (1980). Neuronal activity of the septum following various types of deafferentation. *Brain Res.* 187:353–68.

Vinogradova, O. S., Zhadina, S. D., and Brazhnik, E. S. (1987). Analysis of the organization of background activity of the septal neurons of the guinea pig in vitro. *Neirofiziologiia* 19:586–95.

Volpe, B. T., and Petito, C. K. (1985). Dementia with bilateral medial tempo ral lobe ischemia. *Neurology* 35:1793–7.

Voskuyl, R. A., and Albus, H. (1985). Spontaneous epileptiform discharges in hippocampal slices induced by 4-aminopyridine. *Brain Res.* 342:54–66.

Walker, A. D., Johnson, H. C., and Kollros, J. J. (1945). Penicillin convulsions. The convulsive effects of penicillin applied to the cerebral cortex of monkey and man. *Surg. Gynecol. Obstet.* 81:692–701.

Wallen, P., Grillner, S., Feldman, J. L., and Bergelt, S. (1985). Dorsal and ventral myotome motoneurons and their input during fictive locomotion in lamprey. *J. Neurosci.* 5:654–61.

Walmsley, B., Edwards, F. R., and Tracey, D. J. (1988). Nonuniform release probabilities underlie quantal synaptic transmission at a mammalian excitatory central synapse. *J. Neurophysiol.* 60:889–908.

Westbrook, G. L., and Lothman, E. W. (1983). Cellular and synaptic basis of kainic acid-induced hippocampal epileptiform activity. *Brain Res.* 273:97–109.

Whishaw, I. Q. (1987). Hippocampal, granule cell and CA3–4 lesions impair formation of a place learning-set in the rat and induce reflex epilepsy. *Behav. Brain Res.* 24:59–72.

Whishaw, I. Q., and Sutherland, R. J. (1982). Sparing of rhythmic slow activity (RSA or theta) in two hippocampal generators after kainic acid CA3 and CA4 lesions. *Exp. Neurol.* 75:711–28.

White, J. C., Langston, J. W., and Pedley, T. A. (1977a). Benign epileptiform transients of sleep. Clarification of the small sharp spike controversy. *Neurology* 27:1061–8.

White, W. F., Nadler, J. V., Hamberger, A., Cotman, C. W., and Cummins, J. T. (1977b). Glutamate as a transmitter of hippocampal perforant path. *Nature* 270:356–7.

Wiener, N. (1961). *Cybernetics.* M.I.T. Press, Cambridge, Mass.
    (1958). *Nonlinear Problems in Random Theory.* M.I.T. Press, Cambridge, Mass.

Wigström, H., and Gustafsson, B. (1981). Two types of synaptic facilitation recorded in pyramidal cells of in vitro hippocampal slices from guinea pigs. *Neurosci. Lett.* 26:73–8.
    (1983). Facilitated induction of hippocampal long-lasting potentiation during blockade of inhibition. *Nature* 301:603–4.

Wigström, H., Gustafsson, B., Huang, Y.-Y., and Abraham, W. C. (1986). Hippocampal long-term potentiation is induced by pairing single afferent volleys with intracellularly injected depolarizing current pulses. *Acta Physiol. Scand.* 126–317–19.

Williams, S., and Johnston, D. (1988). Muscarinic depression of long-term potentiation in CA3 hippocampal neurons. *Science* 242:84–7.

Wilson, C. L., Motter, B. C., and Lindsley, D. B. (1976). Influences of hypothalamic stimulation upon septal and hippocampal electrical activity in the cat. *Brain Res.* 107:55–68.

Wilson, M. A., and Bower, J. M. (1989). The simulation of large-scale neural networks. In Koch, C., and Segev, I., eds., *Methods in Neuronal Modeling: From Synapses to Networks,* pp. 295–341. M.I.T. Press, Cambridge, Mass.

Winson, J. (1974). Patterns of hippocampal theta rhythm in the freely moving rat. *Electroenceph. Clin. Neurophysiol.* 26:291–301.
    (1976a). Hippocampal theta rhythm. I. Depth profiles in the curarized rat. *Brain Res.* 103:57–70.
    (1976b). Hippocampal theta rhythm. II. Depth profiles in the freely moving rabbit. *Brain Res.* 103:71–9.
    (1978). Loss of hippocampal theta rhythm results in spatial memory deficit in the rat. *Science* 201:160–3.

Winson, J., and Abzug, C. (1978). Neuronal transmission through hippocampal pathways dependent on behavior. *J. Neurophysiol.* 41:716–32.

Witter, M. P., and Groenewegen, H. J. (1984). Laminar origin and septotemporal distribution of entorhinal and perirhinal projections to the hippocampus in the cat. *J. Compar. Neurol.* 224:371–85.

Wojtowicz, J. M., and Atwood, H. L. (1986). Long-term facilitation alters transmitter releasing properties at the crayfish neuromuscular junction. *J. Neurophysiol.* 55:484–98.

Wong, R. K. S., Miles, R., and Traub, R. D. (1984). Local circuit interactions in synchronization of cortical neurones. *J. Exper. Biol.* 112:169–78.

Wong, R. K. S., Numann, R. E. Miles, R., and Traub, R. D. (1985). Hippocampal pyramidal cells: ionic conductance and synaptic interactions. In Alkon, D. L., and Woody, C. D., ed., *Neural Mechanisms of Conditioning,* pp. 311–18. Plenum Press, New York.

Wong, R. K. S., and Prince, D. A. (1978). Participation of calcium spikes during intrinsic burst firing in hippocampal neurons. *Brain Res.* 159:385–90.

(1979). Dendritic mechanisms underlying penicillin-induced epileptiform activity. *Science* 204:1228–31.

(1981). Afterpotential generation in hippocampal pyramidal cells. *J. Neurophysiol.* 45:86–97.

Wong, R. K. S., Prince, D. A., and Basbaum, A. I. (1979). Intradendritic recordings from hippocampal neurons. *Proc. Natl. Acad. Sci. U.S.A.* 76:986–90.

Wong, R. K. S., and Traub, R. D. (1983). Synchronized burst discharge in disinhibited hippocampal slice. I. Initiation in CA2-CA3 region. *J. Neurophysiol.* 49:442–58.

Wong, R. K. S., Traub, R. D., and Miles, R. (1986). Cellular basis of neuronal synchrony in epilepsy. In Delgado-Escueta, A. V., Ward, A. A., Jr., Woodbury, D. M., and Porter, R. J., eds., *Advances in Neurology, Vol. 44, Basic Mechanisms of the Epilepsies. Molecular and Cellular Approaches,* pp. 583–92. Raven Press, New York.

Wong, R. K. S., and Watkins, D. J. (1982). Cellular factors influencing GABA response in hippocampal pyramidal cells. *J. Neurophysiol.* 48:938–51.

Wyler, A. R., Ojemann, G. A., and Ward, A. A., Jr. (1982). Neurons in human epileptic cortex: correlation between unit and EEG activity. *Ann. Neurol.* 11:301–8.

Yaari, Y., Hamon, B., and Lux, H. D. (1987). Development of two types of calcium channels in cultured mammalian hippocampal neurons. *Science* 235:680–2.

Yaari, Y., Konnerth, A., and Heinemann, U. (1983). Spontaneous epileptiform activity of CA1 hippocampal neurons in low extracellular calcium solutions. *Exp. Brain Res.* 51:153–6.

(1986). Nonsynaptic epileptogenesis in the mammalian hippocampus in vitro. II. Role of extracellular potassium. *J. Neurophysiol.* 56:424–38.

Yakushiji, T., Tokutomi, N., Akaike, N., and Carpenter, D. O. (1987). Antagonists of GABA responses, studied using internally perfused frog dorsal root ganglion neurons. *Neuroscience* 22:1123–33.

Yamamoto, C. (1982). Quantal analysis of excitatory postsynaptic potentials induced in hippocampal neurons by activation of granule cells. *Exp. Brain Res.* 46:170–6.

Yamamoto, C., and Chujo, T. (1978). Long-term potentiation in thin hippocampal sections studied by intracellular and extracellular recordings. *Exper. Neurol.* 58:242–50.

Yamamoto, C., Higashima, M., and Sawada, S. (1987). Quantal analysis of potentiating action of phorbol ester on synaptic transmission in the hippocampus. *Neurosci. Res.* 5:28–38.

Zbicz, K. L., and Weight, F. F. (1985). Transient voltage and calcium-dependent outward currents in hippocampal CA3 neurons. *J. Neurophysiol.* 53:1038–58.

Zipser, D. A. (1985). A computational model of hippocampal place fields. *Behav. Neurosci.* 99:1006–18.

Zipser, D., and Andersen, R. A. (1988). A back-propagation programmed network that simulates response properties of a subset of posterior parietal neurons. *Nature.* 331:679–84.

Zivin, L., and Ajmone-Marsan, C. (1968). Incidence and prognostic significance of "epileptiform" activity in the EEG of nonepileptic subjects. *Brain* 91:751–78.

Zola-Morgan, S., and Squire, L. R. (1986). Memory impairment in monkeys following lesions limited to the hippocampus. *Behav. Neurosci.* 100:155–60.

Zola-Morgan, S., Squire, L. R., and Amaral, D. G. (1986). Human amnesia and the medial temporal region: enduring memory impairment following a bilateral lesion limited to field CA1 of the hippocampus. *J. Neurosci.* 6:2950–67.

(1988). Amnesia following medial temporal lobe damage in monkeys: the importance of the hippocampus and adjacent cortical regions. *Soc. Neurosci. Abstr.* 14:1043.

(1989a). Lesions of the hippocampal formation but not lesions of the fornix or the mammillary nuclei produce long-lasting memory impairment in monkeys. *J. Neurosci.* 9:898–913.

(1989b). Lesions of the amygdala that spare adjacent cortical regions do not impair memory or exacerbate the impairment following lesions of the hippocampal formation. *J. Neurosci.* 9:1922–36.

Zucker, R. S. (1989). Models of calcium regulation in neurons. In Byrne, J. H. and Berry, W. O., eds., *Neural Models of Plasticity*, pp. 403–22. Academic Press, San Diego.

Index

acetylcholine, 6, 7, 19, 20, 21, 24, 44, 55, 86
action potential, 15, 17, 20, 23, 29, 38, 40, 41, 43, 49–51, 89, 96–7, 113, 140, 191–3.
  Hodgkin-Huxley theory of, 101–103
  synchronized, 29, 194–203
afterdepolarization, *see* depolarizing afterpotential
afterdischarge, 31–2, 98, 124, 140, 152–6, 189–91, 197
afterhyperpolarization (AHP), 20, 37, 39, 43, 51, 89, 96, 152, 164, 172, 183–5, 223
amnesia, 9–12, 31–2
amygdala, 7, 10, 31, 227
anoxia, 30
attractor, 176, 179–80, 208, 218
aura, seizure, 31
axon, 4, 5, 19, 57–60, 65
  conduction block, 155–6
  conduction velocity, 106, 134
  initial segment, 86, 99
  model, 74, 104
  output transduction, 106
  spatial distribution of connections, 61–4, 108–109, 133–4
  sprouting, 30
  squid, 88, 101–103

backpropagation algorithm, 209
basket cell, 4, 43, 51, 55
behavioral state, 15
  consummatory, 27
  and EEG, 16–17
  walking, 16
bicuculline, 26, 125, 183, 187, 229
brainstem, influence on EEG, 21–2
burst
  EPSP initiated by, 66
  field potential associated with, 124, 130, 134, 142, 152, 189, 191
  intrinsic, 37–43, 89, 96–7
  partially synchronized, 70–3, 140–51, 164

synchronized, 69–71, 119–56, 182–7
transmission, cell-to-cell, 67, 121–4

cable equation, 77–8, 91–3
calcium
  conductance, 20, 37–8, 89–90, 96, 154
  -dependent K conductance, 20, 39, 89–90, 96
  -free media, 197
  intracellular, 35, 92
carbachol, 19
central pattern generator, xiv, xv, 6, 15, 25
chandelier cell, 4, 43, 60
channel, *see* conductance
chaos, 175–80, 204
cingulate gyrus, 6–7, 10, 12, 21
  sharp waves in, 28
  theta rhythm in, 21, 24
CNQX (6-cyano-7-nitroquinoxaline-2,3-dione), 56, 172, 183, 187
computational model, xiii, 33, 205
conductance
  calcium, *see* calcium conductance
  leak, 75; *see also* membrane resistivity
  potassium, 20, 39–41, 88–90, 101–103
  rate functions, 93–4
  sodium, 88–90, 101–103
  synaptic, 46–57, 85–7; equations, 94–5; excitatory (glutamate), 86–7; $GABA_A$, 41, 50–1, 55, 57, 77, 86–7, 141; $GABA_B$, 41, 43–5, 87; kainate/quisqualate, 44, 56–7; NMDA, 13, 29–30, 44, 56, 77, 125, 152, 226, 229
cornu Ammonis, 1

déja vu, 31
dendrite, 90–1
  active properties of, 38–9, 41, 88–9, 154–5
  branching rule, 75–6
  current flow in, 74–85
  excitation on, 69, 85–7, 106–108, 202
  extracellular resistance near, 198–200
  inhibition on, 45, 86–7, 106–107